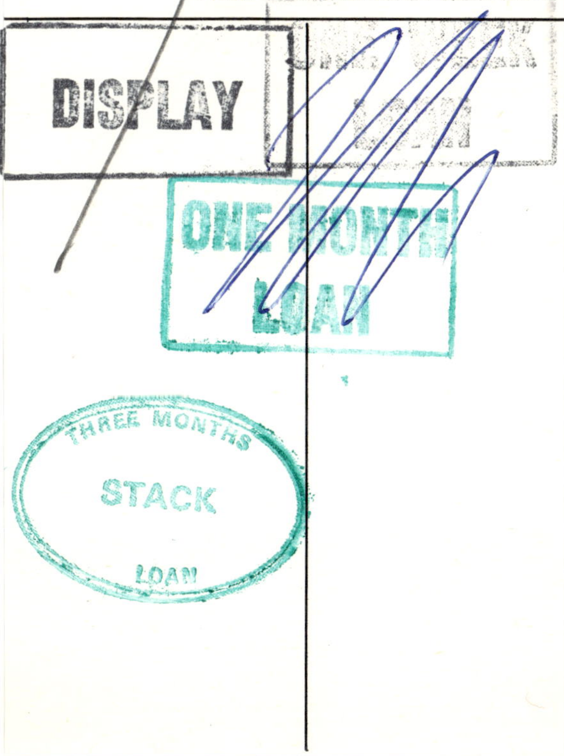
Medical Library
University of Bristol
THIS BOOK/JOURNAL MUST BE RETURNED TO THE LIBRARY BY THE LAST DATE STAMPED BELOW.
DISPLAY
ONE MONTH LOAN
THREE MONTHS
STACK
LOAN

SERVICE AND EDUCATION IN MEDICAL GENETICS

BIRTH DEFECTS INSTITUTE SYMPOSIA

Ernest B. Hook, Dwight T. Janerich, and Ian H. Porter, editors: MONITORING, BIRTH DEFECTS, AND ENVIRONMENT: The Problem of Surveillance, 1971

Ian H. Porter and Richard G. Skalko, editors: HEREDITY AND SOCIETY, 1972

Dwight T. Janerich, Richard G. Skalko, and Ian H. Porter, editors: CONGENITAL DEFECTS: New Directions in Research, 1973

Hilaire J. Meuwissen, Richard J. Pickering, Bernard Pollara, and Ian H. Porter, editors: COMBINED IMMUNODEFICIENCY DISEASE AND ADENOSINE DEAMINASE DEFICIENCY: A Molecular Defect, 1975

Sally Kelly, Ernest B. Hook, Dwight T. Janerich, and Ian H. Porter, editors: BIRTH DEFECTS: Risks and Consequences, 1976

Ernest B. Hook and Ian H. Porter, editors: POPULATION CYTOGENETICS: Studies in Humans, 1977

H. Lawrence Vallet and Ian H. Porter, editors: GENETIC MECHANISMS OF SEXUAL DEVELOPMENT, 1979

Ian H. Porter and Ernest B. Hook, editors: SERVICE AND EDUCATION IN MEDICAL GENETICS, 1979

SERVICE AND EDUCATION IN MEDICAL GENETICS

Edited by

Ian H. Porter

Ernest B. Hook

Birth Defects Institute
New York State Department
of Health
Albany, New York

Proceedings of the Seventh Annual
New York State Health Department
Birth Defects Symposium

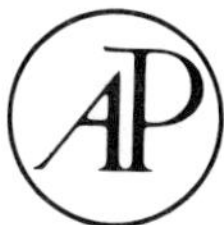

ACADEMIC PRESS *New York San Francisco London*
A Subsidiary of Harcourt Brace Jovanovich, Publishers
1979

ACADEMIC PRESS, INC.
111 Fifth Avenue, New York, New York 10003

United Kingdom Edition published by
ACADEMIC PRESS, INC. (LONDON) LTD.
24/28 Oval Road, London NW1 7DX

Library of Congress Cataloging in Publication Data
Main entry under title:

Service and education in medical genetics.

1. Medical genetics. 2. Genetic counseling. 3. Community health services. 4. Medical genetics—Study and teaching. I. Porter, Ian H. II. Hook, Ernest B., Date [DNLM: 1. Genetic counseling. 2. Hereditary diseases—Prevention and control. 3. Cytogenetics. QZ50.3 S491]
RB155.S43 362.1'9'6042 79-12549
ISBN 0-12-562650-9

PRINTED IN THE UNITED STATES OF AMERICA

79 80 81 82 9 8 7 6 5 4 3 2 1

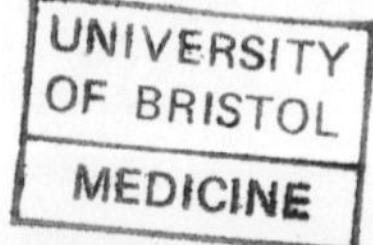

CONTENTS

II. GENETIC COUNSELING AND OTHER GENETIC SERVICES IN THE COMMUNITY

III. ATTITUDES TOWARD GENETIC COUNSELING

IV. EDUCATION FOR MEDICAL GENETICS

CONTRIBUTORS AND PARTICIPANTS

Numbers in parentheses indicate pages on which authors' contributions begin.

Cheryl A. Austein (361), Department of Human Genetics, and Office of Continuing Education, Yale University School of Medicine, New Haven, Connecticut

M. A. Barr (137), Division of Medical Genetics, Thomas Jefferson University, Philadelphia, Pennsylvania

Karlene Brantley (163), Department of Pediatrics, Division of Medical Genetics, Emory University, Atlanta, Georgia

Katherine K. Bucholz (361), Department of Human Genetics, and Office of Continuing Education, Yale University School of Medicine, New Haven, Connecticut

Linda L. Carter (303), Yale University School of Nursing, New Haven, Connecticut

Andrew T.L. Chen (163), Bureau of Laboratories, Center for Disease Control, Atlanta, Georgia

Barton Childs (419), Department of Pediatrics, The Johns Hopkins Hospital School of Medicine, Baltimore, Maryland

Carol L. Clow (337), McGill University-Montreal Children's Hospital Research Institute, Montreal, Quebec

Jessica G. Davis (69), Department of Pediatrics, Cornell University College of Medicine, New York, New York

Mark Degnan, Department of Pediatrics, Division of Medical Genetics, Albany Medical College, Albany, New York

Robert J. Desnick (237), Department of Pediatrics, Mt. Sinai School of Medicine, New York, New York

Richard A. Doherty (323), Departments of Pediatrics, Genetics, and Obstetrics, University of Rochester School of Medicine, Rochester, New York

Charles J. Epstein (11, 149), Division of Medical Genetics, University of California, San Francisco, California

Murray Feingold (103), Center for Genetic Counseling and Birth Defect Evaluation, Tufts-New England Medical Center, Boston, Massachusetts

Paul M. Fernhoff (163), Bureau of Laboratories, Center for Disease Control, Atlanta, Georgia; and Department of Pediatrics, Division of Medical Genetics, Emory University, Atlanta, Georgia

Lawrence Fisher (285), Department of Psychiatry, University of Rochester School of Medicine and Dentistry, Rochester, New York

G. R. Fraser (21), Departments of Otolaryngology and Epidemiology, McGill University, Montreal, Quebec, Canada

Marshall F. Goldberg (55, 163), Bureau of Epidemiology, Center for Disease Control, Atlanta, Georgia

Ernest B. Hook (29), Birth Defects Institute, New York State Health Department, Albany, New York

Y. Edward Hsia (303, 361), Department of Human Genetics, and Office of Continuing Education, Yale University School of Medicine, New Haven, Connecticut

L. G. Jackson (137), Department of Medicine/Pediatrics, Division of Medical Genetics, Thomas Jefferson University, Philadelphia, Pennsylvania

Rene I. Jahiel (183), Department of Medicine, New York University Medical Center, School of Medicine, New York, New York

Sally Kelly, Birth Defects Institute, New York State Department of Health, Albany, New York

Felix Leung (303), Yale University School of Medicine, New Haven, Connecticut

Boris Libster (221), Neural Tube Defect Laboratory, Nassau County Medical Center, East Meadow, New York

D. Linn (137), University of California, San Francisco, California

Mack Lipkin, Jr. (285), Department of Psychiatry, University of Rochester School of Medicine and Dentistry, Rochester, New York

Marie-Louise Lubs (85), Department of Pediatrics, University of Colorado Medical Center, Denver, Colorado

James N. Macri (221), Neural Tube Defect Laboratory, Nassau County Medical Center, East Meadow, New York

Joan H. Marks (351), Human Genetics Program, Sarah Lawrence College, Bronxville, New York

A. G. Motulsky (409), Departments of Medicine and Genetics, and Center for Inherited Diseases, University of Washington, Seattle, Washington

Edmond A. Murphy (3), Department of Medicine, The Johns Hopkins Hospital, Baltimore, Maryland

Godfrey P. Oakley, Jr. (55, 163), Bureau of Epidemiology, Center for Disease Control, Atlanta, Georgia; and Department of Pediatrics, Division of Medical Genetics, Emory University, Atlanta, Georgia

Ian H. Porter (253), Birth Defects Institute, New York State Department of Health, Albany, New York

Jean H. Priest (163), Department of Pediatrics, Division of Medical Genetics, Emory University, Atlanta, Georgia

John D. Rainer (295), New York State Psychiatric Institute, New York, New York; and Department of Psychiatry, Columbia University, New York, New York

Vincent M. Riccardi (129), Kleberg Genetics Center, Baylor College of Medicine, Texas Medical Center, Houston, Texas

Marian L. Rivas (107), Division of Medical Genetics, University of Oregon Health Sciences Center, Portland, Oregon

Klaus J. Roghmann (323), Departments of Sociology, Pediatrics, and Preventive Medicine, University of Rochester School of Medicine, Rochester, New York

Peter T. Rowley (285), Department of Medicine, Division of Genetics, University of Rochester School of Medicine and Dentistry, Rochester, New York

Mindy Schok (337), deBelle Laboratory for Biochemical Genetics, McGill University–Montreal Children's Hospital Research Institute, Montreal, Quebec, Canada

Charles R. Scriver (337), deBelle Laboratory for Biochemical Genetics, McGill University–Montreal Children's Hospital Research Institute, Montreal, Quebec, Canada

Dorothy E. Scriver (337), deBelle Laboratory for Biochemical Genetics, McGill University–Montreal Children's Hospital Research Institute, Montreal, Quebec, Canada

S. L. Sklower (237), Department of Pediatrics, Mt. Sinai School of Medicine, New York, New York

James R. Sorenson (273), Department of Socio-Medical Sciences and Community Medicine, Boston University School of Medicine, Boston, Massachusetts

Suzanne Trusler (163), Bureau of Laboratories, Center for Disease Control, Atlanta, Georgia

Robert R. Weiss (221), Neural Tube Defect Laboratory, Nassau County Medical Center, East Meadow, New York

Nancy S. Wexler (75), Commission for the Control of Huntington's Disease, National Institutes of Health, Bethesda, Maryland

Joan S. Wilentz (75), Commission for the Control of Huntington's Disease, National Institutes of Health, Bethesda, Maryland

PREFACE

This volume is based on the proceedings of the 7th Annual New York State Health Department Birth Defects Symposium on the occasion of the Institute's 10th birthday.

For the celebration of such an event, symposium (*sym* meaning together; *posis* meaning a drink) is perhaps an appropriate term for a band of scholars to congregate and make speeches on topics of common interest. In ancient Greece, people would, on special occasions, gather after dinner to drink and converse. Such evenings were called *symposia*. Once at such a gathering given by a clever young Greek play wright,the guests agreed to make speeches on a single topic that interested them all. Socrates was there, and his pupil, Plato, recorded the speeches and called it "*Symposium*." They would both have delighted in Dr. Murphy's scholarly, critical, and witty introduction to these proceedings (which appropriately enough was an address delivered after dinner).

The general theme of this symposium—Service and Education in Medical Genetics—was chosen because service is occupying a progressively greater proportion of the time of clinical geneticists and because of our increasing commitment to teaching not only students and colleagues, but also the public, be they adults or school children.

It is neither surprising nor entirely fortuitous that Dr. Laird Jackson, that same year, also had organized a session for the meeting of the American Society of Human Genetics, sponsored by the National Foundation-March of Dimes, in San Diego, California, with a similar orientation. With his and the National Foundation's concurrence, articles based on presentations given at that meeting are included in this volume: the chapters by Drs. Davis, Epstein (on California's regional services), Feingold, Riccardi, and the editors of this volume.

Not enough is known about the effective ways of delivering genetic services or about the impact of educational efforts, and what is known is scattered in many different places. We hope this volume will help to remedy the situation and provide a useful initial reference for those seeking further information.

The themes addressed in this volume illustrate the diverse concerns of the medical geneticist and the evolution of a specialty, which even ten years ago was predominantly based in research units of medical schools. Changes in technology and in social and medical attitudes have resulted in the involvement of medical geneticists in many new areas. These include, among others, long-range community planning for prevention of congenital and genetic disorders, community satellite centers, cost-benefit analyses, and, of course, prenatal diagnoses of a wide variety of disorders. Involvement with questions of service and education in medical genetics is now no longer limited to medical schools in university centers, but includes state and local health departments and branches of the Federal government. Moreover, many medical geneticists have markedly expanded the horizons involved in genetic counseling and genetic education by including ever larger segments of the general public as their target.

The chapters* in this volume should be useful not only in documenting the methods with which medical geneticists today confront many disorders, and in suggesting the direction of future work, but also in indicating the possible limitations upon such advances. While optimism about that which the future will bring is an important stimulus to the search for solutions to the outstanding questions, this must be tempered by caution, not only about the goals themselves, but about the methods of achieving them.

We acknowledge with gratitude the activities of numerous people who contribute to the smooth running of the symposium and to the production of these proceedings. These include, in particular, Mrs. Luba Goldin, our administrative assistant, Mrs. Ellen J. Heenehan, our editorial assistant, and many other members of the staff of the Birth Defects Institute. We are also grateful to Drs. Robert P. Whalen, our former Commissioner of Health, David Axelrod, our present Commissioner, and Roger C. Herdman, Director of Public Health, for support and encouragement.

*Two papers on hemaglobinopathies were given at the symposium but these manuscripts were not submitted for publication.

I. EPIDEMIOLOGICAL ANALYSIS, POLICY CONSIDERATIONS, AND ECONOMICS

GENETIC INTERVENTION: STRATEGY AND TACTICS

Edmond A. Murphy

Thomas Aquinas wrote that the cause of all evil lies in mistaking means for ends.[1] His worst enemies could not accuse him of being impetuous in reaching his conclusions; yet this principle has a breathtaking audacity about it which suggests that, if it is not a hasty generalization, it must embody an extremely penetrating insight. The more I reflect on it, and the more individual cases I apply it to, the more I am persuaded it is a genuine and fundamental truth. And I am convinced that a major preventive measure lies in longheadedness in the metaphorical sense.

There is some risk that the capacity to manipulate may be mistaken for the major problem in the betterment of society. This euphoric belief has an enduring quality which triumphs over mere experience. The theme is an old one, liberally discussed in this century; and the dire prognostications of the theorists seem to have been amply and repeatedly fulfilled in countless experiences. To a romantic such as me the present situation in clinical genetics provides an irresistible challenge to play Cassandra, with the warm and comforting feeling that the moguls will not pay the slightest attention to it until the grave they are digging leads to a landslide.

In trying to articulate in less rhetorical terms what underlies my misgivings, I find three major fallacies in which the reformers indulge. (These are fallacies of judgment rather than in logic since their logic consists mainly of vast enthymemes like a Swiss cheese or the more pregnant passages in early Wagner.) I shall call them the fallacies of linearity, of infinite divisibility and of participating detachment.

The Fallacy of Linearity

There is an extensive field of mathematics which shows that for most well-behaved functions, any segment small enough can be adequately approximated by a straight line.[2] In the world of inference, this property implies that such a segment may be mistaken for part of a straight line and that the best endowment for making this mistake is a carefully cultivated myopia. The demonstration

---

*This work was supported in part by Grant No. GM19489 from the National Institutes of Health.

ISBN 0-12-562650-9

project is an admirable example. In a collaborative study, it is shown, let us say, that amniocentesis is a reliable method of diagnosing aneuploidies with acceptably small risks to mother and fetus. Or it is shown that the carrier state of Tay-Sachs disease can be diagnosed, not infallibly, but with considerable confidence. From these results are projected a series of wild generalizations: as, that what is reliable and safe in the hands of a small group of international experts will perform as well when the tests are done by the rank and file, including the pharmacist and the village barber; or that what can be done in these diseases can be done in others; or because these things can be done that therefore they should be done; or that after all, many mickles do not make a muckle. For instance, it is an old idea that for recessives in which the carrier state is easily recognized, such as sickle hemoglobin, one can avoid the homozygous state by preventing marriages between carriers. As we know from the study of Stamatoyanopoulos,[3] it is not nearly so simple as that: there is more to be overcome than rational difficulties. But, in any case, the rational preventive measure involves some small limitation in choice of a mate. Now we try to imagine similar constraints being applied simultaneously to all loci: the enormous number of incompatibilities to be tested for, the steadily diminishing concession to romantic attachment, the mounting opportunities for mistakes (both false positive and false negative), in the recognition of incompatibilities. All we could conclude is that certain types of homozygous states can be avoided at a price. It is no trivial issue as to whether the price is worth paying – or, for that matter, how the price is to be assessed. These, surely, are issues which we should consider before all else, yet they are commonly relegated to postprandial chatter, or they emerge brightly but briefly at long intervals, like Halley's comet. Meanwhile, countless myopes wander around muttering that if they had two more technicians and five hundred square feet of extra laboratory space they could screen for galactosemia and Pompe's disease as well.

Of course, all this is obvious, painfully obvious. The economists have been discussing the law of diminishing returns for a long time. Utility theory has emphasized that a man with two million dollars is not twice as rich as a man with one million. There is, even in medical circles, a dim recognition that expenses mount faster than yield; but this is usually ascribed to cumbersome bureaucracy, the rising cost of living, or political corruption rather than to a mistaken perception of a complex logical relationship as a linear one.

As an illustration of non-linearity, it is a commonplace that as the sensitivity of a screening test is increased its specificity falls. To increase the proportion of cases of phenylketonuria diagnosed, we must be prepared to accept more false positive diagnoses. But with each further true positive diagnosis, the price (the number of false positives) becomes higher until to be sure of missing no cases one must include everybody, which destroys the whole purpose of a screening test.

The Fallacy of Infinite Divisibility

It has been known for a long time – in physics, for instance – that the phenomena of small systems are not simply scaled models of those of large systems. It is the journalist rather than the physicist who romances about the analogy between the atom and the solar system. There is little to encourage the belief that what may be the dominant issue at one level of organization will also be the dominant issue at all levels. Allow me a rather naive analogy. A carpenter in training may lavish great care on learning to make table legs, finding out all the mistakes to be avoided; and in time, no doubt, he makes an excellent leg. But in the second year of his apprenticeship he has to make tables, and suddenly unfamiliar features like equality of leg sizes become important. Four individually excellent table legs may be put together to produce a very bad table.

Now, in my analogy I would say that what may determine phenotypes, impose patterns of selection, inform our notions of normality, and shape our eugenic aspirations when one thinks at the level of the single gene, may be something quite different from what we see when we examine the individual as a whole. Two defects may cancel each other out; or it may be that both extremes are harmful and the best genotype demands that of its very nature it should be a mixture, such as a balanced polymorphism or, more generally, a stabilizing selection.

But, of course, there are higher levels of integration. We always talk as if intelligence, a fine artistic sense, a musular physique, bodily beauty are all desirable characteristics which it should be our business to promote. However, I suspect that a society consisting only of university professors might fall apart because of lack of practicality, or from a disinclination to do certain types of jobs – repetitive, non-creative work. On the other hand, there are people who enjoy chopping down trees or applying government regulations. I am saying that what may make for the happiest and most efficient society may be something quite different from what makes any one of us happy as an individual. If we go one step further, and consider the ecology, it is well known that even more disparate values may emerge. Man as a hunter must be clever enough to catch some prey, or he will starve. But if he is too good at it, he may thrive temporarily, but by over-hunting eventually exterminate his prey and again starve. It could be argued that the time is running out on the reprieve which the agricultural revolution gave us. Perhaps our farming has recently been over-efficient.

The Fallacy of Participating Detatchment

In several different fields of scholarship – in philosophy, in metamathematics, in analytical psychology, for instance – essentially the same principle emerges. One cannot from entirely within a system rationally select one part which is to govern. To be sure, in any system one part may acquire a stranglehold, as happens in a tyranny, for example, But, except on the principle that might is right, one can scarcely call rational such a *de facto* concentration of power. *We* may agree that the rulers of a country should be the most intelligent; but this is perhaps a prejudice of the intelligent. The brave might extoll bravery; the kindly, compassion; the virtuous, virtue. And all with some plausbility. But it is evident that any or all of these policies leaves unsolved the criteria by which these excellences are to be judged. So-called intelligence tests are merely an artibrary, and I suspect highly personal, selection of what a few people, mostly middle class European males, say are the components of intelligence. There are those of us who might not agree with Botticelli's conception of the ideally beautiful woman. I need say nothing about the immense literature on what constitutes virtue. What is one man's compassion is another man's sentimentality. It is debatable whether Alexander the Great or Dietrich Bonhoffer was the braver man.

It is easy to degenerate into mere nihilism: to say with Aristotle that all that exists is good, or with Rodin that all that has life is beautiful. Much as one might like to do it, one cannot altogether abdicate the responsibility of having opinions about quality. In this age, tolerance, I suspect, is not a virtue but a vice. But I would mistrust anyone who embraced this responsibility gladly and without pain. Such persons, I would fear, do not understand the momentousness of the issues. They probably think that what they believe is objective and what others believe is subjective. Those elder statesmen who have greatness thrust upon them and give postprandial speeches on eugenics seem somehow to be the principal characters in their own epics. I have found that if you ask people what they regard as desirable in the human race they tend to describe those qualities which they themselves possess or aspire to. If this is a casting of a single vote, then egotistical or not, it is at least in accord with well tried democratic principles. But if a person expressing such an opinion is arrogating to himself the right to prescribe for mankind, then as due process it is to be deplored. The situation is little improved if the opinion is that of a committee, appointed by itself or by others.

Strategic Principles

If I am confronted with the question of how this problem of defining excellence is to be solved, I certainly have no instant prescriptions. Having deplored egotism, I can scarcely have the hubris to parade my own puny opinions as the canons of eternal truth. But I think that I can say in broad terms what we would need to know to deal with the matter.

First we need time, thought and honest endeavor. These issues cannot be solved casually, or rapidly, or in the last few minutes of consciousness each day. The subject is at least as important as many purely technical problems. Yet I know of very little, if any, research support which is provided, or even proposed, for its exploration. This anomaly should certainly be remedied.

Secondly, I conceive of the answer, if one exists, as a truth to be discovered, not a remedy to be devised. Thus, it is to be sought, as any scientific answer is to be sought: not by sheer brute force of empirical fact, nor by democratic systems applied to a claim. Rather we must temper fact by theory and theory by fact. In disputed matters we seek not majority opinion, but consensus: that is, the truth is not promulgated by the man with the loudest voice, the most legions, or the largest research grants, but by a painstaking analysis and a scrupulous *resolution* of difficulties. We have not decided by majority vote that the earth goes round the sun; nor have we left the task to a group of accredited scientists. The consensus was established only when all organized argument based on scientific evidence against this hypothesis collapsed. This particular type of truth is, of course, scientific in nature and not necessarily at variance with some alternative viewpoint, a mystical or poetic one, for instance. However, it would seem that the words used may no longer necessarily have the same meaning in the several conflicting disciplines.

Then, thirdly, it seems evident that one should begin with the ultimate and least emotionally charged ideas. It is easier to agree that the human race should survive, or that purposeless pain is undesirable, than that we do not want more light-skinned or left-handed people. Once we are agreed on some strategic objective we can proceed to tactics. If we value survial of the species and can show that variation is necessary to that end, then we cannot pursue a policy of relentless homogenization. That problem is particularly transparent. I wish to illustrate by it that we have no choice but to meet the constraint of consistency. We cannot wish the end without accepting the means to the end. What is more to the point, we cannot aim for a set of mutually inconsistent objectives.

Let me try to illustrate the problem by considering in somewhat more detail the relationship between two objectives: excellence, and survival of the species. As broad objectives, they would be accepted by almost everybody, though we should expect a few dissident opinions. But converting these nebulous aspirations into concrete terms raises many problems.

What, for instance, do we mean by excellence? We might perceive it as the possession in high degree of some quality which we hold desirable – intelligence or bravery, for instance. But there may be little relationship between abstract quality and the virtue for which it is esteemed. Classical learning is said to ennoble the mind; but it was not Macaulay or Thackery who concerned themselves with abolishing poverty and wretchedness, but Dickens. The chief social value of bravery lies in chivalry; but the physically brave are often very far from chivalrous. The main function of the artist is to communicate insight, but many modern artists have little concern with it, so busy are they with their lofty feelings. We are driven, then, to take something of a utilitarian view of excellence – handsome is as handsome does. The Hollywood notion of ideal femininity may have almost nothing to do with reproductive efficiency; yet, it is the stereotype which lingers in the vulgar mind. The public holds in greatest awe pure mathematicians who number in their ranks some of the most inept and helpless. There are those of us who believe that the surgeon is overrated in the public image of medicine. Our stereotypes of excellence may be very much at variance with the interests of society.

Then consider what we mean by survival of the species. I do not have to underscore the elusiveness of the notion of a species, or the controversies which have waxed as to what the defining criterion may be. It is probably hopelessly naive to imagine that perpetuation of mankind means an endless reproduction, generation after generation, of the same kinds of people as ourselves. There has been much science fiction, dating back to H.G. Wells, which expresses the horror in which our descendants hold us, because of our social crudities and physical infirmities. There seems to be little expression of the converse, although it has been true throughout history that the older generation deplores the deterioration in the younger. We must also reckon with the possibility that mankind two thousand years hence will not be palpably better or worse than we are, merely totally different – as alien from our culture as the Mayan was from that of Christendom. What I mean is that when we seek perpetuation, we may not do so on our terms but may have to be content with biological continuity, even to the point at which we doubt whether what has survived may properly be called the same species.

Let us now take these objectives, excellence and survival, jointly. They are not necessarily easy, or even possible, to reconcile. The Hollywood beauty anxious to preserve her figure by avoiding pregnancy clearly contributes nothing to survival of the species; neither does the dashing hero who gets himself killed in early youth. So much is obvious. But at a more subtle level we must recognize that survival depends on interaction of at least four factors which, it is arguable, are all separate: genetic endowment, environmental pressures, chance, and the inventiveness of the free intellect. (I state the issues in these terms because I am somewhat anxious to avoid the stale and unilluminating tautology that all that is not genetic is environmental.) For one thing, the introduction of intellect, the notion that there is coherent purpose possible in some aspects of the system, paves the way for the introduction of a cybernetic element, commonly ignored totally in the biological interpretation of the system.

Now let us suppose, averaging over all possible states (which disposes of the random element), and ignoring the intellectual component for the time being, that for a given environment there is a unique optimal phenotype. Then, trivially, any other phenotype will be suboptimal, although perhaps not very much so. We also will suppose that what is best suited to one environment will, in general, not be best suited to others. We could think of the optimal phenotype as being something like a mathematical function of the environment. Now environments do change, and while they change relatively quickly, the genetic structure of the population also changes, but relatively slowly. Selection will therefore mean that the genotype lags behind the ever-changing optimum. But environmental changes can also be catastrophic. The stock market provides a useful analogy. A rapid change may bankrupt the speculator who has bought only the stock at the current highest price. The precaution, as wise investors know, is to diversify – not, that is to say, to buy indiscriminately, but to choose soundly in different areas. That may not be the way to get rich; but neither is it the quickest way to get poor. The moral is that there is survival value in variety as well as in excellence; indeed, corporately, variety is an excellence. And the analogy carries over with remarkable precision to the gene pool. A narrow preoccupation with the current performance of phenotypes may deprive the pool of that variety which is its insurance against extinction when the environment changes and performances also change. Two things strike me about the genetic structure which has evolved in the higher organisms. First, there are elaborate mechanisms – recombination, for instance – which provides for prodigious diversification of types; and it requires no elaborate documentation to show how great a variation actually exists[4,5] – indeed, it is probable that each individual is completely distinctive. The other and even more remarkable feature in the genetic structure of higher organisms is the extraordinary obstacles which stand in the way of those who would tamper with the composition of the gene pool. To select out from the gene pool all the genes of a particular type, genes which at present we might suppose uncompromisingly harmful, would be a formidable undertaking. But when we attempt to select not for genes but for phenotypes, where for multifactorial traits there may be many combinations which may give the same phenotype, the problem becomes vastly more complicated. In the wild state, where selection is not a matter of artificial manipulation but rather a spontaneous clash with the environment, in the face of these obstacles and the elaborate protective and cybernetic processes, selection must be a very unwieldy business. The Jeremiahs continually deplore the amount of rubbish in the gene pool. It may be salutary to recognize that so complex a system, which seems consecrated to maintaining the present state and to resisting all change, must after all have a selective advantage.

REFERENCES

1. T. Aquinas, cited by Lunn, A., *in* Come What May, Little Brown, Boston, 1941.
2. C. Lanczos, Applied Analysis, Prentice Hall, Englewood Cliffs, New Jersey, 1964.
3. G. Stamatoyannopoulos, *Excerpta Medica*, 1974.
4. H. Harris, D.A. Hopkinson and E.B. Robson, *Ann. Hum. Genet. 37*, 237, 1974.
5. S.H. Boyer, *Nature 239*, 453, 1972.

THE PREVENTABILITY OF GENETICALLY DETERMINED BIRTH DEFECTS*

Charles J. Epstein

As the material presented elsewhere in this volume clearly indicates, genetic counseling is certainly not what it used to be! While all, or at least most of us, undoubtedly consider the changes that have occurred in recent years to be for the better, there are, I believe, potential internal contradictions and conflicts that must be addressed. These are of particular concern when the public health implications of genetic counseling are being considered and when such considerations are used as the basis for seeking public financial support for genetic services. We should all carefully consider the growing disillusionment with the "War Against Cancer" which promised much but still has far to go in realizing the expectations that were generated when the funds to support it were being sought.

My first specific concern is with the current "official" definition of genetic counseling.[1] It is not that I disagree with it – having myself participated in its formulation and attempted to secure its full implementation in the genetic counseling services with which I am associated. Rather, it is that this definition is clearly *not* a public health oriented one and is, to some extent, antithetical to such an orientation. From the public health point of view, the desirable outcome of any medical program is the maintenance of health and the prevention of disease. While both mental and physical health are encompassed by the concept of public health, one is not considered to be of importance at the expense of the other. However, in our definition of genetic counseling, the emphasis is very strongly on improving the psychological state of those who are being counseled. Thus, we insist that they be able to

> "understand the options for dealing with the risk of recurrence (and) choose the course of action which seems appropriate *to them* in view of their risk and their family goals and act in accordance with that decision." (Italics mine.)[1]

---

*This work was supported in part by grants from the National Institutes of Health (GM-19527), the National Foundation-March of Dimes, and the Maternal and Child Health Service (Project No. 445). The author is an Investigator of the Howard Hughes Medical Institute.

ISBN 0-12-562650-9

Viewed from the vantage point of medical practice, this is a highly enlightened approach, one which attempts to allow, indeed to force the patient or family to take responsibility for its own decisions and future. From the public health vantage point, on the other hand, it allows and even lends support to the possibility that the eventual outcome will be an abnormal child who will then impose a considerable burden on both the family and the public, the latter in the form of public assistance for treatment and care. Of course, in many, perhaps most, instances of high risk the family's decision will be to avoid taking the chance of an unpleasant outcome, and both the private and public interests will be simultaneously served. But this is clearly not always the case, and it is here that our insistence on non-directive and supportive counseling, as embodied in the part of the definition quoted above, gives primacy to the private over the public interests.

Again, I want to indicate that I am not opposed to our present definition of counseling and am not arguing for a shift to a more directive approach (although I personally feel that non-directiveness is not always achievable nor necessarily always desirable). Rather, I am trying to emphasize the fact that, unlike in earlier times in this country and in other countries at this time,[2] family oriented genetic counseling in North America is not primarily prevention oriented and should not, therefore, be "sold" to the public in this guise. Prevention will often be the outcome, but this is neither explicit nor implicit in the definition. We must be honest with both ourselves and others about what we really are trying to do. Otherwise, we may some day have cause to regret such statements as:

> "Genetic counseling services which educate the public about the nature and risks of genetic disease and which are intended to assist those families affected by genetic disease to understand and cope with the disease can be *cost effective* and beneficial preventive services." (Italics mine.) (From Section 1, SB 873, California Legislature, 1977, which provides for funding of non-physician genetic counselors.)

When it becomes necessary to justify counseling as being cost-effective we are likely to find ourselves in real difficulty!

In earlier papers which avowed that the purpose of genetic counseling is to prevent genetic disease,[3] I espoused a very broad view of genetic counseling, one which included within its purview newborn screening, prenatal diagnosis, and even the administration of anti-Rh immune globulin.[4] One reason for doing so was to emphasize the expansion of counseling from a relatively passive, basically proband initiated process of calculating and quoting odds to one which actively sought to prevent genetic disease in a prospective manner. As our current carrier screening and age-related prenatal diagnosis programs well illustrate, active approaches to genetic disease prevention are not necessarily in conflict with the more recent definition of counseling, as long as entry into the programs and the ultimate decisions about what to do remain in the hands of those being counseled. Similarly, these programs are not fundamentally in conflict with a public health orientation toward prevention, since entry into them is most often stimulated by the desire to prevent a known and unwanted outcome. The same cannot, however, be said for newborn screening programs. Entry into them is nearly always compulsory, and there is very little option (even though it would undoubtedly rarely be exercised) not to treat an affected individual once he is detected. In this instance, the public, as represented by the State, has decided that public health concerns *are* of more importance than individual freedom of choice, and the general mood, at least for the present, is to agree. I dwell on this to emphasize that the public *does* see prevention as an essential goal and is willing, under appropriate circumstances, to make it mandatory. In other publicly supported programs it has, thus far, been possible to mandate public support without mandating participation, but this distinction, however obvious to us, may not always be obvious to others. Therefore, we will need to encourage public legislation in the genetics area to be more in the following form than in a prescriptive or proscriptive form.

> "The Legislature, therefore, finds that in order to make amniocentesis *available* to women with high risk pregnancies so that affected fetuses can be *discovered*, it is necessary to establish the *availability* of amniocentesis in at least two medical centers in California. . . .
>
> "The participation by any individual in this program shall be wholly voluntary and shall not be a prerequisite for eligibility for or receipt of any other service or assistance. . . ." (From AB 1336, California Legislature, 1975).

Although the intent is clearly to prevent the birth of abnormal children and the program is justified on the basis of cost effectiveness, neither participation nor a specific cause of action if an abnormal fetus is detected are required.

These comments about prenatal diagnosis and screening are not intended as a discussion of legislation concerning genetic matters but, rather, to bring us to the principal point of this paper – the preventability and prevention of genetic disorders. In this context, my concern with the current heavy emphasis on prenatal diagnosis and screening is that we may be restricting our own view of what constitutes prevention and may thereby be misleading others. I must confess that I have already fallen into this trap. In one of the articles on counseling to which I referred earlier,[4] I attempted to estimate the effects of various forms of genetic counseling in reducing the incidence of genetically determined disorders. Genetic counseling was divided into three types: proband oriented counseling (which I termed "genetic counseling of the past"), proband oriented counseling plus limited prenatal diagnosis and screening (termed "genetic counseling of the present") and all approaches that might be reasonably foreseen for the future (termed "genetic counseling of the future") (Fig.1). The genetic disorders were divided into three conventional categories – chromosomal, monogenic (which included Rh incompatibility caused hemolytic disease) and polygenic. The third

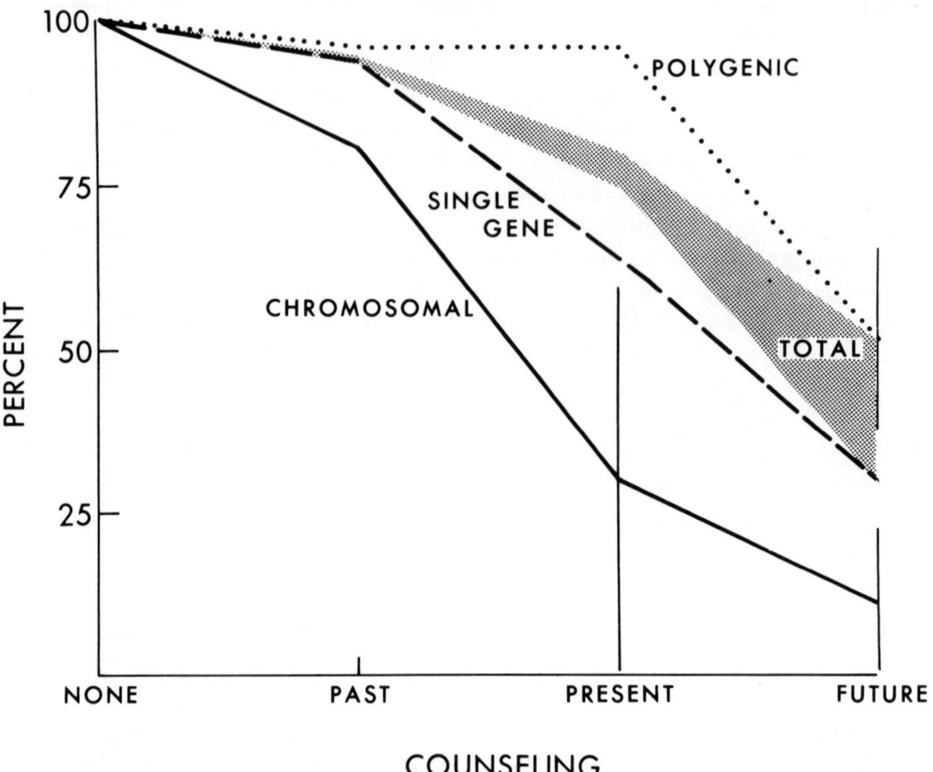

Fig. 1. Estimates made in 1971 of the impact of genetic counseling on the total incidence of genetically determined birth defects. The projected overall reduction was 30% to 50% of basal rates without any form of genetic counseling.

(Reprinted from C.J. Epstein, *in* Birth Defects and Fetal Development: Endocrine and Metabolic Factors, K.S. Moghissi (Ed.), courtesy of C.C. Thomas Co., publishers.)

group, for which I now prefer the term "multifactorial", included congenital malformations and diabetes but not mental illness nor the host of other later onset disorders which have genetic components. The essence of the calculations was that the expected overall reduction in the incidence of these birth defects would be only 7% if proband oriented counseling without prenatal diagnosis and screening were used, would be 18 to 25% if the latter techniques as then employed were added, and could reach 50 to 70% if all approaches then visualizable were used.

Success was expected to be greatest with the chromosomal disorders which, in principle, can be completely prevented by the universal practice of prenatal diagnosis and selective abortion. The monogenic disorders were considered to be the next most amenable to reduction in frequency, mostly because of the potential elimination of Rh induced hemolytic anemia of the newborn, but in part also because of the effectiveness of newborn screening and of carrier screening coupled with prenatal diagnosis in eliminating some of the more common hereditary metabolic disorders. The component of the monogenic disorders considered least amenable to prevention were those in which the defects are structural and have no known metabolic basis, and the same reasoning that applied to these was also applied to the multifactorial disorders such as congenital heart disease which could not be visualized *in utero.*

Depending on how the figures are viewed, the overall conclusion is either an encouraging or a sobering one. A significant proportion, as high as 50%, of genetically determined birth defects are *not* preventable by any foreseeable form of genetic counseling. For those aiming at total prevention of such abnormalities, this is not very encouraging. However, if the same figures were looked at in a reciprocal manner, the incidence of birth defects might be reducible by as much as 70%. This is clearly a very significant achievement particularly when the nature of the conditions which can now and may in the future be presented is considered.

These calculations are now six years old, and much of importance has since occurred, some of which could not have been anticipated. Approaches considered for the future are already in the present. For example, neural tube defects can be relatively easily diagnosed *in utero* by determination of the amniotic fluid α-fetoprotein concentration,[5] and can be screened for, in part, by assay of maternal serum α-fetoprotein;[6] more subtle chromosome aberrations are detectable by newer techniques for prophase and prometaphase banding;[7] possession of specific HL-A antigens and Ia antigens can be correlated with increased susceptibility to a variety of disorders;[8] direct fetal visualization is a reality,[9] and the newer methods for sonography promise greater ability to visualize internal structures such as the heart, kidney, and brain;[10] fetal blood can be directly sampled and its various components analyzed;[11,12] deleted genes can be searched for by molecular hybridization.[13] It may, if we consider only these additional approaches, be possible to reduce the calculated figures to a lower level than had been previously calculated, but even so, some entitites such as "nonspecific" mental retardation are likely to remain quite intractable.

However, although in preparing this paper it was originally my intention to do so, I have, for several reasons, chosen not to recalculate the figures. First, I no longer trust myself, or for that matter anyone else, as a crystal ball gazer. Too many things are occurring which may have as yet unrecognized profound effects on our approach to genetic disease. Second, I am not really certain of what to include under the heading of genetically determined birth defects. The chromosomal and monogenic disorders are easy to deal with. The common congenital malformations ascribed to multifactorial etiologies are, by convention, also included, but as the debate over the etiology of neural tube disorders indicates,[14] it is not always easy to tell what is or is not genetic. Beyond that, the decisions become more difficult, especially as the disease becomes more common. Undoubtedly, this situation will become clarified with time as specific disorders of defined genetic etiology are separated from the heterogeneous groups of disorders which, for want of a better way, are treated as though they were one (see, for example, the recent identification of familial peptic ulcer disease associated with hyperpepsinogenemia[15]). Third, partially but not wholly related to the preceding is the difficulty in deciding just how common each genetic disorder or group of disorders is. This applies not only to those which are less well defined, but also to monogenic conditions and, to some extent, chromosomal abnormalities as well. Consider, for example, the UNSCEAR (United Nations Scientific Committee on the Effects of Atomic Radiation) estimates published in 1966 and the British Columbia figures which appeared in 1974.[16] The estimate for autosomal dominant conditions has dropped from 0.95% to 0.08% of liveborns, for autosomal recessive conditions from 0.21% to 0.11%, and for chromosomal abnormalities from 0.42% to 0.20%. On the other hand, the estimates for congenital malformations have risen from 2.5% to 4.3% and for "other multifactorial" conditions from 1.5% to 4.7%. Overall, the British Columbia estimate of 9.4% of liveborns having a genetic disorder is almost twice the 5.6% estimated by UNSCEAR.

However, the principal reason for not attempting to recalculate the figures is that I question the meaningfulness of doing so, and this brings me back to the trap to which I alluded earlier. On rereading the earlier paper,[14] it became clear that preventability referred, in most instances, to the prevention of the birth of an affected individual primarily by utilization of prenatal diagnosis and selective abortion and potentially, in the case of the multifactorial disorders and possibly of some others as well, by environmental manipulation. Treatment, while considered to be useful for conditions such as phenylketonuria which are not presently diagnosable prenatally, was considered to be distinctly secondary and perhaps even undesirable. Thus, I went so far as to state that

> ". . . given acceptance of abortion as a way of handling genetic problems, it might well be preferable to ensure the birth of a normal child rather than to seek the birth of a treated or treatable but genetically abnormal one."

I now find that I have more difficulty with this approach than I did in 1971, not because I altogether disagree with it, but rather because I am concerned that it may lead to an improper placement of emphasis – with what is possible being stressed over what is reasonable. To state it more specifically, while prevention of birth defects by prenatal diagnosis is a powerful approach to many types of problems, concentration on this method to the exclusion of others leads to a narrowness of approach which runs the danger of neglecting other important modalities.

What then do we mean by prevention and preventability? The prevention of genetically determined birth defects can be approached at three levels: prevention of the appearance of the disease or defect *per se* in a genetically abnormal or predisposed individual; prevention of the birth of the genetically abnormal or predisposed individual; and prevention of the occurrence and/or propagation of mutations leading to genetic abnormality. Precedents for each of these approaches now exist and are worth briefly considering.

Prevention of the appearance of the disease or defect – in other words, prevention at the phenotypic level – is practiced more often than perhaps we realize. Numerous examples, which need not be belabored here, exist for avoidance of environmental factors, whether foods, drugs, or physical agents, that convert an abnormal but essentially innocent genotype into an abnormal phenotype. Similarly, there are many instances in which the administration of hormones, vitamins, clotting factors and the like is used to replace or stabilize or activate missing or otherwise defective gene products or metabolites. The second of these examples may seem suspiciously close to therapy and is, in fact, therapy by any conventional definition. Without wishing to do semantic violence, the point I want to make is that therapy and prevention should not be considered mutually exclusive or contradictory concepts. Therapy, while it cannot correct the intrinsic genetic abnormality or, in the case of multifactorial conditions, alter the genetic predisposition, can in many instances prevent these abnormalities and predispositions from being realized as disease.

A further extension of the concept of therapy as prevention might be derived from the prospective screening and early treatment of persons at risk for such conditions as the several hereditary forms of malignancy. However, mention of this last possibility will, I am sure, immediately bring a question to mind. Is this or any type of treatment, even if we are willing to consider it as a form of prevention, preferable to prevention by some other means which would obviate the need for therapy altogether? To return to the statement quoted earlier, would we, considering all that is involved, prefer to treat a child with phenylketonuria if prenatal diagnosis were actually feasible? Stated as a matter of preference I am sure that many of us would not, but I also do not believe that this is the proper question to be asking. Rather the question ought to be whether, in this case, newborn screening and early treatment would be an acceptable strategy for preventing symptomatic phenylketonuria even if some other more positive means, such as prenatal diagnosis, were available. Given its present widespread utilization and

and apparent success, it would be difficult to argue that it would not be. From this line of reasoning, which can be extended to many situations, I am led to conclude that matters of preference and of the relative merits of one approach over another should not lead to the making of absolute distinctions with regard to whether therapeutic modalities are valid means for preventing the deleterious consequences of genetic aberrations. I believe that in many instances they are and that we would be doing ourselves an injustice in this matter by ignoring them.

If treatment to prevent the appearance of an unwanted phenotype is accepted as a means of prevention, and entities that can be so handled as being preventable, what about treatment after the appearance of the abnormal phenotype? For example, what about the surgical treatment of a cleft lip? It would certainly be difficult in this case to equate treatment with prevention, but I put forward this situation to raise yet another question. Is prevention always the necessary or at least the most desirable outcome? If it could be achieved with only a reasonable amount of effort, I suppose the answer would certainly be "yes". But, if it could not – if the price of prevention becomes too high in either human or economic terms – then it might be better to capitalize on what can be done to correct that which has occurred rather than to feel that we have failed because we have been unable to prevent the condition from occurring in the first place.

The second general approach to prevention – prevention of the birth of individuals with abnormal genotypes – has already been alluded to several times in this paper and does not require detailed discussion here. The various ways of accomplishing this fall into two categories – prevention of the conception of a genetically abnormal fetus and, if conception does occur, prevention of the completion of pregnancy. Included, among other things, are proband oriented counseling, sterilization, artificial insemination, heterozygote screening, and, of course, prenatal diagnosis. It is to this approach that we have looked and continue to look for most of what we consider to be in the nature of prevention.

The third approach is difficult to evaluate in terms of its ultimate impact on the incidence of genetic disease. In theory, the ultimate way to prevent genetic disorders would be to prevent new mutations (and here I use the term mutation to include all genetic abnormalities including gross chromosome aberrations) and to eliminate or reduce in frequency those which already exist. The ability to bring about a reduction of the existing load of mutations, one of the objectives of the eugenics movements of earlier years, seems very distant, if not impossible, and even its desirability is open to great question. On the other hand, the notion of preventing the occurrence of new mutations has come very much to the fore in recent years, particularly with the tremendous expansion of interest and activity in the area of environmental mutagenesis. Because of the frequency with which they now arise as new genetic accidents, the potential effects of this approach, if it should ever become realizable, are likely to be greatest for the chromosomal disorders. However, unless an environmental mutagenic catastrophe is otherwise destined to occur, the effects of controlling environmental mutagens would be much less with regard to the relatively rare occurrence of new autosomal (dominant) and X-linked mutations. It should also be noted that environmental manipulation would not alter the fact of the preventability of chromosome disorders, but it would shift their prevention from the level of the fetus and selective abortion to that of preventing the aberration from ever occurring. Although the theoretical statistics of preventability would not change appreciably – and it is important to realize that they would not – the means for attaining them would. This could, in turn, have tremendous implications for the actual degree of prevention that can be achieved in practice.

Conclusions

This paper has ranged over a variety of subjects, and in concluding it seems appropriate to recapitulate the major points that have been made. Although a frequent outcome of genetic counseling is the prevention of genetic disease, prevention is *not* a specific goal of genetic counseling as presently defined. Consequently, proband oriented counseling should not be equated with prevention. However, the public *is* interested in the prevention of genetic disease and must be given a realistic appraisal of what is and can be accomplished. Means are currently available to reduce significantly the incidence of genetic abnormalities but because of the rapidity with which changes are occurring, care should be exercised in being too definite about what the future is likely ot bring. Many forms of prevention, including some which might be considered as therapy, are presently in use and under development. Flexibility of approach must be preserved, and we should not fall into the trap of placing undue emphasis on any single method. What may be preferable in theory might not turn out to be preferable in practice.

Tremendous progress has already been made in the prevention of genetic disease, and greater achievements are likely in the future. Therefore, in seeking public financial support for our endeavors, we should emphasize what our capabilities actually are and not promise more than we can actually deliver. In these times of great public concern with the spectors raised by the spectacular advances in molecular genetics and "genetic engineering", I believe that only a policy of honesty to both ourselves and the public will permit us to retain the trust of the society which we attempt to serve. This will, in turn, make it possible for us to preserve the interests of our individual patients and families while, at the same time, coming as close as possible to achieving society's goal of reducing the burdens of inherited disorders and of preventing genetic disease.

REFERENCES

1. Ad Hoc Committee on Genetic Counseling, *Am. J. Hum. Genet. 27*, 240, 1975.
2. W. Fuhrmann and F. Vogel, Genetic Counseling, 2nd ed., 51, 1976.
3. C.J. Epstein, *in* Early Diagnosis and Prevention of Genetic Diseases, L. N. Went, C. Vermeij-Keers and A.G.J.M. Vander Linden (Eds.), Leiden Univer-

sity Press, pp. 110-128, 1975.
4. C.J. Epstein, *in* Birth Defects and Fetal Development: Endocrine and Metabolic Factors, K.S. Moghissi (Ed.), C.C. Thomas, pp. 268-299, 1974.
5. D.J.H. Brock, *Br. Med. Bull. 32*, 16, 1976.
6. U.K. Collaborative Study on Alpha-fetoprotein in Relation to Neural-tube Defects, *Lancet 1*, 1323, 1977.
7. J.J. Yunis, *Science 191*, 1268, 1976.
8. H.O. McDevitt and W.F. Bodmer, *Lancet 1*, 1269, 1974.
9. M.J. Mahoney and J.C. Hobbins, *N. Engl. J. Med. 297*, 258, 1977.
10. J. Bartley, M.S. Golbus, R.A. Filly and B.D. Hall, *Clin. Genet. 11*, 375, 1975.
11. Y.W. Kan, M.S. Golbus, R.F. Trecartin, R.A. Filly, C. Valenti, M. Furbetta and A. Cao, *Lancet 1*, 269, 1977.
12. M.J. Mahoney, F.P. Haseltine, J.C. Hobbins, B.Q. Banker, C.T. Caskey and M.S. Golbus, *N. Engl. J. Med. 297*, 968, 1977.
13. Y.W. Kan, M.S. Golbus and A.M. Dozy, *N. Engl. J. Med. 295*, 1427, 1976.
14. I. Leck. *Br. Med. Bull. 30*, 158, 1974.
15. J.R. Rotter, J.Q. Sones, C.T. Richardson, D.L. Rimoin, I.M. Samloff and R.B. McConnell, *Clin. Res. 25*, 325 A, 1977.
16. B.K. Trimble and J.H. Doughty, *Ann. Hum. Genet. 38*, 199, 1974.

LONG-TERM GENETIC CONSEQUENCES OF ADVANCES IN TREATMENT AND PREVENTION OF HEREDITARY DISEASE

G.R. Fraser

The more I have thought during the past five years concerning the questions touched upon in the title of this paper, the more I have felt like an explorer on a voyage of discovery with no charts whereby to steer. In fact, the future is completely unknown territory in this respect, and any long-term effects of whatever we do today in the realm of treatment and prevention of hereditary disease depends on so many factors that the final results can only be surmised rather than defined.

The kind of concern about such activities which was expressed by some commentators was well summarized by Dr. Bentley Glass, who in 1972[1] seemed overwhelmed by gloom as he contemplated the man of tomorrow beginning his day "by adjusting his spectacles and his hearing aid, inserting his false teeth, taking an allergy injection in one arm and an insulin injection in the other, and topping off his preparations for life by taking a tranquilizing pill". I should like to make it clear at the onset that I do not share this particular vision of the future; nor do I think, with all the many changes and modifications in our thinking on this subject which have taken place since 1972, that this is now a generally accepted view, if indeed it ever was. This is not to say that I am not sometimes overcome by even more apocalyptic visions of the future, but these have little to do with our present activities in the field of treatment and prevention of hereditary disease. Of these visions I shall speak briefly later.

I think that the problems under discussion may best be considered under two very distinct headings – that of Mendelian disease and that of the much wider spectrum of multifactorially determined conditions, many of them common, where complex hereditary factors contribute to a predisposition which may only be manifested as overt disease after long-term exposure to the appropriate environmental influences. The first category has the advantage that the problem is amenable to simple mathematical treatment and a particularly clear example is afforded by the autosomal dominant form of retinoblastoma which accounts for most of the bilateral cases of this condition.

A little more than a century ago, advances in surgery first led to survival of a small number of infants with this condition which had previously been fatal (with rare exceptions due to spontaneous regression of the tumors). It was then noted

ISBN 0-12-562650-9

that some of the offspring of these survivors had similarly affected children who clearly would not have been born had it not been for the advances in medical treatment which had saved the lives of their parents. This is a very simple example of what might be termed a dysgenic effect of medical treatment, and it may be shown that, whatever the mechanism of Mendelian inheritance, autosomal or X-linked, dominant or recessive, the prevalence of the disease will stabilize when a new equilibrium is reached at $x_1 = \frac{x_0(1-f_0)}{1-f_1}$ where x_0 is the original prevalence and f_0 and f_1 are the relative fitnesses of persons with the disease before and after treatment is instituted. Assuming that f_0 is zero and f_1 is 0.5, $x_1 = 2x_0$ and the prevalence of the disease is eventually doubled. It should be noted that the time span required for this doubling is very long. It may be of the order of a century for autosomal dominant disease, several hundred generations for autosomal recessive disease and an intermediate period in the case of X-linked recessive disease. Furthermore, this is under the assumption that the treatment is implemented universally in the human population rather than in small economically privileged minority groups.

Again the present trend in preventing the birth of infants with certain types of recessive Mendelian disease will tend to have a dysgenic effect in the sense that the strategy of antenatal diagnosis with selective abortion may lead to reproductive compensation whereby a child who would not have had offspring because of his disease may be aborted and replaced by a healthy heterozygote who will pass on the mutant allele to future generations. More extensive mathematical treatments of these dysgenic tendencies are presented elsewhere.[2] Here, only examples will be presented to illustrate the order of changes which may be expected to occur. In the case of autosomal recessive disease where homozygous abnormal fetuses are aborted and replaced by healthy children, whether heterozygous or homozygous normal, the ratio of the new to the old equilibrium frequencies, of the abnormal allele responsible for the disease, under the assumptions that the balancing mechanism is new mutation and that every couple has two children, may vary in a range between 1.02 and 1.22. The exact figure will depend on the proportion of the population which is subjected to this strategy. For the lower figure (1.02), this is 1/8 corresponding to retrospective counseling where the only reason for monitoring second and subsequent pregnancies is that the first has ended in the birth of an affected child, while the higher figure (1.22) corresponds to prospective counselling where the parents are identified by screening to be heterozygous pre-reproductively and the whole population is, therefore, subjected to this strategy. It should be remembered again that these new theoretical equilibrium values are only attained after many generations, and that the incidence of the disease at birth, as opposed to the gene frequency, invariably decreases under the application of this strategy.

In the case of lethal X-linked conditions, the frequency of the gene in males and hence the incidence of the disease will be 1/3 of the original value where the strategy is that of prospective selective abortion of males, whether it is possible to make the diagnosis of the disease in the fetus or not. This is because even though all carrier mothers may be detected by screening in this situation, one-third of cases of the disease will be due to fresh mutations and hence be born of mothers who are not carriers. In these circumstances, when all males are aborted the incidence of heterozygous females will increase by 50 percent of its original value (4μ where μ is the mutation rate) in each generation, but when a diagnosis of the genotype can be made and only affected fetuses are aborted this incidence will increase only to a new equilibrium value of 6μ over a number of generations. Where the diagnosis is retrospective and it is assumed that each couple has two children, the ratios of the final to the original incidence of the disease in males are 0.90 and 1.32 depending on whether the genotype of male fetuses can be determined or not, and the corresponding ratios for the prevalence of heterozygosity in females are 1.25 and 1.90.

Taking into account all the assumptions which have been built into these calculations and the length of time taken to reach these new equilibrium values, I do not feel that these dysgenic trends can be regarded as disastrous or even dangerous.

Of course, the long-term genetic effects of medical treatment are not restricted to Mendelian conditions and I should like now to turn to the broader definition of hereditary disease to which I alluded previously. As an illustration, I should like to consider the common congenital malformations. In the majority of cases, these are not Mendelian but are determined by complex interactions of genetic and environmental factors. Improvements in surgical treatment have led to the survival to reproductive age of an increased number of infants with potentially lethal conditions such as spina bifida aperta and congenital heart disease and the incidence of similar conditions among their offspring is increased by an order of magnitude to 3-5 percent. Thus, the incidence of these conditions at birth will increase because of these changes though, in the case of spina bifida aperta at least, this tendency will be counter-balanced by the introduction of antenatal detection and selective abortion. Indeed, a dramatic decrease may occur because it is probable that within a few years antenatal screening programs for this condition will be introduced. It should be noted also that, in general, any increase in the population prevalence of these conditions, because persons reproduce who would previously have died, will occur mainly in the first generation after treatment is introduced, and that such an increase will tend in the long term towards a limit of perhaps 10 percent of the initial incidence at birth.[3]

These types of long-term effects due to medical intervention in the case of non-Mendelian disease are by no means restricted, however, to congenital malformations and, in fact, they are by no means all of recent origin. Improvements in the prognosis of those with infectious disease have been occurring for some time and, long before the antibiotic era, the mortality of children and young adults with such diseases as pneumonia, pulmonary tuberculosis and puerperal sepsis decreased substantially. With the advent of antibiotics these improvements became dramatic. Since susceptibility to infections of all types is determined by hereditary factors, there has of necessity been a relaxation of selection for some

TABLE 1

Dysgenic and Eugenic Implications of Present and Some Future Possibilities of Prevention and of Treatment, and of Some Technological and Sociological Changes Affecting Reproductive Patterns, in the Case of Diseases Determined by Mendelian Inheritance. (D = Dysgenic; E = Eugenic)

	Autosomal Dominant Inheritance	Autosomal Recessive Inheritance	X-linked Recessive Inheritance
Treatment			
Increased fertility	D	D	D
Prevention			
Avoidance of marriages between heterozygotes by premarital screening		D	
Counseling leading to reproductive restraint	E	E	E
Early diagnosis	E		
Improvements in heterozygote detection		E	E
Artificial insemination by donor[1]	E	E	E
Antenatal diagnosis and selective abortion of affected fetuses	E	D	D D-all males
Artificial insemination by husband using X-chromosome bearing sperm (future)			D
Genotypic gametic selection (future)	E	E	E
Others			
Break-up of isolates and increase in out-breeding		D[2]	
Reduction of heterozygote advantage		E	E
Lowering of parental age at reproduction	E	E	E
Increase in mutation rate due to radiation and chemical agents	D	D	D

[1] Where the father is affected or a carrier.

[2] This dysgenic effect may be compensated by enhancement of hybrid vigor determined by complex interactions of alleles at many loci at which the average level of heterozygosity will increase.

time against the genes determining these susceptibilities which must therefore be increasing in frequency. The results of this increase are entirely unknown. Since their possessors are at present in no danger of succumbing to the diseases in question, other effects of these genes may be of greater importance, and we have no means of knowing what these are. Thus, it is entirely possible that genes which determine susceptibility to tuberculosis, for example, may also contribute to the determination of favorable attributes, resulting in a net eugenic effect under present circumstances. In passing, it should be noted that the same may be true of alleles which in homozygous form cause autosomal recessive Mendelian diseases. Thus, the increase of the frequencies of these alleles, which may be regarded as dysgenic in one sense, as discussed above, may be eugenic in another. In other words, we cannot define a Manicheistic dichotomy between "good" genes and "bad" genes in this context.

Advances in medicine and public health have, in general, led to considerable increases in the expectation of life. In part, this has been due to specific treatments which have led to the survival to reproductive age of persons who would otherwise have died, before reaching this age, of infectious diseases or of conditions such as, for example, juvenile diabetes; in part it has been non-specific and due to improvements in nutrition and in the general conditions of life. Whatever their modalities, such advances have led to profound changes in the genetic composition of those who survive to reproduce and, hence, of the population. Perhaps those components of these advances which involve the treatment of the degenerative and neoplastic diseases of middle and old age are not of such great importance in this connection, since reproduction has been little affected by such diseases.

I should like now to revert to Mendelian disease and to consider this problem in a more general context. The effects of medical treatment and prevention of hereditary disease cannot be viewed in isolation from changes which are occurring in the patterns of reproduction in human society. In Table 1 some of the factors which need to be taken into account are set out.

Apart from the effects of treatment which have already been discussed, prevention of Mendelian disease is by no means restricted to antenatal diagnosis and selective abortion. It is imperative, if our civilization is to survive in a recognizable form, that an attitude towards reproduction which will stabilize or even reduce population size be generally adopted. Within this context of quantitative limitation with its implication of a greater sense of responsibility towards reproduction, qualitative considerations will acquire more importance. Thus, counseling may be increasingly sought and acted upon, and in this connection such developments as early diagnosis, for instance in the case of Huntington's chorea, and improvements in heterozygote detection may lead to reproductive restraint. It should be noted that if identification of heterozygosity in both members of a couple is followed by abandoning marriage plans. this technically leads to a dysgenic effect since an increased number of heterozygous children will be born following the marriage of each member of the couple to another person who is not heterozygous for that particular allele.

Another technique of which increasing use may be made in the future is artificial insemination by a donor. This is particularly applicable where the husband is suffering from a dominant disease such as retinoblastoma or is at high risk for Huntington's chorea, or where he suffers from an X-linked disease such as hemophilia. It is also an effective method of preventing the birth of affected offspring where the marriage partners are both heterozygous for alleles which cause autosomal recessive disease. The use of this technique may also come to be regarded as more appropriate because of increasing problems with the alternative solution of adoption as the number of available infants becomes smaller. Inhibitions about donor insemination, which is widely used as a treatment for male infertility, may also decrease with changing ideas about the significance and exclusivity of biological parenthood as part of a general realignment of attitudes towards reproduction.

I should like now to say a few words about future prospects. We will be increasingly called upon to guide couples to have a modest number of healthy offspring and, in my opinion, the strategy of antenatal diagnosis and selective abortion, with its attendant strains and stresses on patient and physician alike, can only be regarded as a temporary expedient. Medicine in common with other branches of applied knowledge, does not stand still and, although I would not hazard a guess about the techniques which will be in use in a hundred or in a thousand years, it is safe to say that they will be very different from those in use today.

The idea has unfortunately been voiced in some circles that there is little difference in principle between selective abortion in the third trimester of pregnancy and infanticide after postnatal identification of the same disease. I believe that this is sophistry and that introduction of these types of solutions would represent a retrogressive step from the point of view of our attitude towards the value of human life which represents one of the saving graces of our civilization. I would rather hope that progress will occur at the other end of pregnancy, possibly by gametic selection, especially of sperm. Thus, once the problem of separating sperm into X- and Y-chromosome-bearing classes with retention of their fertilizing power is solved (and this time cannot be far distant), artificial insemination with the appropriate fraction of the husband's sperm will provide an elegant solution to the problem of X-linked disease which would be unlikely to offend ethical susceptibilities. For instance, in the case of hemophilia, carrier females could be fertilized with X-chromosome-bearing sperm, while the wives of affected males could have only unaffected sons by the use of Y-chromosome-bearing sperm, thus avoiding the birth of carrier daughters. Possibly, in the more remote future, gametic selection of a more refined type may enable fertilization to be effected by sperm of a given genotype; for example, the class bearing the allele for normal β-globin chain production derived from a male who is heterozygous (AS) for sickling. Of course, I do not know how this could be achieved and I mention it only as a possibility. To attempt an historical analogy, Archimedes might have conceived of the possibility of Man flying or even traveling to the moon but he could not have been expected to have had any conception of the details of the structure of a Boeing airplane or an Apollo spacecraft.

In the final part of Table 1, the possible effects of other trends which we are seeing in connection with changes in our society are set out. Thus, in principle, the elimination of malaria should have a eugenic effect in that the advantage of sickling heterozygotes will be eliminated and this will lead to a reduction in frequency of the sickling gene. The break-up of isolates and the disappearance of geographical barriers to mating will have a dysgenic effect in the same way as avoidance of marriage by heterozygotes for the same mutant allele causing autosomal recessive disease, as discussed above; there will be a reduction in elimination of the mutant allele by the death of homozygotes. This break-up of isolates may, however, be expected to have a compensatory favorable genetic effect by enhancement of hybrid vigor, as indicated in the table. A very important phenomenon which forms part of the changing patterns of reproduction we are witnessing is the lowering of parental age. This should have a eugenic effect in reducing the frequency of mutations, but this tendency is being counterbalanced to some extent by increases due to pollution of the environment by radiation and chemical agents which form an inescapable by-product of our technological civilization. In passing, although I am not dealing specifically with chromosomal aberrations, this reduction in parental age is having a dramatic effect in decreasing the incidence of these in view of the well-known positive correlation between their incidence and maternal age.

Thus, even in the case of Mendelian disease, the demographic, social and medical changes which we are witnessing today interact with each other in a very complex way and the total resultant of these changes is almost impossible to define. How much more complicated is the situation with respect to the impact of medical treatment of non-Mendelian disease. It is simply impossible to state how advances in treatment are affecting the gene pool of Man in general and, as I have pointed out previously, the more significant changes are probably not the dramatic and obvious ones exemplified by recent changes in the treatment of retinoblastoma but subtler ones such as those induced by modifications of the morbidity and mortality patterns of diseases such as tuberculosis.

I feel, therefore, that I have been dealing with an artificial problem. Every act of medical care has both short-term and long-term consequences. In some cases these long-term consequences are social and economic and may be confined to the lifetime of the treated patient; in others they may be genetic and may affect future generations in ways which we cannot properly foresee. Francis Bacon wrote at the beginning of the 17th century "Men must pursue things which are just in present, and leave the future to the divine Providence".

I think that in the context under discussion this might be interpreted as indicating to us that we should concern ourselves with the problems of our patients and of our patients' immediate families without undue worry about the possible effects of our actions on future generations. While I am myself far from convinced about the protection to be expected of the divine Providence, I do, in fact, have sufficient faith in our descendants to believe that they will be able to deal better than we can, and using methods which we cannot even imagine now, with any untoward results of our activities in the areas under discussion, including modifications in the biological legacy which we leave to them.

There is an all-important proviso in connection with the mention of apocalyptic visions of the future with which I began this paper. This is that our generation leaves to our descendants an intact physical legacy so that they may be able to continue to develop the scientific and technical approaches which we have initiated. Thus, I think that our primary responsibility to future generations is to do all that lies in our power to protect our civilization from the very real physical dangers that threaten it, including pollution, exhaustion of natural resources, war and over-population which could lead to its complete impoverishment, or even collapse, and to the cessation of progress in any field for an indefinite period of time.

If we can achieve this, then I believe that our descendants will be grateful to us and will forgive us for any results, of the type I have been discussing, of our activities in the field of medical care with which they may have to contend. In conclusion, therefore, I feel that we can continue, within the framework of the medical tradition which has been bequeathed to us by our own ancestors, to accomplish our duties towards our present day patients by the exercise of the maximum of tact, understanding and wisdom of which we are capable and without any attempt to introduce coercive or directive measures which might lead to the fulfillment of William Blake's prophecy,

> "Children of the future age,
> Reading this indignant page
> Know that in a former time
> Love, sweet love, was thought a crime."

REFERENCES

1 B. Glass, *Perspect. Biol. Med. 237,* 1972.
2. G.R. Fraser, *Amer. J. Hum. Genet. 24*, 359, 1972: G.R. Fraser, *J. Génét. Hum. 20,* 185, 1972.
3. E. Matsunaga, *Hum. Genet. 31,* 53, 1976.

GENETIC COUNSELING AND PRENATAL CYTOGENETIC SERVICES: POLICY IMPLICATIONS AND DETAILED COST-BENEFIT ANALYSES OF PROGRAMS FOR THE PREVENTION OF DOWN SYNDROME

Ernest B. Hook

INTRODUCTION

Until relatively recently, at many centers, genetic services – especially genetic counseling but also cytogenetic diagnosis – was viewed as exempt from the fee-for-service concept. This has had some unfortunate consequences in that it has, I believe, inhibited rapid expansion of prenatal cytogenetic services. In late 1975, after the widespread publicity given to the results of the U.S.A. collaborative study of amniocentesis,[1] there was an abrupt increase in demand for prenatal cytogenetic diagnosis. Centers which did not charge for their services – or charged only a nominal amount – in many instances could not get internal institutional support for expansion.

At the same time, many centers were receiving (and continue to receive) subsidies from outside sources for provision of services; for example, from the Birth Defects Institute or the National Foundation-March of Dimes. These subsidies could not increase as rapidly as the demand for services did, and, moreover, some centers receiving subsidies could not charge by virtue of contractual agreements with the external agencies. Moreover, many genetic centers which did bill for services often were not billing for their total true cost, but for only a fraction of this. This may have been not only because of a subsidy but also because the true costs were often underestimated. Indeed, since genetic services have traditionally been provided at academic institutions, where, at least in the recent past, the financial aspects of delivery of clinical services were rarely considered, the true costs of services provided were only guessed at, and frequently the amount estimated was much too low. When demand for service was low and clinical cytogenetics could be done primarily by a research laboratory subsidized by grants or general institutional support, this probably did not make much difference. But the directors of such laboratories were often neither practically nor psychologically able to expand suddenly to meet an increased demand for services compared to the directors of commercial laboratories.

Quite separate from this is the fact that individuals who receive genetic services which are subsidized in whole or in part are often unaware of this fact. In

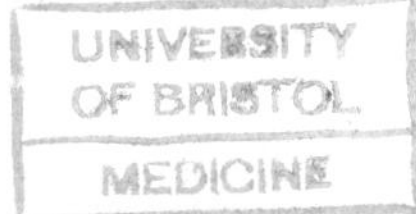

ISBN 0-12-562650-9

psychiatry – which is the field of medicine providing the closest analogy to genetic counseling – even for services which may be completely subsidized, at least some token payment is frequently requested by the provider so that the patient or client will take the service more seriously. Whether this policy would be as useful in genetic counseling for this or other reasons is a separate issue. But I believe those who receive subsidized services both for laboratory work and for counseling should at least be aware of the extent and source of the finances for the services they are receiving that otherwise are taken for granted.

REIMBURSEMENT FOR GENETIC SERVICES THROUGH MEDICAID

In the spring of 1977, in attempting to get an approved Medicaid fee for genetic services in New York State, I encountered some indirect adverse consequences of the absence of such a policy. After extensive discussion with a number of individuals, I had made an estimate of the average cost to centers for prenatal diagnosis of $250 – this for the *laboratory* service only – including all equipment amortization, overhead, etc. But at a meeting with the economist who initially reviewed this figure for approval, the copies of the bill received by a friend of his were produced. His friend had been charged only $150 for cytogenetic analysis of amniotic fluid cells. This service had been provided by a small unit which was probably heavily subsidizing its services from internal institutional sources, but that point was not made evident to the patient. It was with some difficulty that I managed to convince the economic reviewer that this was a subsidized and probably anomalous figure; eventually he approved $200 as the reimbursable fee – in part because one commercial laboratory which had the economies of scale was charging that figure. I still believe this figure is unrealistically low. Genetic counseling was approved at a rate of $30/hour; lower than what many centers may charge, but at least on a par with what Medicaid reimburses for psychiatric counseling.

As this example illustrates, it is important to attach or stamp a fair economic value upon genetic services. As for any other clinical service, the failure to do so may have broad and perhaps inadvertent consequences.

SOME ISSUES BEARING ON QUALITY ASSURANCE

This immediately bears on another issue: defining the appropriate "providers" for genetic services. This question arose in considering reimbursement approval for genetic counseling under Medicaid. As of November 1977 there were no existing standards, requirements, examinations, qualification statements, or professional definitions as to who or what is a "genetic counselor". Until such are defined – and it appears it will be a long time before the American Society of Human Genetics will establish certification in this area – it will be very difficult to extend reimbursement to *individual counselors* within Medicaid at least, except perhaps by defining genetic counseling as a subspecialty of clinical medicine and as a part of the practice of physicians with subspecialty training in genetics. (In the absence of such standards for individuals, an advisory committee has been set up to establish standards for *centers* providing genetic counseling services. See the appendix.)

COST-BENEFIT ANALYSIS: INTRODUCTION

Another question, raised by some of those considering approval of reimbursement for the charges for prenatal genetic services, was the "cost-benefit" one. This is an appropriate question perhaps for mass screening for phenylketonuria at birth, for example, or for screening disorders in an entire population. But for third party reimbursement through Medicaid or other sources, I feel it is an unfair question in one sense, if the procedure is one that is regarded as "medically indicated". For example, if the Cesarean section operation were a new procedure would it be reasonable to seek to justify this procedure on a cost-benefit basis before allowing it to be reimbursed? As another example, psychotherapy is now reimbursable through Medicaid as well as by many insurance companies but, to my knowledge, this has not been based upon cost-benefit considerations, but on the fact that this is a medically warranted procedure. (Genetic counseling is essentially very similar to some types of psychotherapy.) Operationally, prenatal diagnosis is usually regarded as "medically indicated" if it is "generally accepted" that a physician should offer the prospective mother this option if she is at sufficiently "high" risk to have an affected child whose diagnosis might be made prenatally. The question is, who is to decide what is a sufficiently "high" risk and what criteria are to be used? Some suggest the risk of the procedure should be balanced against the risk of having an affected child which could be diagnosed prenatally – a policy which appears sensible but is hard to implement with accurate and appropriate data. The risks of the procedure vary greatly with a number of extraneous factors, such as the experience and knowledge of the obstetrician performing the procedure and, I believe, are very difficult to estimate precisely.

The results of the U.S.A. collaborative study suggest that, *in the hands of an experienced and knowledgeable obstetrician*, the risks are likely to be less than 1%.[1] But this "balancing" of risk and benefits – to the extent that it can even be attempted – should be done by the woman involved, not her own physician, and women may vary greatly in their choice as to what risk of an affected infant and risk of procedure is acceptable.

Eventually, I suspect physicians will find that they will have to discuss with *every* (pregnant) woman the risks and benefits and alert her to prenatal diagnosis, assuming the laboratory resources are there to meet this potentially high demand.

It may be argued that such a policy is not "cost-effective". But from a cost-benefit viewpoint it might be hard to justify any therapeutic (not just preventive) service for individuals who are not now nor likely to be economically productive in the future. I am sure that many who are contemplating eventual retirement would view such a prospect with dismay, and a dismay whose magnitude is proportional to age. While one may happily embrace cost-benefit analysis in considering services that avoid births of defective individuals who will not make economic contributions, such analyses are, in one sense at least, not too far removed from those of the Patagonians of Tierra del Fuego at the time of Darwin, who did their own rough cost-benefit analyses when they gave preference to the survival of hunting dogs over their aged relatives when the latter could no longer actively contribute to the food supply.[2]

For this and analagous reasons that may be readily imagined, I find cost-benefit considerations somewhat repugnant and believe they should not have to be invoked in defending reimbursement for genetic services. But I have found they cannot be ignored in discussions with policy makers concerning subsidation of genetic services, among other reasons.

COST-BENEFIT ANALYSIS: DEFINITIONS

With this justification in mind, I suggest one approach that may satisfy the economic reviewers in various jurisdictions concerning subsidization for women of "sufficiently high" risk and a mechanism for deciding, in fact, what a "sufficiently high"risk is for provision of support.

From the perspective of possible public *subsidization* of these costs, one must consider alternative social goals, and the boundary points of risk boundaries for subsidization associated with each. If society's goal is complete avoidance ("prevention") of all future Down syndrome livebirths irrespective of cost, then there can be no minimum risk or age boundary for eligibility and all costs should be subsidized. On the other hand, if the goal is the maximum prevention of Down syndrome without economic *loss* to society, then one may define one type of risk boundary: the "program break-even risk". If the goal is maximum total economic savings to society, associated with prevention of Down syndrome, one may define another type of boundary, the "marginal break-even risk". Both program and marginal break-even risks may be expressed as a rate per 1,000 livebirths of Down syndrome. As the risk of Down syndrome increases markedly with maternal age, we may associate a program and marginal break-even *age* with the program and marginal even risks respectively.

The difference between the program and marginal break-even points may be illustrated as follows. Let us assume that there exists a subsidized program for all women whose risk of a Down syndrome livebirth is over 8%, about the rate observed at age 49. Assume such a program results in economic savings to society, which appears quite likely (see below). Suppose one lowers the boundary age for inclusion by one year to age 48. The costs per woman participating are fixed, but the economic benefits will drop because the rate of Down syndrome is lower in the group just made eligible. As one lowers the age for inclusion progressively by single year intervals, eventually one reaches a point where the costs of including all women of the *age just added* are exactly balanced by the benefits

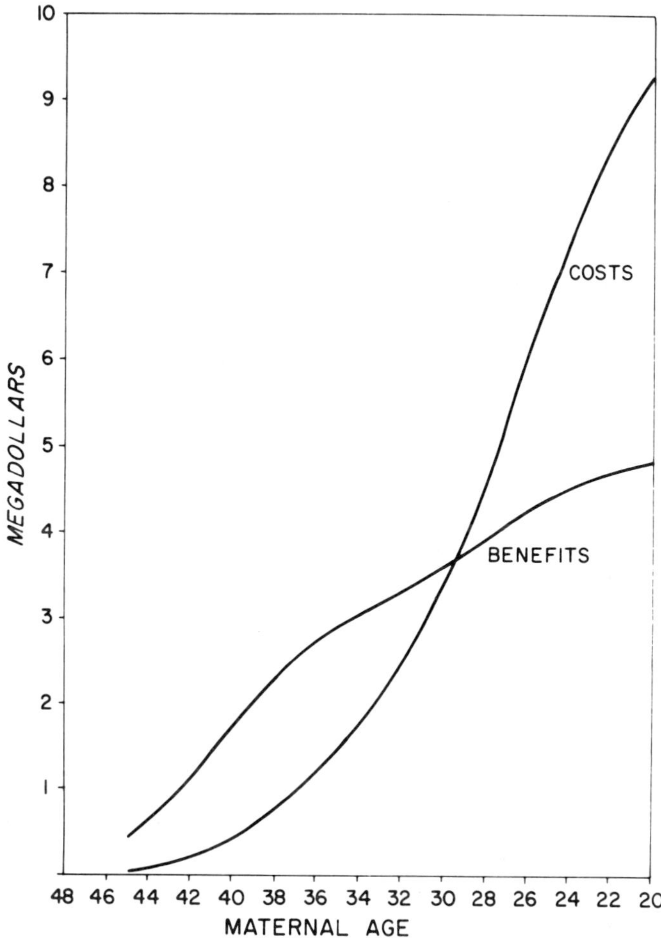

Fig. 1. Graph illustrating costs and benefits in megadollars (millions of dollars) for programs with varying maternal age criteria. The calculations are based on the distribution for New York State livebirths in 1974, and assume choice is proportional to the square root of risk, with 100% utilization at age 49. (The value of c used is \$365, d = \$100,000, b = 3, t = \$1,000, a = 0.5.*) The horizontal axis refers to the *minimum* maternal age criteria for any program. Thus the values for costs and benefits given at age 40 (about 0.3 and 1.6 megadollars respectively) are for a program in which all pregnant women *at* or *over* that age are included. The marginal break-even age is the age at which the net difference between costs and benefits is at a maximum, here at about age criterion 36. Lowering the age below that point results in progressive diminishment of net "social profits", until total costs equal total benefits, which occurs at about age 29, the approximate program break-even age in this formulation.

*See Table 1 for definitions of these variables.

from the participation of women at that age. This occurs at the *marginal* break-even age and risk. But society will still benefit economically because of the participation of all women *over* that age. (This may be re-expressed by noting that society will *lose* money – *i.e.*, lose potential economic benefit – for every woman over the marginal break-even point who does *not* elect prenatal diagnosis.) Thus, the maximum economic gains to society are derived from a program whose boundary for subsidization is the marginal break-even point. If one lowers the age for subsidization of costs *below* the marginal break-even point, losses incurred by participation of those below this point will initially be more than balanced by gains from those above. But eventually one will reach a point at which these gains and losses exactly balance. This is at the ***program break-even*** age and risk. (See Figure 1 for graphs illustrating these concepts.)

VARIABLES IN COST-BENEFIT ANALYSIS

To determine the program and marginal break-even points and ages, one needs extensive data on the variables that contribute to the benefits and costs. Definitions of these variables and their ranges are listed in Table 1. The values for c and t in this formulation may be readily estimated from available data. The values for a and b are more uncertain but these are, in any event, more "nuisance" variables which – within a wide range of plausible values – make relatively little difference to the derived figure for the marginal break-even risk (see below).

The biggest difficulty is in estimating d, the lifetime cost to society of a Down syndrome birth in today's money that may be averted by the program, and thus may be regarded as "benefits". There are many reasons why this cost is difficult to determine – not least because of possible future changes in medical procedures and social attitudes that cannot be anticipated now. For example, changes in special education for retarded individuals and in treatment for congenital heart defects are likely to occur, but the magnitude and direction of the future costs of these is unpredictable for affected individuals. The mortality rate of Down syndrome improved markedly from the 1950's to the 1960's, for example,[3] so that many more affected individuals are now surviving to middle age than previously. The presence of presenile dementia in such individuals may involve significant special costs for the care of affected aged individuals.[4]

After some estimate of future cost is reached, the next issue is discounting this cost to today's money. To illustrate what economists mean by a "discounted" figure, consider an individual with Down syndrome who lives 50 years and whose net cost to society is \$10,000/year in 1977 dollars. Assume *no inflation* whatsoever. While the total lifetime costs to society are \$500,000, the cost today of an annuity which would pay \$10,000/year for 50 years is much lower. This would be even less than \$200,000 because 5% interest on \$200,000 would provide an annuity paying \$10,000/year forever. This consideration illustrates what economists mean when they say future costs must be discounted to today's money. A dollar saved 10 years from now may only be worth 60 cents in today's money, even ignoring inflation.

There are formulas for discounting costs, but their application may be quite variable. When money – at least government money – is "tight" and there is financial stress, then the discount factor may be much higher than when tax monies are readily available. For various jurisdictions, I believe the discount factor should be correlated with, if not equal to, the interest the jurisdiction has to pay on bonds that it issues.

Another pertinent issue in determination of costs is whether reproductive "compensation" occurs, *i.e.*, whether or not the Down syndrome fetus is "replaced" by the parents with a subsequent infant with normal genotype. Paradoxically, if "replacement" occurs, the lifetime costs of a Down syndrome fetus is lower than if "replacement" does not occur. In calculations involving the assumption of replacement, one must subtract the costs of education and care of the individual with normal genotype from those of the Down syndrome individual. But then one must *add* the difference between the earnings of the average individual with normal genotype and those with Down syndrome – a difference that may be considerable if honestly cost-accounted and the calculation does not count "make work" government subsidies for the retarded as "earned income".

Moreover, it may not be widely recognized that there are likely to be marked regional differences attributable to factors involving "replacement" since, for example, individuals with normal genotypes are more likely to migrate from their home states than those with Down syndrome. (This is an additional reason why I believe subsidization for prenatal diagnosis should be, optimally, the responsibility of the federal government.)

Conley and Milunsky[5] considered most of these factors in estimating lifetime costs based upon data available to them in 1972, and trends projected as of that data (except for inflation). (See Table 1.) This is probably the most complete estimate ever attempted. The cost of living has increased about 50% since then, so these projected lifetime costs should probably be increased as well, to allow for the inflationary changes since they made their estimate. (See Table 1 footnote.)

THE MARGINAL BREAK-EVEN RISK: FORMULA AND DERIVATION

The formula for the marginal break-even risk[6] may be approximated as $y = \frac{c}{d}$ but is formally equal to the slightly lower figure $y = \frac{c}{(1\text{-}a)(d\text{-}bt)}$. Those readers wishing to avoid technical details may wish to skip this paragraph in which the derivation of this formula is presented. The marginal break-even risk y is, by definition, that risk of Down syndrome in livebirths such that offering amniocentesis to all women at that risk will result in economic benefits equaling economic costs. For every 1,000 livebirths to women with this risk there will be 1,000 (y) cases of Down syndrome averted, and thus an economic benefit to society of 1,000 (y) (d) where d is the economic benefit from aversion of a single case We must deduct from d, however, the costs of pregnancy terminations associated

TABLE 1

Variables to be Considered on Cost-Benefit Analysis of Prenatal Cytogenetic Diagnoses

Variable	Symbol	Plausible range	Most likely value (1978)*
Lifetime costs to society of Down syndrome livebirth	d		
replacement:		(?) \$75,000 – \$300,000	\$150,000 (\$225,000)*
non-replacement		(?) \$50,000 – \$200,000	\$100,000 (\$150,000)*
Costs per person of prenatal cytogenetic diagnosis (including amniocentesis, ultrasound, laboratory fee)	c	\$250 – \$500	\$375
Spontaneous fetal death rate after usual time of amniocentesis to women undergoing procedure	a	.02 – .10	(?) .05
Ratio of number of Down syndrome cases diagnosed at 16-18th week to number expected at livebirth	b	1.1 – 1.5	1.3
Costs of midtrimester pregnancy termination	t	\$300 – \$1,500 and up	(?) \$1,000

*The estimates of Conley and Milunsky for 1972 data are \$150,000 and \$100,000. These should probably be increased by 50% to adjust for increase in cost of living since that time. These estimates are given in parentheses.

with each livebirth case averted. For each such case there were *b* terminations, so economic benefit is 1,000 (y) (d-bt). Regarding costs, for every 1,000 livebirths there were 1,000/(1-a) women who reached the 16th to 18th week of pregnancy who could have had amniocentesis. The per capita costs of participation of each is *c*. Therefore, the total costs of prenatal diagnosis to this cohort would be 1,000 (c)/(1-a). Costs and benefits will be equal when 1,000 (y) (d-bt) = 1,000 (c)/(1-a); *i.e.*, when y = c/(1-a)(d-bt).

ASSUMPTIONS IN DERIVING MARGINAL BREAK-EVEN RISK

The main assumptions made in this derivation are (1) that all women in whom a Down syndrome fetus is diagnosed prenatally will elect to terminate their pregnancy, and (2) the only benefits from pregnancy terminations that result from prenatal diagnosis are those associated with averting Down syndrome. Regarding assumption 2, there will be an economic savings from the diminishment of other conditions diagnosed *incidentally* in prenatal diagnosis, such as trisomy 18 and trisomy 13, among others, and the rare neural tube defect detected by alpha-fetoprotein determination of amniotic fluid drawn for investigation of cytogenetic disorders. Regarding assumption 1, some women in whom a trisomy 21 fetus is diagnosed elect not to terminate their pregnancy. A recent survey of all North American prenatal cytogenetic centers listed in the National Foundation-March of Dimes directory indicated that by July 1, 1978, there were at least 22 women in the United States and Canada in whom a Down syndrome fetus had been diagnosed but the mother had elected not to terminate the pregnancy. In New York State, where the "denominator" data are available, the proportion of such women among those in whom a Down syndrome fetus has been detected to date was about 4% (2/47 = 4.3%, 95% confidence interval 0.5% - 14.5%).

These two factors, which have not been considered in the main formulation, tend to balance each other out.*

---

*Another assumption is that risk is purely a function of maternal age. There are, of course, women with risks of a Down syndrome much higher than that associated with their age, including those who are trisomy 21 mosaics or translocation-21 carriers (or married to men with these conditions). They have risks of a Down syndrome livebirth that may be 10% or even greater, depending on the condition involved. In addition, empirically, for younger women with ostensibly normal chromosomes married to unaffected husbands, who have had one 47, trisomy 21 child, the recurrence risk is 1%. the same risk of a woman aged 41. The proportion of such women with increased risks because of these factors in the general population, however, is quite low, perhaps no more than 0.2%, and exclusion of this group of women would not make any significant change in the marginal and program break-even risks and ages calculated here for the general population. (Counseling and subsidies should, of course, be based on known risk, if this is greater than that associated with the maternal age in any specific case.)

MARGINAL BREAK-EVEN RISKS

In Table 2, there is a list of marginal break-even risks associated with a range of possible values for *a, b, c, d,* and *t* in Table 1. The reader may calculate how close, in general, the approximation of c/d is to c/(d-bt)(1-a). The maternal ages associated with the marginal greak-even risks may be derived from formulas which give risk by maternal age.[6,8,9] (see Table 3).

As may be seen, a plausible marginal break-even maternal age is about 36 (for d = $100,000, c = $400, relatively conservative values) and is lower for most other situations considered. It is coincidental that this coincides roughly with the age (⩾ 35) at which many physicians regard the pregnant woman as being at "high risk" of having an affected child. The marginal break-even age, I emphasize, is almost entirely independent of demographic considerations (once economies of scale are achieved). That is, it is independent of (1) the *number* of older mothers, and (2) the *proportion* of older women among those pregnant. These variables, however, are highly pertinent to calculation of the program break-even risk, and their estimation makes such calculations more difficult and subject to greater uncertainty. (Some data on demographic variables appear in Tables 4 and 5.)

PROGRAM BREAK-EVEN AGE: DERIVATION AND SOME METHODOLOGICAL CONSIDERATIONS

Those readers who wish to avoid technical details may skip this section in which the method of deriving the program break-even age is presented.

This may be done most easily by considering again a program only for mothers age 49 and assuming this is the highest maternal age. The costs of such a program will be $(n_{49})(c)/(1\text{-}a)$ where n_{49} is the number of livebirths expected to women aged 49 at delivery. The benefits of such a program will be $(n_{49})\ (y_{49})\ (d\text{-}bt)$ where y_{49} is now the expected rate of Down syndrome in livebirths to women age 49. (The other variables are as defined above.) If these two expressions are equal, then 49 is the program break-even age. It is, of course, highly likely they are not equal and that costs are much less than benefits. One may then add in the results for age 48 as well; *i.e.*, the costs for a program for women age 49 and 48 are $(c)\ (n_{49} + n_{48})/(1\text{-}a)$ and the benefits are now $(d\text{-}bt)\ (n_{49}y_{49} + n_{48}y_{48})$. If for criterion age 49 costs are less than benefits but at criterion age 48 they are greater, then the program break-even point is at some point during the 48th year. If this condition does not hold, one just repeats the procedure for age 47, 46, etc.

The variable n_i adjusts for the differing number of pregnant women at each age in the population (see Table 4).

The model above assumes all women to whom services are offered will elect them. This is not likely to be the case, for reasons discussed in detail elsewhere.[6] Women with a higher risk (and higher age) are more likely to elect services than the remainder of the population. Therefore, we must revise both sides of the equation, introducing a *choice-age* (or a *choice-risk* function) which gives the likelihood that a woman with risk y at age x will elect prenatal services. Since one needs only the relative likelihoods at each age for those purposes, one may assume 100% utilization at age 49.* (For determination of actual program costs and benefits and not just the program break-even age, however, one should know the absolute likelihoods of a choice to elect amniocentesis.) Assume the choice age function is given by f_i. Then the expressions should be rewritten by multiplying costs and benefits by f_i at each age *i, i.e.*, for a program at age 48 the costs are:

$$\frac{(c)(n_{49})(f_{49}) + (c)(n_{48})(f_{48})}{(1-a)}, \text{ the benefits } (d-bt)[n_{49}y_{49}f_{49} + n_{48}y_{48}f_{48}].$$

This general form of the formulation for the program break-even age may be expressed as that value of *k* such that:

$$\sum_{i=k}^{49} \frac{(c)(n_i)(f_i)}{(1-a)} = \sum_{i=k}^{49} (d-bt)(y_i)(n_i)(f_i)$$

(If we denote the left hand expression as C_k and the right hand expression as B_k (costs and benefits for a program with eligibility criteria at age k respectively) then the approximate program break-even age is to the *nearest* (*lowest truncated*) year that value of k for which $C_{k+1} < B_{k+1}$ but $C_k \geqslant B_k$.)

Now the equation above may also be rewritten (but see below) by factoring out *a, b, t, d* and *c* as

$$\frac{c}{(d-bt)(1-a)} = \sum_{i=k}^{49} (y_i)(n_i)(f_i) \Big/ \sum_{i=k}^{49} (n_i)(f_i)$$

The new left hand expression is, however, the marginal break-even risk, whereas the expression on the right is an equation which is a function of *k*, the program break-even age. It becomes possible to readily plot one as the function of the other, knowing only the values of n_i, f_i and, of course, y_i at each age *i*.

That is, in any jurisdiction in which the latter functions are known, one may express the program break-even age as a function of the marginal break-even risk. This is particularly useful for heuristic purposes (see Figure 2). In the figure are plotted data for New York State livebirths for 1974, where in one case (the upper curve) f_i is a constant; *i.e.*, the choice-risk age function for amniocentesis is assumed to be *independent* of mother's age and all women are *equally* likely to elect amniocentesis, and in the lower curve for $f_i = h\sqrt{y_i}$; where *h* is a con-

*It is worth elaborating on this point, which may not be obvious. If 10% of all eligible women would elect prenatal diagnosis if offered, no matter what their risk, *i.e.*, irrespective of age, the program break-even age would be the same as if 100% of all eligible women would elect prenatal diagnosis irrespective of age. The total costs and benefits of the latter program would be 10-fold higher than the former one, but the associated break-even ages would occur at the same point.

TABLE 2

Variation in Marginal Break-even Risks (MBR) and Marginal Break-even Ages (MBEA) as a Function of Change in Contributory Variables*,****

	d	c	b	t	a	MBR	MBEA
Variation in d:	$ 50,000					7.57×10^{-3}	39.2
	100,000	$350	1.3	$1,000	0.05	3.73×10^{-3}	36.3
	150,000					2.48×10^{-3}	34.6
	200,000					1.85×10^{-3}	33.4
Variation in c (and d):		$300				3.04×10^{-3}	35.4
		350				3.73×10^{-3}	36.3
	$100,000	400	1.3	$1,000	.05	4.27×10^{-3}	36.8
		450				4.80×10^{-3}	37.3
		500				5.34×10^{-3}	37.8
		300				2.12×10^{-3}	33.9
		350				2.48×10^{-3}	34.6
	$150,000	400	1.3	$1,000	.05	2.83×10^{-3}	35.1
		450				3.18×10^{-3}	35.6
		500				3.54×10^{-3}	36.1
Variation in b (and d):			1.3			3.73×10^{-3}	36.3
	$100,000	$350	2.0	$1,000	.05	3.76×10^{-3}	36.3
			3.0			3.80×10^{-3}	36.4
	$150,000	$350	1.3	$1,000	.05	2.48×10^{-3}	34.6
			2.0			2.49×10^{-3}	34.6
			3.0			2.51×10^{-3}	34.6

Variation in t (and d):	\$100,000	\$350	1.3	\$ 500	.05	3.71×10^{-3}	36.3
				1,000		3.73×10^{-3}	36.3
				2,000		3.78×10^{-3}	36.3
	\$150,000	\$350	1.3	\$ 500	.05	2.47×10^{-3}	34.6
				1,000		2.48×10^{-3}	34.6
				2,000		2.50×10^{-3}	34.6
Variation in a (and d):	\$100,000	\$350	1.3	\$1,000	.025	3.64×10^{-3}	36.2
					.05	3.73×10^{-3}	36.3
					variable f_1**	3.70×10^{-3}	36.2
					variable f_2***	3.86×10^{-3}	36.4
	\$150,000	\$350	1.3	\$1,000	.025	2.41×10^{-3}	34.5
					.05	2.48×10^{-3}	34.6
					variable f_1**	2.43×10^{-3}	34.5
					variable f_2***	2.50×10^{-3}	34.6

*The ages given are those of the mother at the time of amniocentesis.

**Values of f_1 (a) with age are 20-24 = .019; 25-29 = .022; 30-34 = .030.
35-39 = .041; 40-44 = .061; 45-49 = .105.

Solutions for MBR are iterative.

***Values for f_2 (a) with age are twice those of f_1 (a). Solutions are iterative. (See text)

TABLE 2 (Continued)

Variations in Marginal Break-even Risks (MBR) and Marginal Break-even Ages (MBEA) as a Function of Change in Contributory Variables*,****

****Adjustments in maternal ages associated with rates of Down syndrome: The published rates of Down syndrome in livebirths are presented for mother's age at last birthday at time of delivery of the child; *i.e.*, at "truncated" ages. Of course, most women listed at age x are somewhere between their x^{th} and $x+1^{st}$ birthday. The actual average age of women whose truncated ages is x at delivery varies between about x + 0.4 and x + 0.6 years, depending on x. At the older ages, because of the rapid drop in fertility, the average age is about x + 0.4. At the very young ages, in which there is a steep increase in fertility, the average age is about x + 0.6, and for the ages at which fertility is highest, the average age is about x + 0.5. This presentation considers for the most part those mothers whose average maternal age at delivery is between x + 0.4 and x + 0.5 years where x is the truncated age. Conception (dating from the last menstrual period) occurs on the average 280 days (or .77 years) earlier than age at delivery; *i.e.*, at about (x-1) + .63 to (x-1) + .73 years in women whose age at delivery is x + 0.4 to x + 0.5 years. Amniocentesis occurs usually somewhere between the 16th and 18th week of gestation, somewhere about .42 years after conception, *i.e.*, at about age (x-1) + (.63 + .42) to (x-1) + (.73 + .42) years, or x + .05 to x + .15 years. A numerical example may help illustrate this. Women whose truncated age is 40 at delivery have an average age at conception of about 39.63 years, an average age at amniocentesis about 40.04 years, and an average age at delivery of 40.4 years. Women whose truncated age is 25 years at delivery have an average age at conception of 24.73 years, an average age at amniocentesis of 25.15, and an average age at delivery of about 25.5 years.

Note that the average exact age at amniocentesis is very close to the truncated age at delivery. Because of this coincidence, published data on the rate of Down syndrome at delivery by truncated ages (at delivery) are almost exactly those for the expected rates of Down syndrome in livebirths to mothers who have these exact ages at amniocentesis. (This is *not* the case if we were to analyze comparisons of truncated ages for both situations, as has been done in Table 3.) Analysis of marginal and program break-even ages should use – to the extent possible – actual ages rather than truncated ages. But, because coincidentally the truncated age at delivery (x) is so close to the mean age at amniocentesis (x + 0.5 to x + .15), the adjustment required is a trivial one of small magnitude and has not been done in Tables 2 and 4. In general, if the correction is not made, the derived break-even ages will be about 0.1 year lower than they actually should be. Given other sources of uncertainty, this is such a minor correction it has not been made here.

TABLE 3

Rates of Down Syndrome per 1,000 Livebirths by Single Year Interval Age 20-49 From Three Studies[6,8,9]

Maternal age in years	Rate in livebirths, maternal age at delivery			Rates in livebirths, maternal age at amniocentesis (derived)		
	Massachusetts	New York	Sweden	Massachusetts	New York	Sweden
20	0.57	0.52	0.64	.58	.54	.65
21	0.60	0.59	0.67	.61	.61	.68
22	0.64	0.65	0.71	.65	.67	.72
23	0.67	0.71	0.75	.68	.73	.77
24	0.70	0.77	0.79	.71	.79	.81
25	0.74	0.83	0.83	.75	.85	.85
26	0.77	0.89	0.87	.78	.91	.89
27	0.80	0.95	0.92	.81	.97	.94
28	0.84	1.01	0.97	.86	1.03	.99
29	0.87	1.07	1.02	.89	1.09	1.04
30	0.90	1.13	1.08	.92	1.15	1.10
31	0.93	1.21	1.14	.95	1.27	1.16
32	1.15	1.38	1.25	1.22	1.50	1.34
33	1.55	1.69	1.47	1.71	1.86	1.64
34	1.98	2.15	1.92	2.18	2.37	2.14
35	2.53	2.74	2.51	2.79	3.02	2.79
36	3.22	3.49	3.28	3.55	3.85	3.65
37	4.11	4.45	4.28	4.53	4.90	4.76
38	5.24	5.66	5.60	5.77	6.24	6.23
39	6.68	7.21	7.32	7.36	7.95	8.15
40	8.52	9.19	9.57	9.39	10.13	10.65
41	10.86	11.71	12.51	11.97	12.90	13.92
42	13.85	14.91	16.36	15.26	16.43	18.21
43	17.66	19.00	21.39	19.46	20.94	23.81
44	22.51	24.20	27.96	24.81	26.67	30.27
45	28.71	30.84	36.55	51.44	33.99	40.68
46	36.61	39.28	47.79	31.64	43.29	53.19
47	46.68	50.04	62.47	40.34	55.14	69.53
48	59.52	63.75	81.67	65.59	70.25	90.90
49	75.89	81.21	106.76	83.83	89.49	118.82

Footnote: All ages are those at last birthday; *i.e., truncated*. The expected rates in livebirths for women at the time of amniocentesis assume an 0.4 year differential between amniocentesis and livebirth. Therefore, they are obtained by multiplying the following constants: Massachusetts 20-31; 1.018; Massachusetts 33-49: 1.102; Sweden 20-31: 1.021, Sweden 33-49: 1.113; New York 33-49: 1.102. (For 20-30 for New York State, since a linear not a 1st degree *exponential* equation was used, 0.02 was *added* to each of the rates in the interval.) See references 6,8,9 for data in New York, Sweden, and Massachusetts, respectively.

TABLE 4
Livebirths: By Single Year Maternal Age Interval

Maternal Age	New York State 1974	1975	1976	1977	Maternal Age	U.S.A. 1975	1976
<15	649	634	636	589	<15	12,642	11,928
15	1,739	1,720	1.602	1,521	15	33,450	31,851
16	3,821	3,721	3,486	3,650	16	74,138	71,204
17	6,215	6,057	5,842	5,938	17	119,682	112,438
18	8,835	8,786	8,206	8,482	18	162,281	153,795
19	11,216	11,069	10,647	10,818	19	192,687	189,456
20	12,737	12,298	12,311	12,364	20	207,891	204,753
21	14,156	13,644	13,358	13,640	21	216,818	214,747
22	15,415	14,725	14,305	14,661	22	221,662	222,290
23	16,807	15,950	15,520	15,939	23	225,125	225,753
24	17,545	16,278	16,219	16,440	24	222,180	224,059
25	18,328	17,159	17,025	17,131	25	217,680	220,013
26	18,575	17,464	17,001	17,246	26	208,515	208,599
27	18,844	17,038	16,550	16,893	27	197,780	196,240
28	13,902	16,431	15,984	16,129	28	184,371	181,146
29	11,832	11,714	14,943	14,888	29	128,440	166,132
30	10,598	9,985	10,526	13,571	30	106,576	113,934
31	9,260	8,372	8,490	9,196	31	88,782	89,801
32	7,270	7,824	7,438	7,636	32	77,649	76,031
33	5,462	5,724	6,226	6,382	33	57,225	64,212
34	4,459	4,441	4,655	5,479	34	45,268	47,918
35	3,603	3,555	3,594	3,990	35	35,724	36,132
36	2,837	2,752	2,899	2,980	36	26,932	28,090
37	2,330	2,232	2,223	2,308	37	21,986	21,599
38	1,845	1,826	1,749	1,801	38	17,520	17,364
39	1,421	1,329	1,260	1,276	39	13,247	12,477
40	978	998	883	911	40	10,150	9,247
41	654	641	614	577	41	6,615	6,400
42	456	463	379	432	42	4,665	4,406
43	278	269	244	243	43	3,041	2,777
44	153	126	146	123	44	1,848	1,553
45	93	70	74	69	45	922	782
46	50	35	34	22	46	411	414
47	17	11	22	12	47	190	155
48	8	5	4	11	48	78	64
49	2	2	3	0	49	27	28
⩾50	0	0	2	1	⩾50	*	*
NS	62	55	75	43	NS	*	*
Total	242,452	235,403	235,177	243,392	Total	3,144,198	3,167,788

*Data on these categories are not readily available from United States vital statistics sources. NS = not stated.

TABLE 5

Proportion Livebirths in Percent by Five Year Maternal Age Interval

	New York State				U.S.A.	
Maternal age	1974	1975	1976	1977	1975	1976
< 15	0.27	0.27	0.27	0.24	0.40	0.38
15-19	13.13	13.32	12.66	12.49	18.52	17.64
20-24	31.62	30.97	30.49	30.01	34.78	34.46
25-29	33.61	33.90	34.66	33.81	29.79	30.69
30-34	15.28	15.44	15.88	17.36	11.94	12.37
35-59	4.96	4.97	4.99	5.08	3.67	3.65
40-44	1.04	1.06	0.96	0.94	0.84	0.77
45-49	0.07	0.05	0.06	0.05	0.05	0.04
$\geqslant 50$	0.00	0.00	0.00	0.00	*	*
NS	0.02	0.02	0.03	0.02	*	*
Total	100.00	100.00	100.00	100.00	99.99	100.00
Total livebirths	242,452	235,403	235,177	243,392	3,144,198	3,167,788

*Data on these categories are not readily available from United States vital statistics sources. NS = not stated.

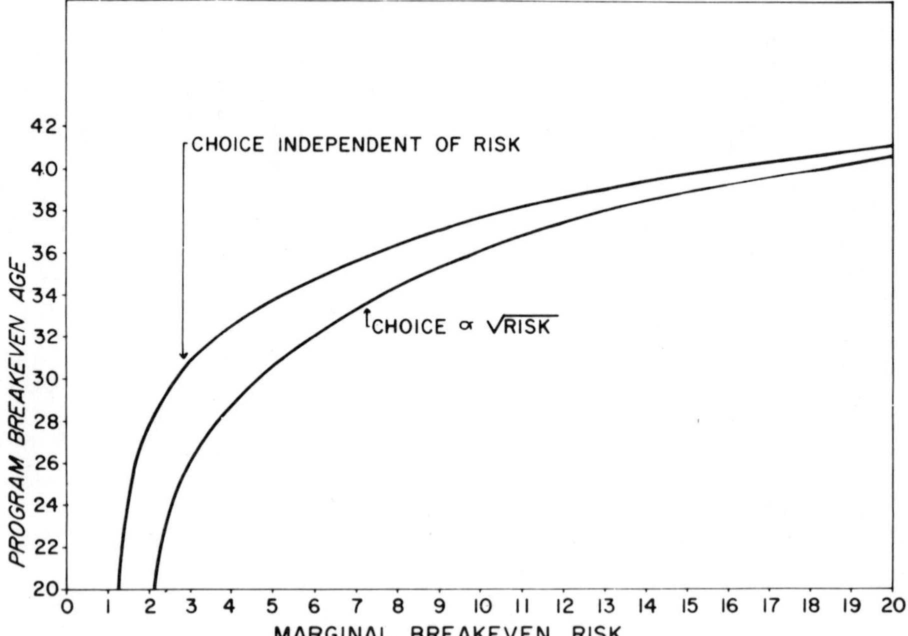

Fig. 2. Graphs illustrating program break-even age as a function of marginal break-even age. The upper curve gives values for choice as a constant over varying ages, the lower curve gives the values for choice proportional to the square root of maternal risk. (The values plotted are for New York State births for 1974, assuming d = \$100,000, c = \$365, b = 3, t = \$1,000, and a = .05. As noted in the text, while a is not, in fact, constant with age, the formulation is robust to any plausible variation of fetal death with maternal age (see Table 6). If the curves were plotted with a as a function of age, as in Table 6, there would be only trivial alterations from the values given here. The graph was drawn before it was realized that 1.3 was a more appropriate value for b than 3.0 (see *e.g.*, reference 7), but in view of the results in Table 2, this difference in b makes only a trivial difference in the results derived.

stant; *i.e.*, where the choice to participate is proportional to the square root of the risk at age *i*, so that a woman with 1% risk (age 41) is about three times more likely to elect the procedure than the woman with 0.1% risk (about age 30).

Recent observations suggest that currently, at age 40 and over, there is not much variation in perception of risk; that is, that in this age bracket the risk is perceived simply as "high". But below age 40 there appears to be a gradient in the choice-risk function. Therefore, an analysis is also presented here assuming that choice is constant from age 49 to age 40, and proportional to the square root of the risk (normalized to the risk at age 40) below 40. The results are intermediate between those derived assuming a constant choice-risk function and those derived assuming a function involving proportionality to the square root of the risk over the entire age span (see Table 6). (Both relative and absolute choice-risk functions are, of course, likely to vary over time with changes in awareness, interest, and availability of prenatal diagnosis.)

There is one mathematical difficulty with this formulation, however. By factoring *a, b, c, d,* and *t* out of the summation signs we have implicitly assumed that these are constants, *independent* of age. This is likely to be not far from the case for all but *a*, the fetal death rate. This variable, however, is known to vary significantly with maternal age. It becomes possible to redo the formulations not with *a* as a constant but as a function of age *i*. The calculations indicate that the formulation is relatively robust to changes of *a* with age, so that the formulation which assumes *a* is constant results in a good approximation (see Table 6).

In fact, in calculation of the marginal break-even risk, the variability of *a* with age also poses a slight problem, but this may be handled readily by iterative methods. For example, one may initially *estimate* the marginal break-even age *i*, and initially use for *a* the value at the age *i*, $\bar{a}_i$. Then one may calculate

$$y' = \frac{c}{(d-bt)(1-\bar{a}_i).}$$

Because y' is a risk, it is associated with a specific maternal age i'. If the value of a_i associated with i' is in fact a_i, then y' (i') is the marginal break-even risk (age). If not, one repeats the process by substituting in the equation for the marginal break-even risk for *a* the value a_i', the fetal death rate associated with age *i* and then calculating:

$$y'' = \frac{c}{(d-bt)(1-a_i'),}$$

and then determining if a_i' is the appropriate fetal death rate for i'' the maternal age associated with y''. Repetition of this iterative process will eventually result in reaching stable marginal break-even risks and ages.

PROGRAM BREAK-EVEN AGES

The results (Table 6) indicate that for a population with maternal age distribution of the one having livebirths in the U.S.A. in 1975, the values of the program break-even age are between about 28 and 33 assuming choice is independent of risk (which is highly unlikely) and between about 22 to 30 if choice is proportional to the $\sqrt{\text{risk}}$. (The higher values are for high per capita

TABLE 6

Program Break-even Ages (PBEA) for Various Values of *c,d* Choice Risk Functions, and *a**,**,***

		PBEA
c = \$300, d = \$100,000, b = 1.3, t = \$1,000, c/(d-bt)= 3.040×10^{-3}		
choice constant	a = .025	30.8
	a = f_1 (Age)	30.9
	a = .05	31.0
	a = f_2 (Age)	31.2
choice proportional $\sqrt{risk}$	a = .025	27.3
	a = f_1 (Age)	27.4
	a = .05	27.6
	a = f_2 (Age)	27.7
choice constant 49-40, proportional $\sqrt{risk}$ below 40	a = .025	28.3
	a = f_1 (Age)	28.4
	a = .05	28.5
	a = f_2 (Age)	28.6
c - \$350, d = \$100, b = 1.3, t = \$1,000, c/(d-bt) = 3.54×10^{-3}		
choice constant	a = .025	31.9
	a = f_1 (Age)	32.0
	a = .05	32.0
	a - f_2 (Age)	32.2
choice proportional $\sqrt{risk}$	a = .025	28.6
	a = f_1 (Age)	28.7
	a = .05	28.8
	a = f_2 (Age)	29.0
choice constant 49-40, proportional $\sqrt{risk}$ below 40	a = .025	29.6
	a = f_1 (Age)	28.7
	a = .05	29.8
	a = f_2 (Age)	30.0

TABLE 6 (Continued)

Program Break-even Ages (PBEA) for Various Values of *c*,*d*, Choice Risk Functions, and *a**,**,***

		PBEA
$c = \$400$, $d = \$100{,}000$, $b = 1.3$, $t = \$1{,}000$, $c/(d-bt) = 4.053 \times 10^{-3}$		
choice constant	$a = .025$	32.6
	$a = f_1$ (Age)	32.7
	$a = .05$	32.8
	$a = f_2$ (Age)	33.0
choice proportional $\sqrt{\text{risk}}$	$a = .025$	29.7
	$a = f_1$ (Age)	29.8
	$a = .05$	29.9
	$a = f_2$ (Age)	30.2
choice constant 49-40, proportional $\sqrt{\text{risk}}$ below 40	$a = .025$	30.7
	$a = f_1$ (Age)	30.9
	$a = .05$	31.0
	$a = f_2$ (Age)	31.2
$c = \$300$, $d = \$150{,}000$, $b = 1.3$, $t = \$1{,}000$, $c/(d-bt) = 2.017 \times 10^{-3}$		
choice constant	$a = .025$	27.8
	$a = f_1$ (Age)	27.8
	$a = .05$	28.0
	$a = f_2$ (Age)	28.1
choice proportional $\sqrt{\text{risk}}$	$a = .025$	22.1
	$a = f_1$ (Age)	22.2
	$a = .05$	22.6
	$a = f_2$ (Age)	22.7
choice constant 49-40, proportional $\sqrt{\text{risk}}$ below 40	$a = .025$	23.7
	$a = f_1$ (Age)	23.8
	$a = .05$	24.1
	$a = f_2$ (Age)	24.2
$c = \$350$, $d = \$150{,}000$, $b = 1.3$, $t = \$1{,}000$, $c/(d-bt) = 2.354 \times 10^{-3}$		
choice constant	$a = .025$	29.0
	$a = f_1$ (Age)	29.0
	$a = .05$	29.1
	$a = f_2$ (Age)	29.3

TABLE 6 (Continued)

Program Break-even Ages (PBEA) for Various Values of *c*,*d*, Choice Risk Functions, and *a**,**,***

		PBEA
choice proportional $\sqrt{risk}$	a = .025	24.5
	a = f_1 (Age)	24.6
	a = .05	24.9
	a = f_2 (Age)	25.0
choice constant 49-40. proportional $\sqrt{risk}$ below 40	a = .025	25.8
	a = f_1 (Age)	25.9
	a = .05	26.1
	a = f_2 (Age)	26.2
c = \$400, d = \$150, b = 1.3, t = \$1,000, c/(d-bt) = 2.690×10^{-3}		
choice constant	a = .025	30.0
	a = f_1 (Age)	30.0
	a = .05	30.2
	a = f_2 (Age)	30.3
choice proportional $\sqrt{risk}$	a = .025	26.1
	a = f_1 (Age)	26.2
	a = .05	26.4
	a = f_2 (Age)	26.5
choice constant 49-40, proportional $\sqrt{risk}$ below 40	a = .025	27.2
	a = f_1 (Age)	27.3
	a = .05	27.4
	a = f_2 (Age)	27.6

*Ages are at time of amniocentesis.

**f_1 (age) and f_2 (age) are as in Table 2.

***See also 4th footnote to Table 2 on the relationship of PBEA to precise maternal age.

costs, c = $400 and low benefits per case, d = $100.000, the lower values are for c = $300, and d = $150,000. Further details appear in Table 6.)

For New York State, in which mothers are slightly older than in the entire U.S.A. average, the values are about a half year older.

Thus, it appears quite likely that, using plausible estimates of the variables involved, that society could subsidize prenatal diagnosis for pregnant women over 30 without incurring economic loss.

CONCLUDING REMARKS

As implied above, the economic considerations presented here are irrelevant to the moral and ethical aspects of pregnancy termination, decisions which each pregnant woman must make for herself. However, as long as the procedure is legally available and ethically acceptable to some part of the population, the economic *consequences* of prenatal diagnosis and the issues discussed here are a legitimate part of community health planning. But even these economic implications involve implicit assumptions about how decisions concerning health needs should be met, how limited resources should be spent, and the pertinence of cost-benefit analysis. There is always a difficulty in drawing any risk boundary for provision of service or subsidy. Optimally, I believe genetic counseling and prenatal diagnosis should be available to any woman who seeks them.

ACKNOWLEDGMENTS

In calculation of the values of the program break-even ages considered in various models analyzed, Barry Noon, Scott Lamson, Philip Cross, and Linda Gulotty, among others, provided invaluable help. The manuscript is expanded from an address given at a Symposium of the meeting of the American Society of Human Genetics in October, 1977, in San Diego, sponsored by the National Foundation-March of Dimes.

REFERENCES

1. The NICHD National Registry for Amniocentesis Study Group, *J.A.M.A.* *236*, 1471, 1976.
2. C. Darwin, The Voyage of the Beagle (Chapter 10, Tierra del Fuego), *in* Darwin for Today – The Essence of His Work, S.E. Hyman (Ed.), Viking Press, New York, p. 35, 1963. (This rather poignant description notes ". . . it is certainly true that when pressed in winter by hunger, they kill and devour their old women before they kill their dogs; the boy being asked by Mr. Low why they did this, answered, 'Doggies catch otters, old women no.' " The further details Darwin provides are even more unpleasant.)
3. G. Tarjan, R.K. Eyman and C.R. Miller, *Am. J. Dis. Child.* *117*, 609, 1969.
4. L.L. Heston and A.R. Mastri, *Arch. Gen. Psychiat.* *34*, 976, 1977.

5. R. Conley and A. Milunsky, *in* Prevention of Genetic Disease and Mental Retardation, A. Milunsky (Ed.), W.B. Saunders Co., Philadelphia, 442-445, 1975.
6. E.B. Hook and G.M. Chambers, *in* Numerical Taxonomy on Birth Defects and Polygenic Disorders, D. Bergsma, R.B. Lowry, B.K. Trimble and M. Feingold, (Eds.), Birth Defects Original Article Series, Vol. 13, No. 3A, Alan R. Liss, Inc., New York 123-141, 1977.
7. E.B. Hook, *N. Engl. J. Med. 299*, 1036, 1978.
8. E.B. Hook and A. Lindsjo, *Amer. J. Hum. Genet. 30*, 19, 1978.
9. E.B. Hook and J. Fabia, *Teratology 17*, 223, 1978.
10. E.B. Hook, *Lancet 1*, 1053, 1978.

APPENDIX

Guidelines for "Genetic Centers" Established by the Advisory Committee to the Birth Defects Institute*

Requirements concerning staff and facilities:

1. Clinical Geneticist: An M.D. with appropriate training and experience in genetic *diagnosis* and counseling. Boards (or board eligibility if less than seven years out of medical school) in a specialty involving primary patient care, and two years specialized full time training, or equivalent in clinical genetics are required.
2. Cytogeneticist: Ph.D. or M.D. degree with appropriate training and experience in clinical cytogenetics. (Full time total of two years training, minimum. Equivalent experience must be documented.)
3. Laboratory with permit by the New York State Department of Health for cytogenetics (unrestricted), or one meeting equivalent standards.

The following additional items are recommended:

4. Additional staffing may include one or more Associate Genetic Counselors who are persons with at least Bachelor's degree education in biological science, social work or nursing, and additional training and experience in clinical genetics (Master's Degree). Their duties will include follow-up of families, especially in relation to prenatal diagnosis.
5. Close association with a University Medical Center.
6. Biochemical Genetics Laboratory. Recognizing the wide range of biochemical tests which may be called for in clinical and prenatal diagnosis, this laboratory need not be expected to cover all tests. However, regular arrangements should exist with other laboratories for appropriate backup.
7. Association of individuals with documented experience and skills in dysmorphology.

---

*The guidelines are those established as of February 15, 1978, slightly revised from the preliminary draft drawn up in November 1977. Members of the Advisory Committee are Robin Bannerman, M.D., W. Roy Breg, M.D., Richard Erbe, M.D., Laird Jackson, M.D., and Dorothy Warburton, Ph.D. Ernest B. Hook, M.D., participates as a non-voting rapporteur, and Ian H. Porter, M.D. (ex-officio), as Director of the Birth Defects Institute.

8. Genetic Clinic: A recognized clinical facility in which patients and families are seen for genetic diagnosis and counseling with an appropriate system of record storage and retrieval. (Note: Appropriate record storage and retrieval is, of course, an absolute requirement. A fixed clinical facility for provision of diagnostic and counseling services is not an absolute requirement.)

In extraordinary circumstances a center may not meet all criteria stated above (*e.g.*, the required board eligibility or certification of an individual) but may still be able to provide high quality genetic counseling services. Centers which provide documentation of equivalent qualifications may be considered for approval as well.

PRENATAL SCREENING FOR ANENCEPHALY-SPINA BIFIDA: SOME EPIDEMIOLOGIC PROJECTIONS FOR A NATIONAL PROGRAM

Marshall F. Goldberg
Godfrey P. Oakley

Introduction

In June 1977, the results of the United Kingdom's study on prenatal screening for neural tube defects appeared in the *Lancet*[1] and thereby established the medical efficacy of maternal serum alpha-fetoprotein (MS-AFP) for the detection of anencephaly-spina bifida (ASB). In a country with limited health resources and approximately 3 times the U.S. incidence of ASB, MS-AFP screening represented a major breakthrough in preventive care; indeed, the United Kingdom is seriously considering screening as a part of routine obstetrical care.[2]

For the United States, where MS-AFP is currently being performed in only a few centers, the U.K. collaborative study provided valuable data regarding the best time for screening and the optimal detection rate for anencephaly (AN) and spina bifida (SB). With the addition of data derived from various sources in the United States, it became possible to forecast the impact of mass screening on the prevention of ASB in this country. Whether such screening ever becomes widespread in the United States is certainly open to speculation; however, considering that some 5,000 individuals with ASB are born each year, it seems reasonable to assume that mass MS-AFP screening could become a reality in the United States.[2]

We utilized a multiphasic screening model for ASB and constructed a series of population-based projections for some of the possible outcomes for a mass screening effort. In so doing, numerous assumptions about the screening model itself and the resultant projections were necessary. By varying certain technical traits and participant factors within each of the projections, we also addressed some of the epidemiologic variables that would undoubtedly influence the overall effect of such a program in the United States.

The Target Population

Before doing the various projections in our study, it was necessary to define the target population to be screened – *i.e.*, the number of ASB cases and normal fetuses one might expect to find in a mass screening program and to estimate the annual incidence of ASB for the entire country. Since precise data for the United

ISBN 0-12-562650-9

TABLE 1

Estimated Incidence of Anencephaly and Spina Bifida (ASB) for the United States Population, by Race and Defect

	Incidence of ASB (Per 10,000 Total Births)[a]		
Race	Anencephaly	Spina Bifida	Total
White	8.46	9.82	18.28
Other	3.21	3.89	7.10
Total	7.47	8.70	16.17

[a]Based on Atlanta race-specific rates from the Metropolitan Atlanta Congenital Defects Program, 1968-1975, and incidence figures from the Birth Defects Monitoring Program 1970-1975 (see Appendix); total births include live births and fetal deaths.

TABLE 2

Expected Cases of Anencephaly and Spina Bifida (ASB) for Total United States Births, 1975,[a] by Race and Defect
(n = 5,137)

	Expected Number of Cases of ASB[b]		
Race	Anencephaly	Spina Bifida	Total
White	2,180	2,530	4,710
Other	193	234	427
Total	2,373	2,764	5,137

[a]Includes 2,551,996 live births plus 24,309 fetal deaths for whites and 592,202 live births plus 5,487 fetal deaths for others (U.S. Natality and Mortality Statistics, NCHS, 1975).

[b]Based on adjusted Atlanta race-specific rates (see Appendix).

States were lacking, we derived national incidence figures for ASB from adjusted race- and defect-specific rates provided by our Metropolitan Atlanta Congenital Defects Program. This method of adjustment, which also accounts for geographic variations in ASB incidence, is discussed in the Appendix. The adjusted rates derived for the entire country, subsequently, were consistent with a slightly higher incidence of SB over AN as well as a higher incidence of ASB among whites compared to other races, as shown in Table 1.

The estimated race-specific rates for ASB were next applied directly to the total population of singletons and twin U.S. births for 1975 (n = 3,177,994) to ascertain the number of fetuses with ASB that would be expected.[3] The total number of affected and unaffected live and stillborn infants in that year thus constituted our target population. As seen in Table 2, an estimated 5,137 cases of ASB occurred in that year with 4,710 (or 91.7%) in white infants. Regardless of race, we assumed that ASB did not occur among twin births since our screening model operationally treated this group as if it were free of these defects.

The Multiphasic Screening Model for ASB and Its Underlying Assumptions

The ASB screening model that we used was based partly on the U.K. experience[1] and partly on the work of Macri and his associates[4] in this country. Essentially, the model consisted of a multiphasic screening process which began with the MS-AFP testing of an unselected target population and concluded with a highly selected group of women who had either 2 positive MS-AFP results and an abnormal sonogram, or had 2 positive MS-AFP results and a positive amniotic fluid alpha-fetoprotein (AF-AFP). As shown in Figure 1, we envisioned 5 phases for the screening model.

The first phase of screening called for an initial MS-AFP determination in the target population at 16-18 weeks gestation. Data from the U.K. study[1] indicated that the ability to detect AN and SB (all cases, open and closed) was maximum at this stage. The proportion of ASB cases that would be detected or the number of normal gestations with a positive result is a function of the test's cut-off for an abnormally elevated MS-AFP – *i.e.*, its sensitivity and specificity. This is discussed further below.

Following a positive MS-AFP result in the initial phase of screening, we presumed that a repeat test for the second phase would be performed since data from the U.K. study[2] and Macri *et al.*[4] indicated that 30-40% of the normal gestations would retest negative. Hence, we assumed in our model that about one-third of the normal pregnancies would be eliminated by a negative retest, thereby enhancing the overall specificity of the MS-AFP assay. In the absence of any firm data, we also assumed that about 1% of the ASB infants and twin gestations would be removed from further screening due to some biologic variation in maternal serum AFP elevations. Since an MS-AFP could be completed within 72 hours,[2] it was likewise presumed that the timing of a repeat MS-AFP would fall within the same 16 to 18 week screening interval.

Target Population
Phase I
MS-AFP
(16-18 weeks)
Phase II
Repeat MS-AFP
(Phase I positives)
Phase III
Sonography
(Phase II positives)
Twins
Miscalculated
gestational ages
(underestimation)
Anencephalics
Phase IV
Amniocentesis
(AF-AFP)
Phase V
Selective Abortion
(Phase IV positives)

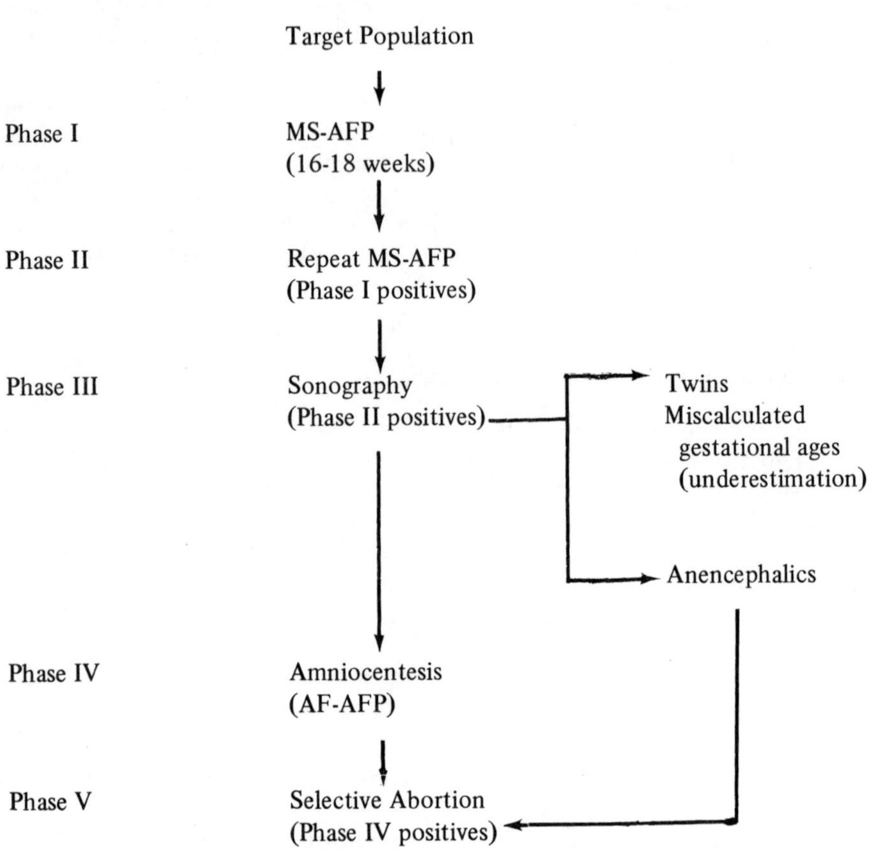

Figure 1.

Because of its well established role in detecting twins and anencephalic fetuses, as well as estimating gestational age, sonography constituted the third phase for gravidas with 2 positive MS-AFP results. In our study, we presumed that a careful sonographic examination would detect about 99% of the twins and 99% of the anencephalic fetuses and, in light of Macri *et al.'s* series of 3,672 patients,[4] correct about one-fourth of the false-positive MS-AFP results due to underestimation of gestational age. All of the pregnancies having these sonographic findings would consequently be eliminated from further testing since a twin gestation would usually be sufficient to explain 2 positive MS-AFP results, and the diagnosis of anencephaly would generally be certain enough to warrant a decision about pregnancy termination. A correction in gestational age, likewise, would account adequately for the 2 previous elevations in MS-AFP levels. Finally, it should be noted that, for our screening model, ultrasound was *not* considered sufficiently reliable to detect variants of spina bifida; hence, we presumed that *all* cases of SB would be missed by sonography.

Following 2 positive MS-AFP results and a sonogram negative for the conditions mentioned above, we next assumed that an amniocentesis for an amniotic fluid alpha-fetoprotein (AF-AFP) determination would be appropriate for the fourth phase. At this point in screening, AF-AFP testing might be tantamount to a diagnostic test because relatively few normal gestations would test positive. The exact proportion of normals included here would be a function of the tests' specificity (MS-AFP and AF-AFP), as discussed below.

The final, or fifth, phase of our screening model provided for the selective abortion of gestations deemed abnormal after a positive AF-AFP result. Most of the gravid women reaching this state would base any decision regarding pregnancy termination on 3 sequentially positive AFP results (MS-AFP x 2 and AF-AFP x 1). Those women carrying anencephalic fetuses diagnosed by sonography and 2 positive MS-AFP values would also fall into this fifth and final phase.

Following this overview of the multiphasic screening model depicted in Figure 1, several additional comments are warranted. Amniography was *not* included in our scheme for mass screening because we felt that it was an invasive diagnostic procedure which seemed to offer little more than that provided by a good sonographic examination. Unlike sonography, it also carried the risk of fetal-maternal irradiation and was not readily available for routine use in screening. In addition, the use of a second AF-AFP determination was not shown in Figure 1; in general, we assumed that only 1 AF-AFP result would be needed, or feasible, when the other tests had been completed on or about 18-20 weeks gestation.

Technical Details of Screening

The results of a screening program depend in large measure upon 3 technical details: (1) the *incidence* of the disease in the population being screened; (2) the *sensitivity* of the screening test (the likelihood of the test being positive, given that the subject is affected; and (3) the *specificity* of the test (the likelihood of the test being negative, given that the subject is unaffected).[5] The proportion of those with a positive test who do not have the diseases is the other main concern of a screening program. This proportion is a function of the incidence of the disease in persons being screened and the specificity of the test. As the incidence or specificity decrease, the proportion of those with a positive test who are normal (false positives) goes up.[5]

The model we used has 3 screening tests: MS-AFP, sonography, and AF-AFP. The outcome of a screening program can be affected by the incidence of the disease presented to *each* screening test and by the specificity and sensitivity of each test. To set the stage for our national projections, we show in the paragraphs that follow how the incidence, specificity, and sensitivity interrelate for each test and how variations in these 3 affect the total multiphasic screening program.

1. Maternal Serum Alpha-fetoprotein Screening

Since we were interested in making national projections, we utilized our estimated race- and defect-specific incidence of ASB for the U.S. population (Table 1). Specific figures for estimating the test's sensitivity and specificity were taken from the U.K. collaborative study.[1]

In MS-AFP screening, sensitivity and specificity are very much interrelated and can be arbitrarily established to give priority to a certain aspect of the screening program – *e.g.*, number of ASB cases detected, number of required sonograms and amniocenteses, etc. If one elects to call abnormal or positive, all serum specimens $\geqslant$ 95th percentile (essentially, a specificity of 0.95), the sensitivity for anencephaly is 0.88 and that for spina bifida 0.78.[1] Of the women initially screened, 3.6% would require sonography and 2.2% would subsequently require amniocentesis. At a cut-off corresponding to the 95th percentile, it is noteworthy that 2 positive MS-AFP results have raised the incidence of ASB by 23-fold to 3.7% for women who undergo sonography in the next phase.

Entirely different results occur if the MS-AFP cut-off is at the 99th percentile. The specificity becomes essentially 0.99 and the sensitivity drops to 0.84 for AN and to 0.59 for SB.[1] On the other hand, the percentage of women screened who require subsequent sonograms and amniocenteses is reduced to 0.9% and 0.4%, respectively. The incidence of ASB for women who undergo sonography, however, is 13% – an 80-fold increase, which reflects the higher specificity of this more restrictive cut-off (only 1% of the gravidas with unaffected fetuses are included).

The difference in specificity levels represented by 2 cut-offs for the MS-AFP assay can also profoundly affect the ratio of abnormal-to-normal fetuses that are eventually aborted. Indeed, this ratio is 5 times higher when the cut-off is the 99th percentile compared to the 95th percentile, which again highlights the importance of the specificity used in the screening process.

2. Sonographic Screening

The sensitivity and specificity of this test in ASB screening are not known.

Consequently, we assumed that the test had a sensitivity of 0.99 for anencephaly and a sensitivity of 0.00 for spina bifida. We also assumed that no normal fetuses would be diagnosed as abnormal, with careful sonographic technique – *i.e.*, a test specificity of 1.00. Since we remove the anencephalic fetuses prior to presentation for amniocentesis in our screening model, the incidence of ASB is not as high among those for AF-AFP screening as it was for women who undergo sonography. Still the incidence of ASB (primarily SB at this stage) is substantially higher than in the general population – *e.g.*, 3% to 13%, depending upon the MS-AFP cut-off selected, as noted above.

3. Amniotic Fluid Alpha-fetoprotein Screening

Although the AF-AFP detection rate for ASB ranges from 85% to 95%, depending upon the series studied, we utilized a moderate sensitivity level equal to 0.90 for all of the projections in our study. Because of the usually marked differences in AF-AFP values for normal fetuses and for those with ASB,[6] we presumed that the 90% detection rate for the AF-AFP assay would not change significantly within the specificity range of 0.990 to 0.999.

In established laboratories, the AF-AFP specificity should range between 0.990 and 0.999. Where it lies within this range can have a substantial effect on the proportion of normal fetuses with a positive test. For example, if the specificity lies close to 0.990, a woman is 7-8 times as likely to have a normal fetus, given a positive test, than if it approaches 0.999.

In our screening model, the AF-AFP specificity is markedly affected by the MS-AFP cut-off. The more restrictive the cut-off, or the higher the MS-AFP specificity, regardless of the precise AF-AFP specificity level, the higher the ratio of abnormal to normal fetuses with a positive AF-AFP result becomes. If we assume that all women with positive AF-AFP tests will have an abortion, this difference can be important to those persons wishing to minimize the loss of affected fetuses.

Under the best of laboratory and field conditions, occasional difficulties will occur in the interpretation of a positive AF-AFP due, for example, to fetal blood contamination.[6] As a consequence, we have purposely elected a moderate AF-AFP specificity of 0.995 for use in all of our projections.

Participant Factors

The major participant factors that are likely to determine the outcome of any national program can be listed as follows: (1) the proportion of women who come for their first prenatal visit by 18 weeks gestation (Table 3); (2) the proportion of those who come in time and want the test; (3) the proportion of those with 2 positive MS-AFP tests who elect amniocentesis; and (4) the proportion of those with a positive AF-AFP who elect an abortion.

To construct a series of national projections ranging from the theoretic maximum to the most realistic, the target population of 3,177,994 total U.S.

TABLE 3

Cumulative Percent of United States Women
Who Could be Screened with Maternal Serum Alpha-Fetoprotein (MS-AFP),
By Race and Timing of Their First Prenatal Visit[a]

	Timing of First Prenatal Visit (Menstrual Weeks)						
Race	$\leqslant 12$	$\leqslant 15$	$\leqslant 18$	$\leqslant 21$	$\leqslant 24$	Others[b]	Total
White	55.5	75.9	83.8	89.1	92.6	7.4	100.0
Other	38.8	57.0	68.6	77.7	84.6	15.4	100.0
Total	52.2	72.3	80.9	86.9	91.0	9.0	100.0

[a]Based on 1975 live birth data provided by the Natality Statistics Branch, NCHS (includes 42 reporting states and the District of Columbia for which the month of pregnancy prenatal care began was known and recorded).

[b]Includes women who came for their first prenatal visit after 24 weeks gestation, or received no prenatal care.

births for 1975 was stratified primarily by the presumed timing of prenatal care and the willingness of gravid women to participate in a multiphasic screening process. In the first 2 projections (I and II), all of the pregnant women represented in the target population are presumably screened with MS-AFP at 16-18 weeks gestation; in the second 2 projections (III and IV), only those women who actually begin their prenatal care by 18 weeks of gestation are screened (for whites, this is 83.8%, and for other women, 68.6% of those in the target population – Table 3). Lastly, in the remaining projections (V and VI), only those women who begin prenatal care in time *and* are actually willing to undergo a screening process that might involve amniocentesis and possibly abortion are included for MS-AFP testing (for white pregnant women this is estimated to be 41.9% and for others, 34.3% of those in the target population). For the percentages in the latter 2 projections (V and VI), we simply assumed that, at most, only 50% of those women who begin prenatal care in time for prenatal screening would actually decide to participate. This assumption was based on our experience, and that of others, with fetal chromosomal diagnosis among women of advanced maternal age, in which only 30-40 percent of the older gravid had the test performed.

In our projections, we assumed that all of the women with 2 positive MS-AFP results and a sonogram negative for anencephaly or twins would elect amniocentesis for an AF-AFP determination. Actually, were such screening a reality, probably as many as 5% of these women might decline the procedure.[7] However, considering that the risk of ASB at this stage of screening is at least 3%, which is higher than the risk of Down syndrome usually associated with advanced maternal age,[8] we doubt seriously that the refusal rate would ever approach the 20% reported by Koehler *et al.*[9]

And lastly, since the probability of having an affected fetus after 2 positive MS-AFP and a positive AF-AFP was at least 85%, we assumed that women faced with these results, so late in the screening process, would uniformly elect pregnancy termination. As mentioned previously, we assumed that every woman faced with positive MS-AFP results and a sonogram suggestive of anencephaly would do likewise.

National Projections

Each of the 6 projections presented in Table 4 were derived by applying the 2 cut-offs in MS-AFP testing and the screening assumptions about sonography and AF-AFP testing to the target population of total U.S. births for 1975. Presumed groups of women arriving in time for screening and desirous of MS-AFP testing were followed "prospectively" through the various screening phases outlined in Figure 1. At each phase of screening, separate computations were made for the anencephalic fetuses, those with spina bifida, and the normal singletons and twins which would test positive within each racial group.

Projections I and II (theoretic maximums) assume that all of the women in the target group present by 18 weeks of gestation and elect to be screened, and that all of those with indications for sonography and amniocentesis will have these procedures, and lastly, that all of those who have a positive AF-AFP will elect an abortion (Table 4). Of the 3,177,994 gestations screened initially in Projection I, where the MS-AFP cut-off is less restrictive (specificity set at the 95th percentile), 115,232 women would test positive on repeat MS-AFP and require subsequent sonographic examination. In this projection, 71,223 amniocenteses would also be needed. For Projection II, where the MS-AFP cut-off is more restrictive (specificity set at the 99th percentile), fewer positive repeat MS-AFP tests would necessitate only 27,376 sonograms and 12,373 amniocenteses. Although there would be little difference in the proportion of ASB cases detected (87% for AN, 69.5% for SB in I, *vs.* 83.1% for AN, 52.6% for SB in II), there would be a *marked* difference in the number of normal fetuses aborted and the ratio of abnormal-to-normal fetuses involved. As seen in Table 4, 345 normal fetuses would be among the total of 4,331 aborted in the first projection (abnormal-to-normal ratio approximately 12:1). With the enhanced specificity of the second projection, only 54 normal fetuses would be aborted along with the 3,424 cases of ASB (ratio about 63.1).

In Projections III and IV, the target population is based only on those women who actually begin their prenatal care by the 18th week of gestation. Projection III resembles Projection I and Projection IV resembles Projection II, with respect to the MS-AFP cut-offs used. Projections III and IV represent, in our opinion, maximal realistic expectations for a national program. Proportionately, fewer sonographs and amniocenteses would be required in either projection (Table 4). Of particular importance, however, is the impact of more limited participation in the prevention of ASB. As seen in Table 4, one would expect to detect 71.3% of the anencephalics and 57.3% of the spina bifidas in III, but only 68.5% of the AN and 43.4% of the SB cases in IV. As expected, considerably fewer normal fetuses would be aborted in either projection.

Projections V and VI, which take into account both the actual timing of the first prenatal visit and our best estimate of the proportion of women who will want MS-AFP testing represent, in our judgment, a realistic expectation in a field situation (Table 4). Hence, under the circumstances described above, one could expect a national program to reduce the incidence of AN and SB by no more than 36.0%-34.3% and 29.1%-21.7%, respectively (Projections V and VI).

Discussion

No one can know *a priori* what impact a national neural tube screening program would have, were such a program initiated in the United States. Although it is clear that such a program might theoretically prevent the live birth of 75-80% of fetuses with ASB, this theoretic maximum is unlikely to be reached. Some women will not want the test. Even to offer MS-AFP testing, moreover, would require a reordering of how pregnancies are managed – *i.e.*, devising a system to ensure that all pregnant women make their first prenatal visit by 18 weeks gestation. Furthermore, it seems that no screening program conducted on such a

TABLE 4

Projections for a National Prenatal Screening Program for Anencephaly-Spina Bifida

Epidemiologic Variable	Projections for the General Population					
	I	II	III	IV	V	VI
Number of gestations screened	3,177,994	3,177,994	2,571,703	2,571,703	1,285,586	1,285,586
Number of positive MS-AFP x 1[a]	162,887	35,353	131,876	28,667	65,939	14,334
Number of positive MS-AFP x 2[b]	115,232	27,376	93,465	22,287	46,733	11,144
Number of required sonograms	115,232	27,376	93,465	22,287	46,733	11,144
Anencephalics detected by sonography	2,046	1,953	1,689	1,612	845	806
Number of amniocenteses required for AF-AFP[c]	71,223	12,373	57,716	10,063	28,858	5,052
Spina bifidas detected by AF-AFP[c]	1,921	1,453	1,585	1,199	803	600
Anencephalics detected by AF-AFP[c]	19	18	15	14	8	8
Number of normal fetuses having positive AF-AFP[c]	345	54	279	44	140	22
Abnormal-to-normal fetus abortion ratio	11.6:1	63.4:1	11.8:1	64.2:1	11.8:1	64.3:1
Percent of all anencephalics in 1975 birth cohort-detected/aborted	87.0	83.1	71.8	68.5	36.0	34.3
Percent of all spina bifidas in 1975 birth cohort – detected/aborted	69.5	52.6	57.3	43.4	29.1	21.7

[a]First positive maternal serum alpha-fetoprotein.

[b]Second positive maternal serum alpha-fetoprotein.

[c]Amniotic fluid alpha-fetoprotein.

massive scale would be perfect. Even if the screening program outlined in our paper is followed closely, some normal fetuses would still be among the many abnormal ones that were aborted.

The projections, nevertheless, do give us an idea or range of what might be expected. Projections I and II seem highly unrealistic because we assume universal participation will take place. Projections III and IV also seem to be relatively unlikely outcomes, given that a substantial proportion of women are not likely to enter the program even if they do arrive in time for screening. We do believe, however, that Projections V and VI most likely resemble the outcome of an established program. If this is so, then approximately 34-36% of fetuses with anencephaly and 22-29% of those with spina bifida would be detected but at the cost of aborting 1,436 to 1,796 fetuses – 3.5-15% of which would probably be normal.

In program planning, due consideration should be given to certain variables in the screening process (number of sonographies, amniocenteses required, etc.), which would also be important. Here, as in other screening programs, limitations in trained personnel, diagnostic facilities, laboratory materials, and financial resources would greatly influence the screening methods that were employed. To handle the enormous volume of examinations that would be required, adequate laboratory facilities and skilled personnel would have to be available. As seen in our 6 projections (Table 4), the degree of participation and the initial MS-AFP cut-off would appear to be crucial in this regard.

Finally, it is appropriate to ask, based on our projections, whether the prenatal detection of only one-third of those in the target population is sufficiently high to warrant such a mass screening effort. Anencephaly and spina bifida are among the most common severe birth defects.[10] The 800 cases of SB that could be prevented are numerically superior to the 250 cases of phenylketonuria (PKU), the 500 or so cases of congenital hypothyroidism, or a like number of Down syndrome infants born to women $\geqslant 35$ years old, which occur annually in the United States. Screening programs for these three defects are already in progress throughout the country. In addition, AF-AFP is now being offered to gravid women with a positive family history for ASB; however, if all of these women were screened and elected abortion following a positive result, only 125 cases of SB (out of a possible 2,764, Table 2) would be prevented. Although a national program for neural tube screening based on MS-AFP would not be perfect, it could still have a major impact on the overall incidence of ASB and obviously a profound effect on the proportion of families who are destined to have infants with ASB. In light of the above, we hope that the discussions concerning a national screening program will continue and that our projections will stimulate others to think seriously about the overall effects of such an undertaking.

ACKNOWLEDGMENTS

The authors thank Mrs. Joyce J. Kendrick, Mrs. Mary A. Brown, and Mrs. Faye Williams for their assistance in the preparation of this manuscript. In addition, the statistical support and advice provided by Mr. Levy M. James and Dr. Peter M. Layde is gratefully acknowledged.

REFERENCES *

1. Report of U.K. Collaborative Study on Alpha-Fetoprotein in Relation to Neural-Tube Defects, Maternal Serum-Alpha-Fetoprotein Measurement in Antenatal Screening for Anencephaly and Spina Bifida in Early Pregnancy, *Lancet 1,* 1323, 1977.
2. W. Check, *J.A.M.A. 238,* 1441, 1977.
3. National Center for Health Statistics, Monthly Vital Statistics Report, Vol. 25, No. 10, Supplement, December 20, 1976.
4. J.N. Macri *et al.*, Maternal Serum Alpha-Fetoprotein Screening for Neural Tube Defects: Structure and Organization, elsewhere this volume.
5. M.F. Goldberg and G.P. Oakley, *Am. J. Obstet. Gynecol. 133,* 126, 1979.
6. A. Milunsky and E. Alpert, *Obstet. Gynecol. 48*, 1, 1976.
7. N.J. Wald, personal communication.
8. N. Wald, H. Cuckle and G. Stirrat, *Lancet 1,* 495, 1976.
9. S. Koehler *et al., Fifth International Conference on Birth Defects, Excerpta Medica, International Congress Series, 426,* 54, 1977.
10. Center for Disease Control, Congenital Malformations Surveillance Report, October 1976-September 1977 (issued March 1978).

*Editors' note: We call attention in particular to the article by Dr. Macri and associates in Section II – Genetic Counseling and Other Genetic Services in the Community.

APPENDIX

Estimation of national (crude) rates of ASB was made from 3 data sets: (1) race-specific ASB rates from the Metropolitan Atlanta Congenital Defects program, 1968-1975; (2) total number of reported cases and race-specific number of births in each U.S. census division, reported through the Birth Defects Monitoring Program (BDMP), 1970-1975; and (3) race-specific number of live births in each U.S. census division from U.S. vital records data.

First, assuming that the Atlanta race-specific rates represent "true" rates in Census Division 3 (the South Atlantic), an expected number of cases in the BDMP for all races was calculated. The ratio of reported to expected number of cases in Division 3 yielded an estimate of the rate of ascertainment in BDMP, assumed to apply to both "white" and "other" race categories in each census division. Inflation of the number of BDMP reported cases in each division by the reciprocal of the ascertainment rate yielded the number of BDMP cases adjusted for under-ascertainment. Application of the Atlanta rates to BDMP race-specific births in each division provided expected numbers of total cases. The ratio of the "adjusted observed" to the expected number of cases in each division was assumed to represent a geographic effect relative to Atlanta (and Census Division 3) and applicable to both race categories. Multiplication of this ratio for each division by the Atlanta race-specific rates yielded the estimated rates by division. National race-specific rates were then computed by weighing each derived division rate by the proportion of race-specific live births in each division.

GENETIC SERVICES ECONOMICS: METROPOLITAN NEW YORK EXPERIENCE WITH HEALTH CARE INSURANCE PROGRAMS

Jessica G. Davis

For the past four years I've been concerned with the funding of genetic services in my capacity as a director of a genetics service and as the chairperson of the legal-economics subcommittee of the Task Force on Medical Genetics in the New York City-Greater Metropolitan area. The Task Force is an *ad hoc* group made up of representatives of the local medical genetics community. The group meets several times during the course of the academic year under the auspices of the National Foundation-March of Dimes.

The Task Force meetings provide an opportunity for active participation and interaction of all persons delivering medical genetic services in our area. In addition to its scientific interests the group's activities are varied and include the preparation of comprehensive surveys of all local genetic services and their rate of utilization; the publication of a Newsletter and educational materials; and the drafting of proposals for joint genetic screening and educational programs. The legal-economics subcommittee was formed to enable the membership to keep abreast of all pertinent national and state legislation pertaining to genetic services. The subcommittee's other major concern is the funding of genetic services. Committee members have examined the actual costs of genetic services, the fee structures in the New York Metropolitan area and the types of coverage available. In order to accomplish this, a close working relationship has been established with representatives of Medicaid and third party insurance as well as with the consumer. This report concerns our experiences with third party insurance in the New York City Metropolitan area.

One of the essential components of a modern society is a fully differentiated medical care system. The expressions "health care system" or "medical system" designate the totality of efforts and resources, human and material which a society sets aside for health care problems. The system is amazingly complex. It requires the labor of many types of technical health workers; encompasses hospitals, nursing homes, rehabilitation centers and health departments; includes environmental controls, biomedical research programs, and the pharmaceutical industry as well as insurance companies; large national voluntary health agencies and small areawide planning councils. Since health care is now perceived as a civil

ISBN 0-12-562650-9

right, it interests the federal, state and local governments. Uncounted individuals from all walks of life participate daily in the system. Finally, health care requires vast and increasing expenditures. Advances in biomedical knowledge and their technological application lead to increased demands for health services and in turn to rising costs. Although the allocation of resources tends to be a major issue for health systems planners, most of their difficulties stem from the fact that costs for medical services continue to rise steadily.

There are several alternative ways to deal with this problem. The first is to increase services and allow costs to soar without controls. Clearly this is an inflationary approach and one that could not continue indefinitely. The second is to cut services and reduce costs. Although all of us are in favor of fiscal restraint, if this approach were adopted it would soon prove unacceptable to consumers, vendors and insurers. The third possibility is to manage health systems in such a way that the highest level of care is assured within resource constraints. If one follows this course, it is unlikely that medical costs will decrease because as the capability of a system increases the pressures to use it grow. We have chosen the last option because it is the most flexible and it permits growth. Medicaid and Medicare, the existing federally supported health care programs, and Blue Cross and other third party payment plans are designed to spread the risks and benefits of health system capability. There has been steady decline over the last four decades in direct-fee-for-service payments with a concomitant expansion of third party programs: voluntary and statutory as well as ingenious new combinations of the two.

Let us now consider voluntary health insurance. Voluntary health insurance or health prepayment coverage is designed to protect the individual who contracts an illness or suffers an injury, the insurance covering the resultant hospital and/or medical expenses. It is sold by private companies defined and regulated by state law. Protection is in no sense absolute and varies from individual to individual (and from plan to plan). The consumer agrees to pay a fixed amount of money to an organization which in turn agrees to provide care or medical service of a specified type.

There are two major types of voluntary health prepayment organizations, the private insurance companies and the hospital and/or medical service organizations. The first group is made up of mutual and stock insurance companies. The second group has varied sponsorship with most being organized on some non-profit basis. The best known are the Blue Cross plans. These are community, regional or statewide hospital service corporations operating with the approval of the American Hospital Association. Complementing the Blue Cross plans are the Blue Shield plans, community, regional or statewide medical service corporations sponsored by state or county medical societies and meeting standards set by the Council on Medical Service of the American Medical Association. There are also a large number of independent plans, many of which provide quite comprehensive medical care benefits and, in some cases, hospital service. Included here are employer plans, union plans, community plans comparable to the Health

Insurance Plan of Greater New York and consumer-controlled organizations.

Voluntary health insurance is sold on two different enrollment bases: indivdual (or personal) and group. In order to qualify for an individual plan, a would-be policyholder applies to an insurance company or another prepayment organization for coverage. If accepted – with or without medical examination – the new policyholder (or subscriber) pays premiums directly to the carrier, normally on a quarterly or an annual basis. The premium charges vary according to the benefits involved and the age, sex and occupation of the policyholder.

Group insurance is written on members of a group held together by some mutual interest such as the employees of a common employer or the members of a union. A group insurance contract is issued to a master policyholder, an employer, or union not to the individual members of the group. Eligibility requirements for group insurance policies tend to be broad.

There's no doubt that by increasing the total amount of money available as well as by spreading payments over a much larger portion of the population, health insurance has brought the reality of modern medicine to a far greater number of people than otherwise would have been possible. However, health insurance has also made a substantial contribution to the Pandora's box of medical care difficulties. Inability to establish control over rising costs impedes the extension of benefit coverage to include new techniques and many still uninsured areas of outpatient care such as genetic services. This contributes directly to expensively skewed patterns of utilization. As hospital costs rise hospital demands for higher reimbursement increase. In order to meet these demands, rates will have to increase at consumer expense.

Costs of health services receive serious consideration by all segments of our society. There is scarcely a major collective bargaining conference today in which the issue of improving health insurance benefits does not arise. The phrase "comprehensive" coverage is an almost universally accepted goal but is still not a reality. The higher the individual's educational and employment level, family income and length of employment, the better the coverage an individual will have. The American consumer is groping for the most complete medical coverage available. The consumer wants inexpensive protection against small as well as large expenditures and for care that the individual can initiate. The consumer has become increasingly more committed to the idea of preventive medicine and early diagnosis. Consumers point out that since the form of health insurance inevitably influences patterns of health behavior it should be geared to influence them constructively in a health-inducing direction.

Therein lies the rub! Third party insurers do not now cover nor do they anticipate expending their benefit programs to include preventive services in their regular contracts. Some special new contracts such as the Blues' Premier Physician Care Coverage seem to have a preventive slant. At the present time, third party insurers do not cover genetic services, particularly counseling. The reason that third party insurers do not cover genetic counseling is that they state the procedure is wholly discretionary. The Blues' also believe that any action or inaction taken subsequent to counseling is discretionary. Purely discretionary services are not medically necessary.[1] Why? The Blues feel that services that can be anticipated and are discretionary do not constitute insurance risks. According to the Blues the traditional purpose of prepaid health insurance is to provide for unexpected occurrences. Genetic counseling, along with routine well-baby care and annual physical examinations, are perceived as being in no sense unexpected services giving rise to unanticipated costs. Furthermore, the Blues state that if genetic counseling is offered to all subscribers as a part of a large scale preventive screening program, overall costs will increase. Third party insurers question whether genetic counseling would be cost-effective if applied to the population as a whole. Third party insurers also do not cover geneticists as a specialty group. They view medical and doctoral geneticists as hospital-based and hospital-salaried. Insurers know that most geneticists are pediatricians or internists with a dual specialty in genetics. The salaries of hospital-based personnel are included in the hospital's cost base.[2] Additional charges would lead to an increase in the cost base which third party insurers wish to avoid. The Blues also do not believe it is the responsibility of an insurer to support research efforts so they will not pay for the hospital geneticist engaged in research.[3] Third party insurers will also not pay for genetic counseling given by non-medical personnel such as social workers or associates in genetic counseling.

What then do third party insurers pay for? In those cases when the onset of a genetic disease occurs in later life, such as Huntington disease, and the patient is covered under the Blues, the coverage is the same as it would be for any medical condition. Sometimes if the problem falls into the category of prolonged illness under the Master or Major Medical contract, deductibles and coinsurance are waived for many services. Deductibles and coinsurance are normally required. If the disease occurs prior to non-group enrollment, a waiver of liability can be required exempting that specific condition from coverage permanently or for a limited period of time. The Blues do cover all medically necessary hospitalizations and disease or symptom related medical care. Some services such as visits to physicians' offices are subject to deductibles and coinsurance unless waived, but most diagnostic tests, including buccal smear, cytogenetic studies, metabolic screening tests, sonography, and amniocentesis are partially and/or fully covered. I have also determined that should a couple decide, as a result of genetic analysis and education, to abort the definitely or probably defective fetus, claims for the abortion would be paid under the medical necessity guidelines.

How can change occur? New legal developments may prove helpful. For example, forty-eight states now give wide protection and benefits to newborns. The New York State law (the former Cochrane-Bianchi Bill) states that all health insurance policies with family benefits must provide immediate coverage for the care and treatment of any medically diagnosed congenital defect or birth abnormality including prematurity. I believe that as applications and payments for these benefits increase, third party insurers will reconsider their portion of the funding of preventive genetic services. A recent change in the New York State Medicaid fee schedule to include payments for genetic counseling and amniocentesis may also lead to adjustments on the part of third party insurers. However, as newborn insurance coverage expands, funding for maternal antenatal care lags. Only thirty percent of women who have maternity insurance are covered for prenatal visits. This means that seventy percent are and may be excluded for appropriate genetic services which would have been implemented early in pregnancy. Many recently pregnant couples are also excluded because often maternity benefits do not begin until nine months after the effective date of the policy. We must give more attention and effort to expanding maternity benefits.

Lastly, in medicine it is impossible to determine a line or even a zone of catastrophic expenses by a monetary definition, except at extremes. One family's routine expenses are another's disaster. As effectiveness and cost of care increase, the majority of individuals in this country will require the assistance of an insurance mechanism to cope with what should be routine expenses. Although facts are hard to obtain in the wizard world of insurance accounting, it appears that this can only come about if there is continued interaction between the professional and individuals from the private and public funding sectors. We have made gains in the past years in that the insurance companies in our area now know about genetic services and have funded some services. There obviously is room for improvement and expansion. It is important for us as vendors of genetic services to establish good lines of communication with all consumer groups, third party insurers and public funding agencies. It is only through cooperation that large scale financing and reorganization of health care can be achieved without sacrificing the essential values of highly professional individualized and humane service.

REFERENCES

1. J.L. Thompson and W.M. Greenfield, *in* Genetics and the Law, A. Milunsky and G.J. Annas (Eds.), Plenum Press, New York, p. 293, 1975.
2. *Ibid.*, 291-292.
3. *Ibid.*, 292.

THE HUNTINGTON'S DISEASE COMMISSION: A MODEL APPROACH TO A MULTIFACETED PROBLEM

Nancy S. Wexler
Joan S. Wilentz

The Commission for the Control of Huntington's Disease and Its Consequences was established by Congress in 1976 in response to pleas from families afflicted by Huntington's disease. No new monies were appropriated for the work of the Commission, but the National Institute of Neurological and Communicative Disorders and Stroke was charged with its support, both financially and administratively. The Commission's mandate from Congress was to report on the state of the art of research and care of Huntington's disease patients and to develop a national plan for its alleviation and eventual eradication. This plan was presented to Congress and the President on October 17, 1977, as prescribed by law.

The Commission was composed of six professional and three lay persons chosen for their knowledge and personal involvement with Huntington's disease, as well as their interests in public health problems. To carry out its mandate the Commission appointed 15 work groups in fields of biomedical research and social management. These groups reported on the state-of-the-art of research, care, and treatment of Huntington's disease. They gathered new data, advised on promising leads, and made general and specific recommendations for the National Plan. Guidance and information were also elicited from world authorities on Huntington's disease, leading neuroscientists, geneticists, lawyers, educators, psychologists, and other professional and lay persons.

The Commission held hearings in 11 cities chosen to represent urban and rural regions throughout the country. Over 2,000 persons, Huntington's disease patients and family members, government officials, health care providers, and others testified in person or wrote to the Commission to describe their personal experiences and problems, and to make recommendations.

The Commission had a very specific charge to study Huntington's disease. In fulfilling this charge, the Commission departed from precedents set by previous categorical commissions. It concluded that Huntington's disease cannot be studied in isolation, nor can the solutions to the problems created by Huntington's disease, if they are to be truly effective, concern Huntington's disease alone. The following are passages from the Prologue of the Commission's Report which express the Commissioner's philosophy:

ISBN 0-12-562650-9

A disease which is hereditary, which produces radical physical changes destroying coordination, speech, and self-control as well as profound mental changes – demolishing the power to think or remember or reason – a disease which causes severe mental illness, strikes in the prime of life, and is progressively fatal over 10 or 20 years – is a microcosm of the major health problems the country is facing today. In fulfilling its mandate, the Commission found it necessary to expand the scope of its deliberations to consider the more general problems created by hereditary, neurologic, psychiatric, chronic, and terminal disease.

There is no yardstick to measure human misery. Huntington's disease will not be cured because people suffer more greatly, but because scientists supported by generous funding will struggle to find the answers. Huntington's disease patients will find appropriate care in the community not only because they are needy, but because they stand with other groups – the elderly, those with epilepsy, multiple sclerosis, muscular dystrophy, and others – now demanding a change in long-term care.

The Commission believes that in an era of scarce resources and increasing demands, costly and redundant programs for individual diseases are no longer feasible. Accordingly, the National Plan developed by the Commission adopts a generic rather than a categorical approach, one that is problem-oriented rather than disease-oriented. Recommendations for the control of Huntington's disease and its consequences emphasize the commonalities that unite interests rather than the differences which separate them.

The Commission was an interdisciplinary group chosen because of personal interest in the pursuit of a common goal. After a year's study, it was clear that all those concerned with the amelioration of suffering caused by hereditary, neurological, and neuropsychiatric disorders must find common ground. The territorial behavior that sets one disease sufferer against another must give way to a united approach aimed at achieving compassionate care, treatment, and cure for all these diseases.

Congress has granted the Commission a superb opportunity to review the problems created by one complex and formidable disease. This review has entailed a careful look at the state of the art not only in Huntington's disease but in other genetic and chronic disorders. The Commission has concluded that to generate greater creativity and productivity in biomed-

> ical research, provide a more rational and humane plan of health care management, demonstrate greater fiscal responsibility and cost effectiveness, and recognize the needs of countless sufferers from kindred disorders who have no such privileged voice, its recommendations must go beyond Huntington's disease to address a broader range of fundamental health problems.

I would like to share with you some of the recommendations of the Huntington's Disease Commission which have the most relevance for hereditary diseases in general.

First and foremost among the Commission's recommendations is the need for increased support for a broad program of basic and clinical research in genetics and in the neurosciences. Not only did the Nobel Laureates and other eminent scientists who counseled the Commission make this recommendation, but the most urgent and overwhelming plea from Huntington's disease patients and families across the nation was for increased support of biomedical research. Unfortunately, at a time when genetics and the neurosciences are flourishing as the vanguard of scientific discovery, there has been a serious decline in funds for research. The National Institute of General Medical Sciences (NIGMS), which supports fundamental research and research training in genetics and in molecular and cell biology, could fund only about one-fourth of its approved grants in 1977. It receives only 10 percent of funds appropriated to the National Institutes of Health. The National Institute of Neurological and Communicative Disorders and Stroke (NINCDS), with only one-sixth of the NIH budget, has an even more straitened funding situation. It was able to fund less than one-fourth of approved grants in 1977. Approximately 500 hereditary disorders are neurological. Unfortunately, the heavy emphasis in recent years on generous funding for particular categorical diseases has led to a skewing of research funding. There is a danger that disenchantment with the power of the dollar to buy a cure may lead Congress to try to reduce funding for biomedical research. Education is needed on Capitol Hill to enable Congress to better appreciate the essentially quixotic but crucial role of basic biomedical research. Dollars may not be able to buy a cure, but assuredly, without dollars, there is no hope of treatment or cure.

A second major recommendation of the Commission which has relevance for all hereditary disorders is the necessity for drug companies to develop new drug treatments for small populations of patients. At the moment, the pharmaceutical industry does not find sufficient economic incentives in small patient populations to make it worth their while to invest their considerable resources in talent and facilities to this end. A number of complex factors make drug development a time-consuming and costly process. These include steps to assure the safety and efficacy of drugs, reporting requirements, and a limited lifetime of patents during which companies can recoup their investments. Without sufficient guarantees of returns on investments and profit, drug companies will not undertake research on and development of new compounds.

Most hereditary diseases affect relatively small numbers of patients, even though in the aggregate serious genetic disorders afflict over 12 million Americans. Sufferers from sickle cell disease, cystic fibrosis, Cooley's anemia, and Huntington's disease, to say nothing of Lesch-Nyhan's disease and dysautonomia victims, all find that potential relief through the development of new treatments is effectively denied them through considerations of the marketplace.

The Huntington's Disease Commission met with leaders of the Food and Drug Administration, representatives of the drug industry, the National Institutes of Health, and with prominent clinical investigators to explore this problem. The Report describes six alternatives which could conceivably rectify this situation. These suggestions range from direct and indirect subsidization of new drug development through tax and patent laws to the utilization of NIH to develop new compounds, a precedent for which exists in the National Cancer Institute. The Commission felt the intricacies of the problem were so complex and so intertwined with the economic structure of this country that the Commission did not have sufficient time nor expertise to opt for a specific alternative. Instead, it called for the President to appoint immediately an interdisciplinary Task Force consisting of representatives from the appropriate sectors of the Government, private industry, and consumers to study the problem and make recommendations as quickly as possible.

Huntington's disease takes a slow toll over 15 to 20 years. Ten or more of these years may be spent in chronic care facilities, either a nursing home or state hospital, usually a psychiatric institution. Almost every patient is institutionalized at some point in the course of the illness. Costs of such care are astronomical. One year in a nursing home, at the average projected cost for 1978, is $12,700. Fifteen years of patient support can absorb nearly $200,000 in institutional care costs alone. The direct costs for 15,000 Huntington's disease patients (based on a conservative prevalence estimate of 7 per 100,000) amount to between $110 million and $125 million annually. This figure does not include productivitiy lost, nor the costs of ancillary supports required for good patient care and to maintain a household. They do not include the price of social and emotional upheaval which can lead to additional medical and psychotherapy costs for family members.

Genetic diseases are typically chronic diseases requiring long-term care. And long-term care is the major cause of catastrophic health expenses in the United States today. The Commission found that the middle income family affected by chronic illness has little or no financial protection and is quickly improverished. Private and government financial aid programs are neither designed for the chronically ill nor for the middle income family. Private medical insurance rarely pays long-term care costs. Medicare is geared to the acute hospital system. Medicaid does provide protection against catastrophic expenses, but only for the indigent or near indigent. Certain provisions of Social Security programs developed to aid families in financial need have the effect of discouraging work and splintering families. There is no way that families threatened by hereditary illness can adequately save for children jeopardized by genetic risk. And to mention a further inequity, women with chronic disease who are homemakers are ineligible for Disability Insurance benefits under Title II of the Social Security Act because their labor in the home has not been for wages. Huntington's disease families have frequently been advised by social service personnel to divorce so that the ill spouse becomes indigent – and thus eligible for medical benefits. Needless to say, this economic expedient is psychologically demoralizing to patient, spouse and at-risk children.

The most ominous sign that this sorry condition will persist is the fact that current plans for National Health Insurance, from administrative, Congressional, and private sources such as the National Committee on Health Insurance do not include coverage of chronic illness. A key recommendation of the Commission is that the needs of the chronically ill be addressed in any program of National Health Insurance. These needs demand the inclusion in any insurance program of coverage of the full range of medical, social, and mental health services required by the chronically ill. Until such programs are enacted, the Commission is also recommending that certain alterations be made in the provisions and implementation of programs under the Social Security Act. These changes would benefit all those with chronic disease.

Most people with hereditary disorders do not require institutional care. But for those who do, truly adequate and appropriate care is difficult to find. In most communities, there is no continuum available of facilities and services matched to meet the needs of individuals at all levels of disability. Home help providing domestice chore and companionship services is virtually non-existent. Day care centers which could give meaningful work and recreation to disabled adolescents and adults of all ages are not to be found, and there is, in general, a paucity of respite care programs and appropriate institutional care for most young and middle-aged individuals. The Commission has made specific recommendations for a number of pilot research, care, and treatment programs providing alternative forms of care.

In addition, the Commission has proposed something called a Center Without Walls to facilitate basic and clinical research on Huntington's disease and related disorders. In order to pursue many promising avenues of research, including research on services, access to patients or patient tissues is necessary. Huntington's disease patients and others with relatively uncommon disorders also have need for a clinical facility offering the latest in diagnostic and therapeutic techniques and integrated programs of medical, genetic, psychological, social, and rehabilitative services. Traditional specialized disease centers typically involve a staff of scientists, supporting personnel, equipment, and patients all under one roof. Centers are quite expensive and can be in danger of becoming ossified, depending on the creativity and flexibility of the center director. The Commission felt that "funds should go primarily to support innovative thinking and activity, wherever it may be found, and not spent on accumulations of buildings and equipment. As long as there is a clinical facility providing access to patients, and as long as valuable research is supported, center components do not have to be geographically contiguous."

The Commission's proposal for Centers Without Walls departs from the traditional concept of an "all under one roof" center. Each Center should include a clinical facility for conducting basic and clinical research on patients with Huntington's disease and related disorders – genetic and/or neurological – as well as research on services (speech and physical therapy, mental health, genetic counseling, etc.). The clinical facility, which would serve as the administrative core, would be affiliated with center investigators engaged in basic and clinical research throughout the country. These other investigators would be funded from Center funds and would have access to patients or patients' tissues through the clinical facility. The Center as a whole should function as a demonstration, education, and training model in research, treatment, and care of Huntington's disease patients and those with related disorders. It would stimulate new research and communication, and heighten visibility of those diseases under study, as well as provide a humane service for affected patients and families.

The Commission has also recommended that the Center for Disease Control, in collaboration with the NINCDS, establish a pilot program of Health Services Coordination and Development in order to make optimal use of services that are available in a community and to develop new ones. This program would provide a staff of public health personnel, including genetic associates and "genetic" nurses and social workers, who would be an immediate first line of help for Huntington's disease patients and those with related disorders. If necessary, they would also serve as ombudsman to see that services to which patients or families are entitled are expeditiously provided.

In illnesses such as Huntington's disease, for which there is no effective treatment, no predictive test, and a protracted and terminal course, it is imperative that those affected and at risk receive the most accurate information possible regarding the hereditary nature of the disorder. Voluntary abstention from childbearing is the only possible way currently available to reduce the incidence of the disease. The importance of good genetic counseling cannot be overestimated because only through knowledge can individuals make an informed choice regarding major life decisions. Of equal importance, however, is helping the individual or family to cope with the psychological devastation which can attend learning about an hereditary condition. Emotional trauma can prevent a person from even assimilating the information given. In almost 2,000 letters of public testimony, the psychological impact of the disease, including its hereditary nature, was mentioned more often than almost any other problem created by the disorder. Frequently, genetic counseling was provided by the physician making the diagnosis and consisted of the most minimal facts, delivered in a highly impersonal manner and in a single session. In numerous letters families railed against the failure of the doctor-patient relationship to provide the emotional sustenance necessary to cope with such shattering news. All too often, physicians were unable to provide the necessary emotional support, and mental health professionals were uninformed regarding physical disorders and were perceived by families as being of service only for those with psychological illnesses. Genetic counselors were thought to concern themselves only with risk factors. If the family knew the risks they saw no need for traditional genetic counseling. The troubled family had nowhere to turn. Family members can express this need far more eloquently than I:

> "For many years, my father had been in and out of therapy and hospitalized twice for extreme depression. He also had shock treatment. . . The end result was a diagnosis of HD. . . It took about two months for me to become so severely depressed that I ceased functioning almost completely. I simply couldn't live knowing all I knew about the disease, knowing tomorrow I might be next, thinking the depression that had gripped me was telling me I had it already, thinking my daughter might get it (how do you tell your child?), thinking that since I was single and had hopes of someday remarrying, who would want me?
>
> "Last week my father refused to take his medication and then tried to kill my mother and himself. Today he is again in the hospital. . . It's terrible living with the guilt of wishing your father dead. . . I think the biggest problem was the fact that I had literally no one to turn to. I lived with my daughter alone. My brother couldn't accept the disease and I could not speak to him. My mother was not permitted to be made aware of it, so there was literally no one to talk to, and I was the one who was handling everything dealing with my father, since there was no one else, and I think that it was just too much for one person to attempt to handle. Unfortunately, there was absolutely nowhere to turn."

For families struggling with burdensome and debilitating hereditary disorders such as Huntington's disease, the traditional mode of genetic counseling – explaining the nature of the illness and relevant facts in one or two sessions – will not suffice. Long-term support and sympathetic guidance in coping with the condition must be made available, either through using a team of interdisciplinary professionals or training genetic counselors in the requisite counseling skills and assuring their availability for long-term contact. A cadre of mental health professionals should also be trained in helping individuals cope with hereditary and other chronic conditions which impose particular psychological stress. The Commission has called for the development of a new discipline, "Health Psychology", to emphasize the normative psychological stress response to physical conditions. "Adjustment or coping counseling", "preventive guidance", or "ventilation and education" would be a routine step in the diagnosis, referral, and treatment process of hereditary and other conditions. Counseling sessions should be considered as primary prevention of expectable emotional distress in reaction to medical problems. The Commission has recommended several pilot projects in concert with existing Community Mental Health Centers to determine if this kind of counseling is, in fact, beneficial in limiting or preventing serious emotional disturbances in patients and families affected by Huntington's disease or related disorders.

One of the most serious problems reported in Commission public testimony, a difficulty encountered by sufferers of many different hereditary diseases, was that of misdiagnosis and misinformation. The need for professional, family, and public education was repeatedly emphasized by witnesses. There are a number of factors in medical training and practice which militate against doctors including hereditary disorders in their differential diagnoses. Medical students are instructed in genetics early in the course of their training, divorced from subsequent teaching regarding individual diseases. They are not taught algorithms for differentiating among common presenting symptoms and do not take sufficiently careful family histories. The Commission emphasized that physician awareness must be increased regarding the ubiquitousness of hereditary diseases so that any individual disorder has a greater likelihood of being recognized. In addition to the development and dissemination of specific educational materials on Huntington's disease, the Commission felt that a national clearinghouse for the development and distribution of materials on human genetics in general, genetic disorders, and birth defects would improve treatment and care for all hereditary diseases. Rather than the current fragmentation of information, a central source would be efficient and cost-effective.

The Commission has recommended that such a clearinghouse be established under the auspices of P.L. 94-278, the National Sickle Cell, Cooley's Anemia, Tay-Sachs, and Genetic Diseases Act. The purpose of this Act is to establish a national program of "basic and applied research, research training, testing, counseling, and information and education programs with respect to genetic diseases". Thirty million dollars was authorized annually for fiscal year (FY) 1976, FY 1977, and FY 1978. No new monies were appropriated for the Act in FY 1976, FY 1977. The 1978 Labor-HEW appropriations bill for the first time includes $4 million for Title IV, only 13 percent of the original authorization.

The Commission strongly affirmed that the National Genetic Diseases Act, as one of the first non-categorical pieces of legislation with respect to genetc diseases, is worthy of support. The Commission has recommended that the Act be extended when it expires at the end of FY 1978, and that the full authorization of $30 million be appropriated for FY 1979, FY 1980, and FY 1981. In addition, the Commission concluded that an identifiable administrative unit must be created within the Office of the Assistant Secretary for Health. This office would be responsible for planning, evaluating, and coordinating genetic services and research, monitoring grant review and allocation of funds, establishing program and funding priorities and planning policy with respect to the social, economic, legal, ethical, and psychological problems that are anticipated with the development of new technologies in genetic screening. Input from non-governmental professionals and consumers should be solicited. Only an office at the level of the Assistant Secretary for Health would have the flexibility and authority to establish contacts both within and without the Public Health Service.

I think that we have seen the end of an era in Washington when grant money was plentiful and the "disease of the month club", as it is facetiously called, had easy access to Congress' ear. One potentially positive outcome of diminishing resources is that those concerned with categorical diseases may be pushed to cooperate with each other, and that health care professionals and politicians may be forced to learn a common language in order to spend existing funds wisely. Dollars are becoming scarcer as health is becoming the nation's number one industry. Those who seek to guard the national health must begin to learn the intricacies of the political system, while those empowered to make bold decisions which can have a profound impact on millions of lives must be educated regarding the most judicious uses of their delegated power. Let us hope and let us work toward ensuring that a healthier citizenry is the beneficiary of this dialogue.

CARRIER SCREENING IN HEMOPHILIA AND DUCHENNE MUSCULAR DYSTROPHY: ECONOMICAL AND PSYCHOLOGICAL CONSEQUENCES

Marie-Louise Lubs

Disorders which are due to X-linked recessive genes constitute a particular challenge for the genetic counselor. The inactivation of one of the X-chromosomes during early embryogenesis in females[1] results in a wide range of expression in clinical and laboratory test characteristics in carrier females. With the possible exception of X-linked mental retardation, the two most common severe X-linked disorders are hemophilia A and Duchenne muscular dystrophy. While Duchenne muscular dystrophy is considered to be a high burden disease from a clinical and social standpoint, hemophilia is a disease with high economical burden as well, both for the family and for society.

In a survey of all families in Colorado with cases of severe hemophilia, the yearly cost in 1974 for blood products was estimated as shown in Table 1. It should be noted that the question referred to an average year and the answers did not include special surgery, tooth extractions, etc. The average cost for severe hemophilia was $5,520 per patient, but about 18% of the sample indicated yearly costs in excess of $9,000.

The development of a carrier test based on immunological techniques by Zimmerman *et al.*[2] has made it possible to more accurately predict the risk for female relatives of hemophiliacs with factor VIII deficiency. Figure 1 shows test results from obligate carriers and controls at University of Colorado Medical Center Hemophilia Clinic. With a cutoff point at 0.84 as the ratio of AHF activity to AHF antigen, a total of 91% of carriers could be identified. At that level, the false positive rate among controls was 8%. Even though these results are a considerable improvement over the cold carrier test which consisted of evaluating factor VIII activity along, it is still not good enough for population screening. If we were to screen all women, the results would be as shown in Table 2.:

Among every 5,000 women screened, 401 would test positive, and among those 400 would be false positives.

Fortunately, there are other means of identifying carriers than total population screening. Before progressive genetic counseling became part of hemophilia and muscular dystrophy clinics, identification of a carrier was usually made when her son was diagnosed as having the disease. This made genetic counseling for future pregnancies possible, but since the majority of families have only one

ISBN 0-12-562650-9

TABLE 1

Estimated Yearly Cost of Hemophilia

Yearly Cost	Severely Affected N = 49 %	Mildly Affected N = 19 %
None	0.0	47.4
$< 200	3.9	10.5
$200-1,000	17.7	21.0
$1,001-3,000	27.5	10.5
$3,001-6,000	27.5	0.0
$6,001-9,000	5.9	10.5
$> 9,000	17.7	0.0
Mean Yearly Cost	$5,520	$1,380

TABLE 2

Severe Hemophilia A

Carrier frequency:	1/5,000
Cost of carrier test:	$38
False positive rate	8%
Cost per carrier if all women screened:	$190,000
Falsely identified among 5,000 women:	400

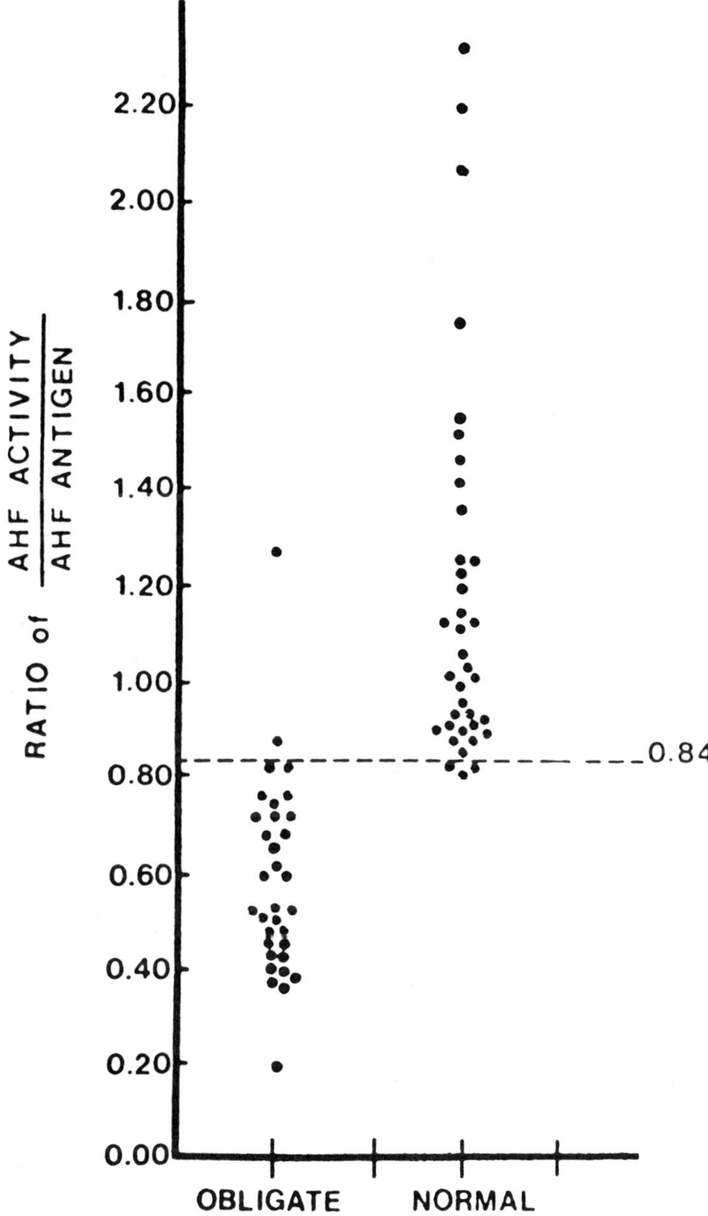

Fig. 1. Ratio of $\frac{\text{AHF activity}}{\text{AHF antigen}}$ in obligate carriers of classical hemophilia and normal controls.

TABLE 3

Proportion Preventable Cases by Type of Ascertainment
(All families have two children)

	Proportion Preventable Cases		
	Retrospective Counseling %	Prospective Counseling %	Screening of All Women %
Duchenne Muscular Dystrophy	8	50*	67
Hemophilia A	11	80*	90

*These are empirical values. If all families have two children in future generations, these values are decreased.

TABLE 4

Mean CPK in Females with a 50% Risk of Being Carriers for DMD

		Mean Value	
Age Group	Number Tested	Log CPK	IU/L
0-10	19	2.11	129
11-20	28	1.89	78
21-30	43	1.85	71
31-40	23	1.87	74
41-50	25	2.01	102
14-50	81	1.84	69

affected son, the counseling did not make it possible to prevent but a few cases. In Colorado, we have been doing what we call prospective genetic counseling whenever possible. By prospective we mean counseling of high-risk individuals before an affected child is born. This is possible in all X-linked disorders, since many females in a family have a relatively high risk. By contacting even distant relatives of an affected male and offering carrier testing, it is possible to identify a large proportion of the carriers in the population. Table 3 shows the optimum prevention possible under three methods of ascertainment for testing and counseling. First, carrier identification and counseling after the first affected child is born. Providing all couples have only two children, one can only prevent 8% of muscular dystrophy and 11% of hemophilia cases. Those represent the second cases in a family. The second column shows empirical data from a near total ascertainment of families in Colorado over a three-year period. In severe hemophilia A, 80% of mothers of affected sons had a positive family history before the birth of the affected son. In other words, by simply taking a family history, these women could have been identified as high-risk individuals by, for instance, their family physician or OB-GYN specialist and referred to specialty clinics for carrier testing. The figure indicates that a relatively low mutation rate is necessary for genetic equilibrium in severe classical hemophilia. This was in good agreement with data obtained in these pedigrees for reproductive fitness of affected males, which was found to be approximately two-thirds of their normal brothers. It should be emphasized that only males over age 45 were included in the reproductive fitness evaluation. With more effective treatment, the reproductive fitness will undoubtedly increase over the next few decades, and at the present time we probably do not have a genetic equilibrium in hemophilia.

In muscular dystrophy, about 50% of mothers had a positive family history at the time of conception of their first affected child. The value is lower due to the fact that a larger proportion of affected are due to a new mutation. The third column, finally, represents preventable cases if the whole population was screened *and* if we had a perfect carrier test. The non-preventable cases all represent new mutations. It is noteworthy that screening in families with positive family history, which is infinitely more cost effective, will identify the majority of carriers in the population.

Carrier detection in Duchenne muscular dystrophy has been a frustrating problem. There are several methods published in the literature, the two most extensively used being creatine phosphokinase levels in blood serum and histological changes in muscle biopsy. Other methods have had limited use, mainly because of very high cost of the techniques and they are, therefore, unsuited for screening purposes. Elevated serum CPK and abnormal muscle biopsy are two highly correlated findings. Since a blood sample is easier to obtain than a biopsy, most muscle clinics use serum CPK to identify the carrier status. Unfortunately, the overlap between carriers and controls is quite considerable and it is rarely possible to exclude an individual as a carrier. The distributions in our laboratory are shown in Figure 2. The carrier data are the result of a collaborative project

LOG CPK IN SERUM OF CARRIERS
FOR DUCHENNE MUSCULAR DYSTROPHY AND CONTROLS
PERCENT
22
20
18
16
14
12
10
8
6
4
2
Adult Controls
N-230
Obligate Carriers
N-90
0.8
1.0
1.2
1.4
1.6
1.8
2.0
2.2
2.4
2.6
2.8
3.0
3.2
75
LOG CPK

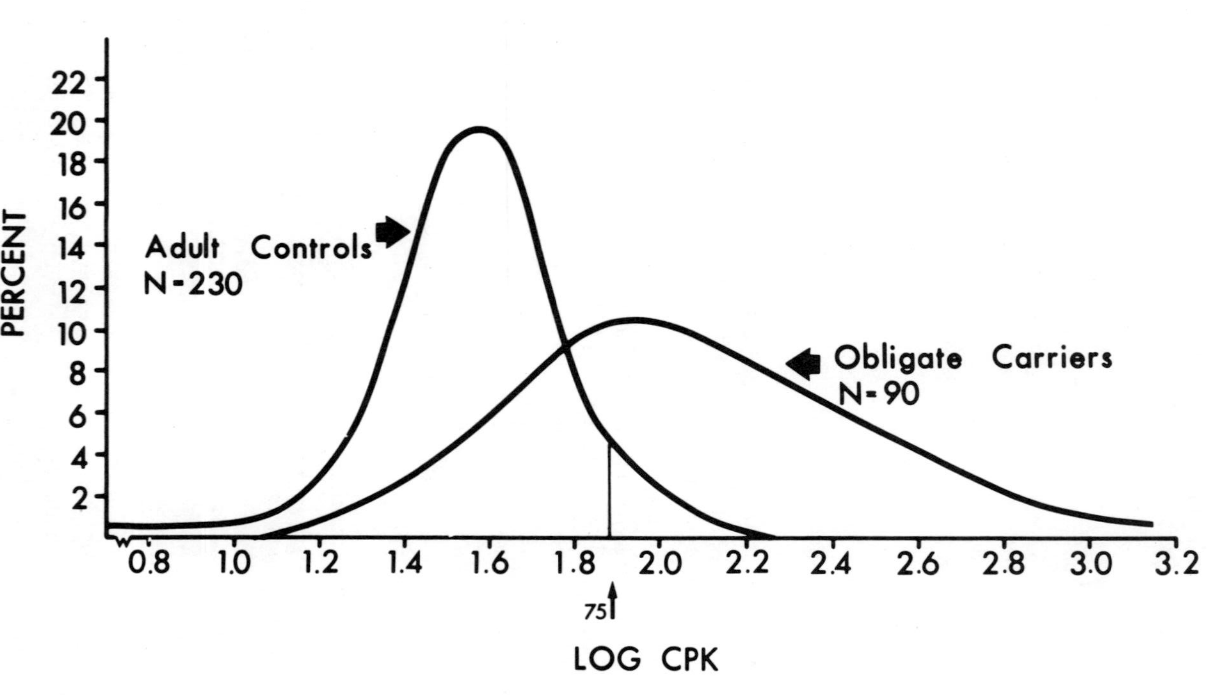

Figure 2.

including five medical centers across the United States.* A total of 90 obligate carriers were evaluated. It should be noted that CPK's are expressed as their log value. This is important since the repeated readings will show a greater standard deviation for higher values than for lower, if expressed as the standard international units/liter. The distributions also appear normal if the values are expressed as the log. The 90% upper limit of normal was found to be 1.88, which corresponds to a value of 76 IU/1.

There has been some question of whether serum CPK is dependent on age. Pediatric controls had somewhat higher levels than adults (Fig. 3). The mean log for adults was 1.57 or 54 IU/L. The age group 11-20 was not different from adults, indicating that puberty is possibly the time when CPK levels decrease in normal controls. Figure 4 shows log CPK levels by age in carriers and controls. The regression on age is so slight as to be of no clinical importance. Preliminary data from our own laboratory indicated that carriers might show considerably elevated CPK values in childhood and decrease later in life compared to the decrease in serum CPK which occurs around puberty. This is shown in Table 4. The table includes data from females with a 50% risk, since no obligate carriers under childbearing age exist. The sample size is small, but the very young children at risk seem to have higher CPK levels than the adult possible carriers. The mean log for girls under age 10 with a 50% risk was 2.11 as opposed to 1.73 for controls in that age group.

In an effort to find other indications of the carrier state, we asked obligate carriers about clinical symptoms of the disease. The results are shown in Figures 5 and 6. Among hemophilia carriers, excessive menstrual bleeding and bleeding at tonsillectomy and tooth extraction seem to be more common, whereas other problems, such as nosebleeds, bruising or bleeding at surgery or childbirth, were not common. It is noteworthy that carriers of mild hemophilia A have equally many carrier symptoms as do carriers of severe hemophilia. In Duchenne muscular dystrophy, there seems to be no good clinical indicator of the carrier state. The subjective opinion of "large calves" was twice as common in carriers as in controls, and we are now investigating this further by obtaining data on height, weight, and calf circumference in carriers and controls.

One additional mode of ascertaining carriers and preventing additional affected children may be from the pediatric well-baby clinics. We asked mothers of affected sons about early signs of the disease. The results are shown in Table 5. It is evident that gross motor developmental milestones are often delayed in boys with muscular dystrophy. If an early diagnosis can be made, a second affected child in the family can be prevented. It would be very useful, for instance, if pediatricians would obtain a blood sample for CPK determination from all boys who do not walk by the age of 18 months. The cost for the test is $2.50 in our

*The collaborators were: K.M. Dumars, University of California at Irvine; P.M. Conneally, Indiana University Medical School; R.M. Greenstein, University of Connecticut Health Center; and W.A. Muir, Case Western Reserve University.

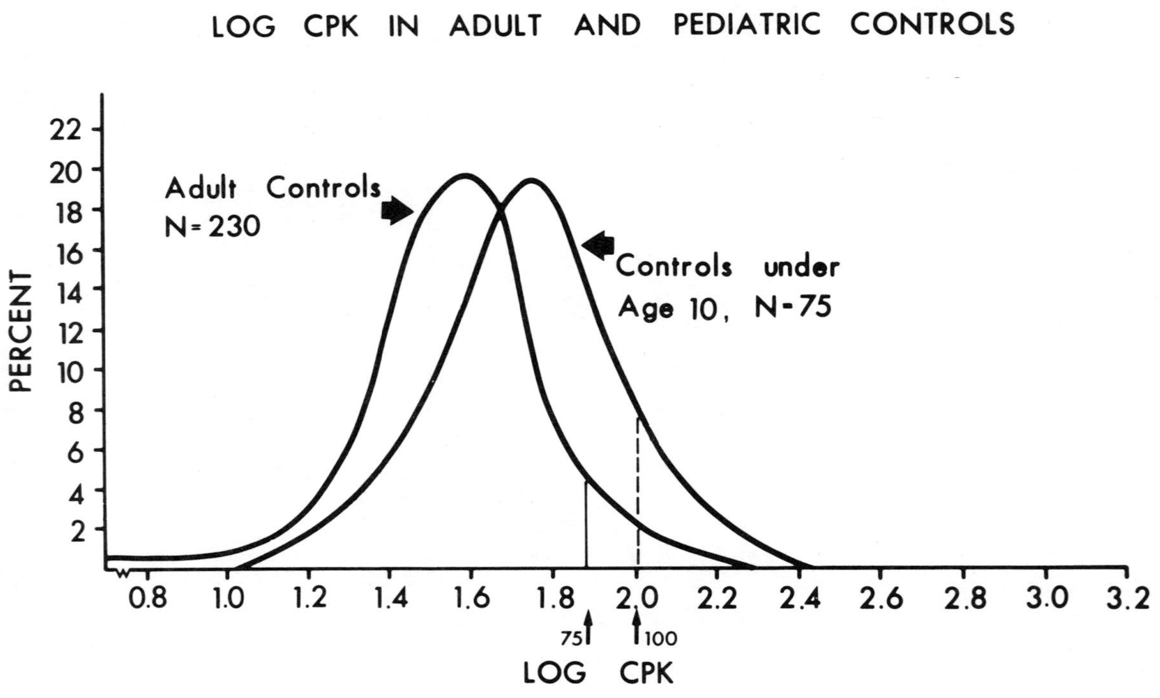

LOG CPK IN ADULT AND PEDIATRIC CONTROLS

PERCENT
22
20
18
16
14
12
10
8
6
4
2

Adult Controls
N=230

Controls under
Age 10, N-75

0.8
1.0
1.2
1.4
1.6
1.8
2.0
2.2
2.4
2.6
2.8
3.0
3.2

75
100

LOG CPK

Figure 3.

LOG SERUM CPK BY AGE IN DUCHENNE MUSCULAR DYSTROPHY
CARRIERS AND CONTROLS - 90% INTERVALS INDICATED
2.79
Obligate Carriers N=90
Controls N=75
Controls N=230
LOG CPK
2.3
2.2
2.1
2.0
1.9
1.8
1.7
1.6
1.5
1.4
1.3
15
25
35
45
55
AGE

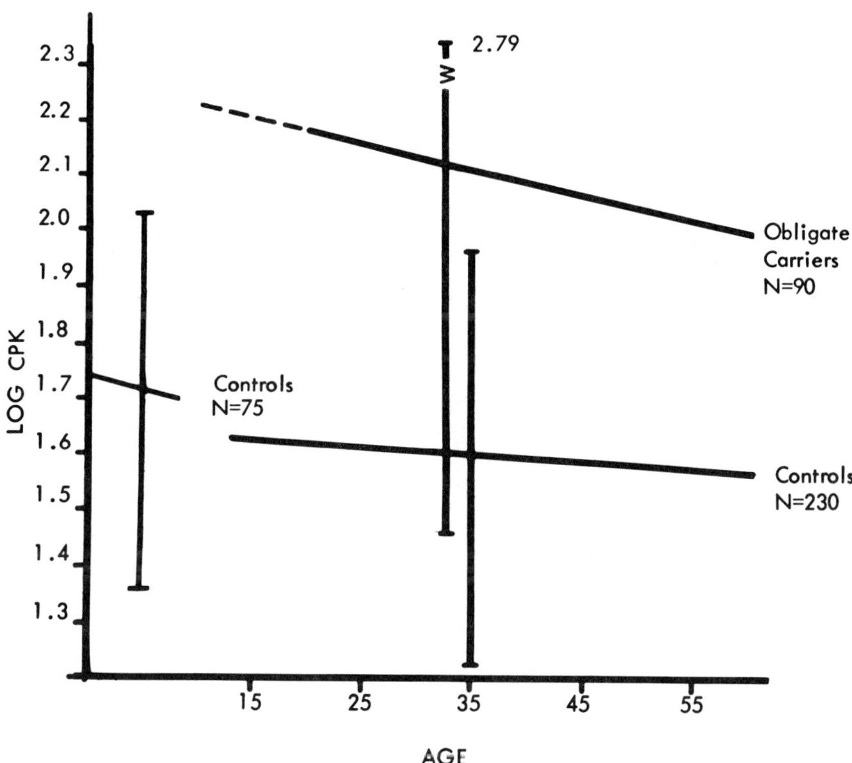

Figure 4.

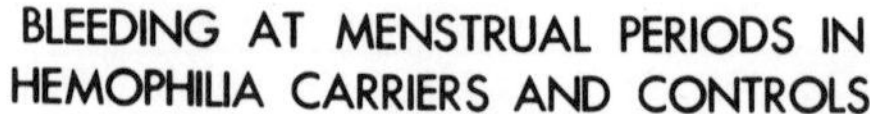

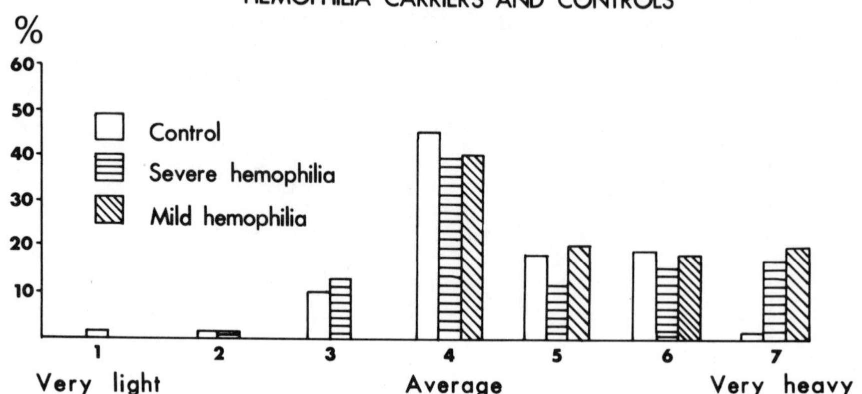

BLEEDING PROBLEMS IN HEMOPHILIA
CARRIERS AND CONTROLS

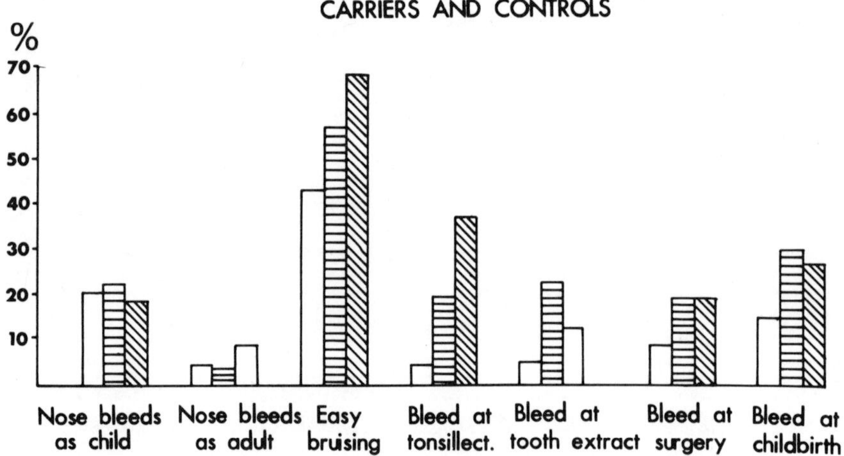

Figure 5.

MUSCLE WEAKNESS IN CARRIERS OF DUCHENNE
MUSCULAR DYSTROPHY AND CONTROLS
%
50
40
30
20
10
Control
Carriers of Duchenne
Pain in legs
Large calves
Unequal calf size
Hard calves
Diff. getting up
Diff. walking upstairs
Leg cramps

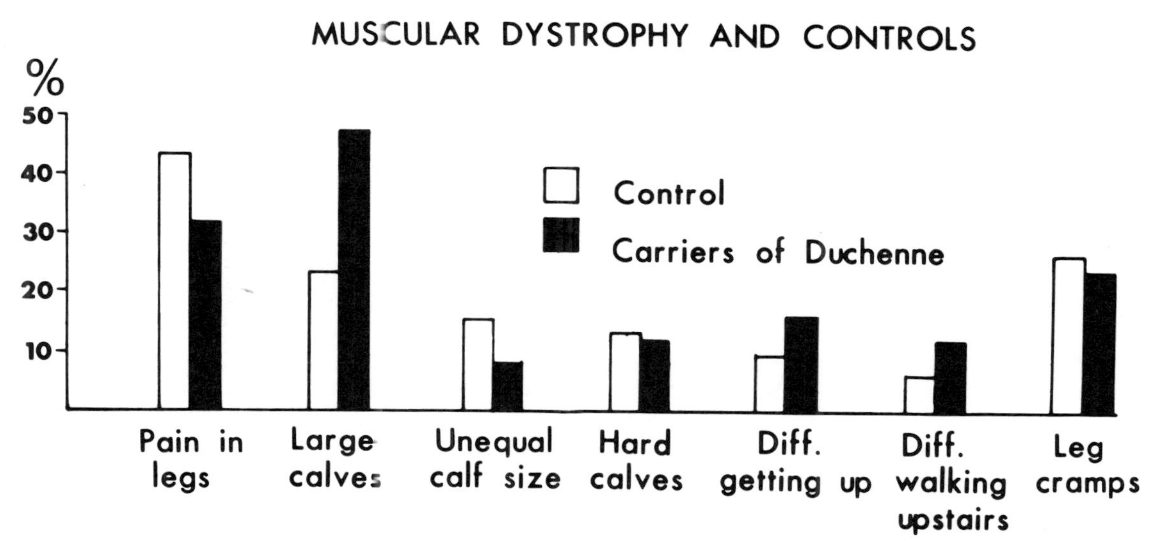

Figure 6.

TABLE 5

Answers About Prevention of Affected Males in Questionnaire III
Individuals in Childbearing Age Only

	Counseled in Person %	Counseled by Mail %
Would you choose to have a prenatal diagnosis of sex?		
No	32.9	29.4
Uncertain	11.0	17.6
Yes	47.9	52.9
Would you abort if the fetus was a male?		
No	25.6	25.0
Uncertain	27.9	33.3
Yes	46.5	41.7

TABLE 6

Early Signs of Duchenne Muscular Dystrophy in 39 Cases

	Affected Boys %	Normal Children %
First sit before 8 months	52	90
8 months or older	48	10
First walk before 12 months	10	50
12-17 months	45	50
18 months or older	45	1
Never could run well	100	

laboratory and, in contrast to carriers, it is 100% diagnostic in affected boys.

Thus, family history, carrier symptoms, carrier tests and early diagnosis of affected males are all tools which may lead to the prevention of affected births. How do carrier females and their spouses feel about their reproductive alternatives once they have been identified as carriers or possible carriers of these disorders? Table 6 indicates how many of the high-risk couples would elect to have prenatal diagnosis of sex. The left column includes couples in the Colorado area who were counseled in person. The right column includes high-risk relatives who were living outside the state and received genetic counseling by mail. Their answers to the first question indicate that about one-half of the couples of childbearing age would elect to have amniocentesis. However, among those who would have the procedure done, only one-half said that they would definitely elect to abort a male fetus and 25% said that they did not think they would abort. This last category, presumably, would want the procedure hoping that the results would be the diagnosis of a female, which would relieve their anxiety for the remainder of the pregnancy. Another question was asked: "What numerical risk of having an affected son is too high for you to take?" The answers are shown in Table 7 divided by the two disorders. First, the answers show that when it becomes possible to identify these disorders prenatally on a routine basis – the great majority of individuals who choose to chance a pregnancy would use this procedure. It also shows the opinion among these families that Duchenne muscular dystrophy is considered a higher burden disease than hemophilia. About one-half of the respondents in muscular dystrophy families consider a risk of 25% too high to take.

What are the attitudes toward a prospective counseling program with a geneticist who contacts the relatives instead of the relatives making the first contact? If the families feel that their privacy is invaded and if their attitude toward the counseling is a negative one, screening of families would obviously not be effective. After the Colorado program, the families were asked whether relatives should be informed about the risk and, if so, who should be responsible for informing them. The results are shown in Table 8. About three-fourths answered that they preferred an active approach from the medical community. About 22% would prefer to be contacted by the parents of an affected child, but if the parents declined to do this, the geneticist or physician should approach the relative. Nobody thought that genetic counseling was useless and should not be given. It should be emphasized that the response rate even in the post-counseling questionnaire, which was mailed, was very high. More than 80% of individuals who had received counseling either in person or by mail, are included. The conclusion, therefore, is that the great majority of individuals in these families think genetic counseling is important for them and would welcome a program such as the one carried out in Colorado.

In summary: It is not economically or technically feasible to screen the population for carriers of hemophilia A and Duchenne muscular dystrophy. However, screening of families which have one case diagnosed is an efficient and inexpensive

TABLE 7

What Risk of Having an Affected Child is Too High to Take?

Risk	Proportion Who Thought Risk Too High	
	Hemophilia	Muscular Dystrophy
1%	2%	7%
5%	4%	11%
10%	9%	29%
25%	20%	49%
50%	49%	67%
100%	78%	91%

TABLE 8

Should Relatives at Risk be Contacted and Told About Their Risk?

	Before Counseling		12-36 Months After Counseling	
It is the physician's or geneticist's *duty to inform* everyone of the risk	23.6	70.8	30.0	74.8
It is the geneticist's *duty to ask* each relative if he/she *wants information* about the risk	47.2		44.8	
It should be *left up to the parents* of the affected child to inform their relatives of the risk	24.9		19.9	
Relatives should *never be contacted*	0.4		0	
No answer	3.9		5.3	

way of identifying the majority of carriers. Additional carriers can be identified by CPK screening by pediatricians of boys who don't walk by the age of 18 months.

The cost effectiveness of a prospective counseling program for X-linked diseases such as classical hemophilia is readily apparent – the prevention of one case every four to six years would pay for such a program in Colorado.

REFERENCES

1. M.F. Lyon, *Nature 190*, 372, 1961.
2. T.S. Zimmerman, O.D. Ratnoff and A.S. Littell, *J. Clin. Invest. 50*, 255, 1971.

II. GENETIC COUNSELING AND OTHER GENETIC SERVICES IN THE COMMUNITY

WHAT SERVICES SHOULD BE AVAILABLE AT A GENETIC COUNSELING CLINIC

Murray Feingold

The following services should be available in a genetic counseling clinic:

1. Diagnostic
2. Genetic Counseling
3. Clinical and Research Laboratory Testing
4. Management
5. Educational

Diagnostic Services

If the genetic counselor is aware of the diagnosis, the genetic counseling will obviously be more accurate. Since many genetic diseases are uncommon, it is important that a physician who is experienced in the diagnosis of these diseases, a syndromologist, be a key member of the genetic team. Having such a person is essential in a genetic clinic that sees multiple disease entities.

An example of the importance of the correct diagnosis is vividly demonstrated in the following case history. An infant who was operated on for tracheoesophageal fistula in the newborn period was noted to have microcephaly, clinodactyly and hypoplasia of the middle phalanx of his index and fifth fingers. Examination of his father and paternal grandmother revealed that they also had microcephaly and similar hand abnormalities. Neither of them, however, were retarded. By obtaining this information we were able to determine that this was an autosomal dominant disease with microcephaly but not associated with mental retardation. The identification of this particular syndrome was of great practical importance when we saw another infant for a pre-adoption physical examination who had the same findings as the family described above. Information was lacking concerning the natural parents and it took many months of discussions with the mother before she agreed to be seen in the genetic clinic. She also had microcephaly and hand abnormalities, as did her brother and father. All three of them, however, were of normal intelligence. We were therefore able to reassure the adopting parents that although the baby had microcephaly it would be very unlikely that she would be retarded.

Great emphasis should be placed on the diagnostic capabilities of a genetic

ISBN 0-12-562650-9

counseling service. Not only can correct genetic counseling be given but an informed prognosis and proper treatment can be outlined for the patient or family.

Genetic Counseling

Every genetic counseling clinic should have an experienced and/or well trained counselor. There is obviously much more to genetic counseling than saying a person's chances of having another affected child are one out of two or one out of four. In our clinic, as in many others, the amount of information retained by the patient is frequently not sufficient for them to make a meaningful decision. Statistics in our clinic indicate that approximately 30 to 40 percent of the patients who were counseled did not either understand the information or did not retain it after a single genetic counseling session. This is in spite of the fact that they are offered adequate time for questioning and after the physician counselor leaves they frequently discuss their genetic counseling with our genetic nurse associate. These statistics have improved since we initiated the policy of sending a letter to the patient which includes the genetic counseling they received. However, whenever possible, I believe that a second counseling session is frequently indicated.

An experienced counselor is aware of the many pitfalls that he or she may encounter when providing genetic counseling. For example, the consultand may be too anxious to comprehend what is told to him. Many psychological reactions may also be taking place in the patient, such as anger, denial, and so on, which limits his understanding of the genetic counseling. Another reason why the patient may not understand the genetic counseling is that he may not be particularly interested in the counseling that is being provided. We frequently take for granted that all patients are interested in the information we are giving them when, in fact, for various reasons, they are not interested in the genetic counseling. Therefore, it is important to be certain that individuals who are seen for genetic counseling actually want this information. Another pitfall is that the counselor does not clearly communicate to the consultand the various risk factors. Either the information is too involved (which is unusual) or the counselor had difficulty in communicating. Tape recording the genetic counseling session is frequently helpful in assessing one's ability to communicate properly.

Other safeguards should also be instituted such as the utilization of the genetic nurse associate who reinforces the genetic counseling. These individuals have training in genetic counseling but less training than those who receive a Masters degree in genetic counseling. Follow-up letters should be sent to all individuals who have received genetic counseling. On follow-up visits we use the so-called "quiz" method and in a very friendly and unpressured fashion the genetic counselor asks the patient what his or her interpretation is of the genetic counseling they received. Depending upon the answer, we can then determine the amount of genetic counseling that was retained or understood by the patient and what areas need to be emphasized.

The role of the individual with a Masters degree in genetic counseling will not be discussed at this time. There are, however, various roles which they can very adequately fulfill but much of this depends upon the local setting, funding, availability of a physician or Ph. D. genetic counselors, and other factors.

Clinical and Research Laboratory Testing

It is not only impossible but impractical and unrealistic for every center to be able to perform all the tests that are necessary to make a genetic diagnosis. However, it is important that the center has the ability to either do such tests or be aware of the laboratories that will accept the necessary specimens. This also includes the ability to perform various clinical tests such as proper x-ray examination that can be interpreted either at the center or by others more versed in this area. If a skin fibroblast study is indicated the genetic center should be able to obtain the skin and if their laboratory does not perform such a study they should take the responsibility of sending it to the proper facility. Performing these tests should usually not be left to the referring physician who may not have the time, ability, or experience to follow through.

Obviously a chromosomal laboratory should be either present in the center or available to the center and a close relationship should exist between them.

Management

The majority of centers do not provide continual management for their genetic patients. In our center we do manage our patients and whenever it is possible we would recommend this approach. Although genetic counselors provide a prognosis concerning genetic disease, many of these counselors have not had the opportunity to follow these patients and their families for a long period of time. For example, we are following over 600 children with Down syndrome and believe we have a much better understanding of the course these children will follow and how their families cope with having such a child. Some genetic counselors believe that since they have seen a large number of families for genetic counseling that they also have a good understanding of the significance of this condition. However, it is not until you follow these children and their parents for many years that you get a total concept of what Down syndrome, or any other syndrome, means to the patient and his family.

Education

The responsibility for educating people concerning genetics is even greater than many other specialty areas because genetics, as it is practiced today, is very new and many people are unaware of its significance and purpose. We must educate our fellow physicians because frequently their medical training did not include genetics. This is done most effectively in the community hospital setting at the medical staff meetings or at various specialty meetings. We must also educate other professionals in the health-care system and fortunately they usually demonstrate a great deal of interest in the field of genetics. There have been many ongoing programs attempting to educate the lay public and one would suspect that everybody would know, for example, all about amniocentesis. However, educating the public is an ongoing process and this is vividly demonstrated to me each week when I see new patients who appear to have an almost total lack of knowledge concerning genetics and the disease that affects them personally.

A genetics center must assume the responsibility of educating the public, other health professionals and physicians.

Ethical Considerations

Should one of the responsibilities of a genetic center include being involved with the various ethical dilemmas that relate to genetic diseases? I personally do not see how those of us who are working in the field of genetics and birth defects can stay away from this issue. In our own hospital we are continually presented with ethical dilemmas which have no easy solutions. However, these same dilemmas also face our patients and their families. Because of the nature of the patients we see, we hopefully have more expertise in this area than most other physicians. We must therefore share this expertise with our patients, their families, and other members of the community who are interested in trying to solve these perplexing and difficult problems.

I would like to conclude with some comments concerning the genetic services that should be available in satellite clinics based on our experience of servicing 11 satellite clinics in Massachusetts and Maine. The answer is relatively simple: all services that are available in a large center should also be available or accessible in a satellite clinic. Our experience indicates that approximately 80 percent of the patients seen in the satellite clinic need not be seen in a larger center. For example, a patient who seeks genetic counseling because her brother has Down syndrome, and is worried about the chances of her own children having Down syndrome, can be very easily counseled in a satellite clinic. When the problem is more complex, then a referral to a larger center is indicated. However, the majority of patients seen in a satellite clinic can be handled locally and the services discussed above should also be available to them.

RECORD KEEPING AND THE DELIVERY OF GENETIC SERVICES*

Marian L. Rivas

Introduction

A thorough genetic work-up is lengthy and costly. It would be difficult to estimate the total direct costs involved in the collection, storage, interpretation and maintenance of patient and family records. In our clinical genetics unit, which is representative of a medical center-based medical genetics unit, three full-time staff members, clinical fellows, and research associates and assistants are involved at one point or another in the writing of information in the records, filling out forms, dictating or writing letters to patients, relatives and/or physicians, searching through patient folders for specific information and/or generating additional information about the family in clinical research studies. In addition, personnel in various supporting laboratories such as the cytogenetic, biochemical genetic, and blood grouping laboratories are also involved in generating, collating, and storing results, and in updating their individual laboratory record systems. There is little doubt that our unit as well as other clinical genetics units have made a major commitment of time and space to the maintenance of a record keeping system.

Surely, this can be said of any patient care system whether it be that of a private family physician or that of a hospital complex; but for clinical genetics, with its focus on the *family unit*, the organization of records presents unique problems – and unique opportunities. How these problems can be minimized and opportunities maximized is the focus of this paper.

The Family History

Patients with a genetic problem, or who are suspected of having one, are evaluated in the context of both personal *and* family history. The information obtained from the family history alone can be quite lengthy. Fortunately, it can be summarized concisely in the standard pedigree format (see Fig. 1a). Information regarding sex, age, name, birth and death dates, birth order, reproductive history, relationship to proband, manifestation of disease, ethnic background,

*Supported in part by the Genetics Study Project (HS 7803-2-080), the Hemophilia Diagnostic and Treatment Center (MC-B-410001-02-0) and the Interregional Cytogenetics Register Contract (No1-HD-32713).

ISBN 0-12-562650-9

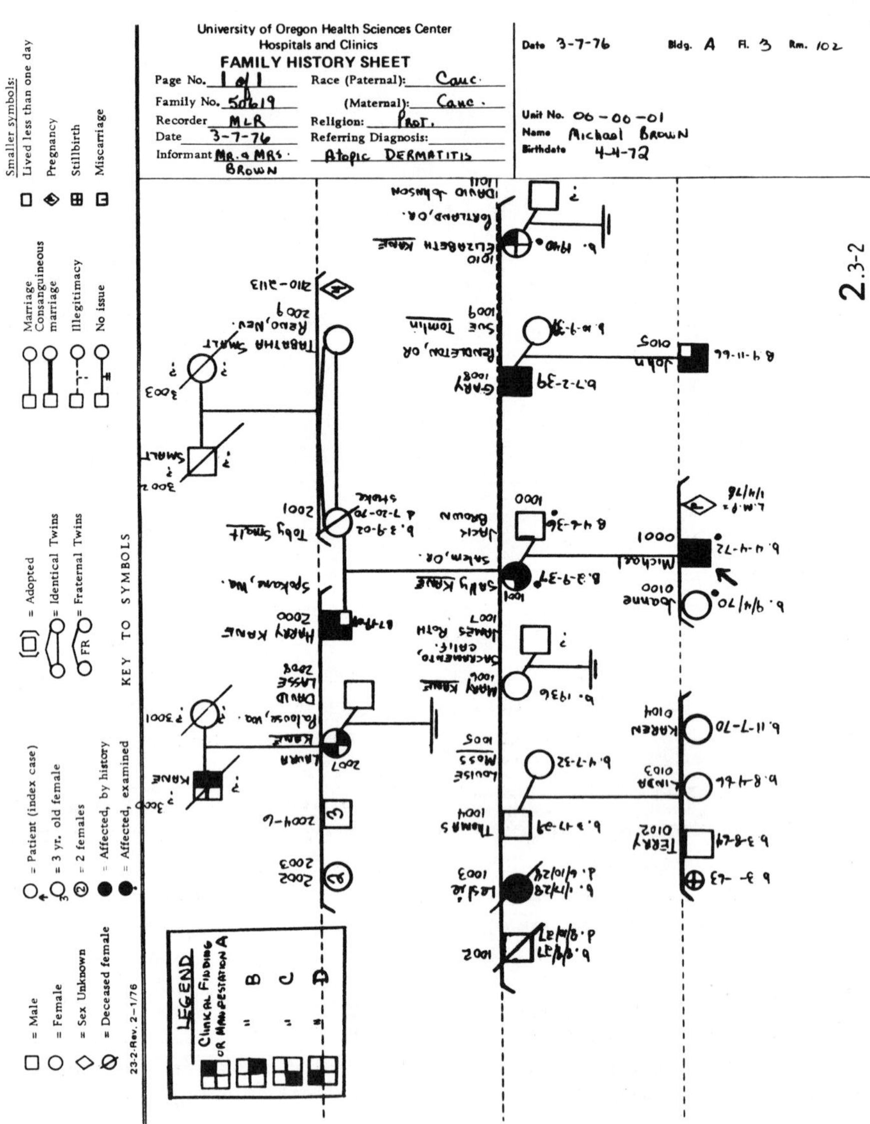

Figure 1a. Pedigree form currently in use at the University of Oregon Health Sciences Center. Front side of form with *simulated* family information; *i.e.*, fictitious entrys for illustrative purposes only.

Page No.________

COMMENTS

Family Name:

RECORD FOR EACH INDIVIDUAL (INCLUDING SPOUSES)

(A) Full Name, Including Maiden Names
(B) Residence Location (County or City) or Place of Death
(C) Age or Age at Death
(D) Health Status or Cause of Death
(E) Consanguineous Marriage
(F) Number, Ages and Sex of Offspring
(G) Birth Order in Sibship
(H) Marriage Order for Multiple Marriages
(I) Abortions and Stillbirths for Females
(J) Illegitimacies where Determined
Identify Propositus (Index Case) with Arrow
(K) Dates of Marriages, Divorces and Separations

Fig. 1b. Pedigree form currently in use at the University of Oregon Health Sciences Center. Reverse side of form with space for additional notes and comments as listed.

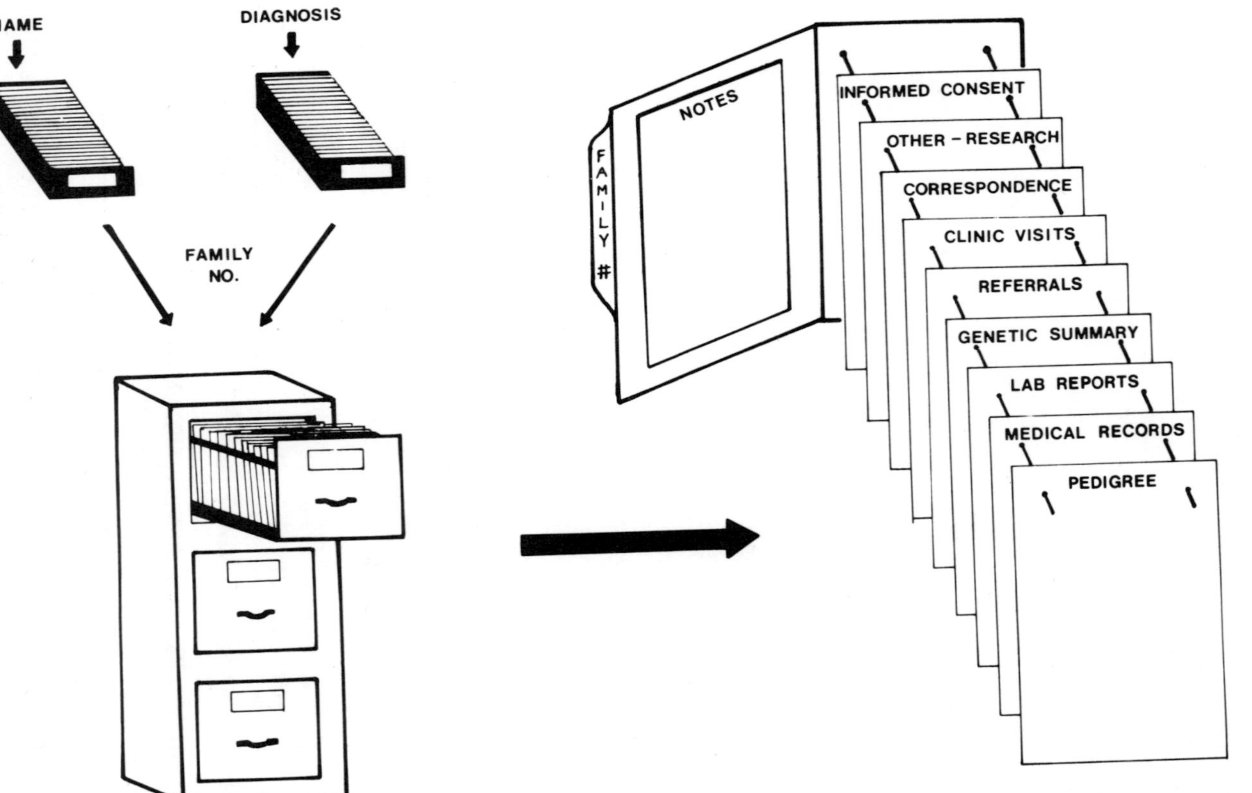

Fig. 2. A manually-linked central genetic record system based on the family folder concept. The central file is organized sequentially by family number; hard-copy family records may be accessed by proband's surname and/or diagnostic files which are cross-referenced with family number. Entries in family folders are securely fastened to minimize loss of contents. Possible inclusions in and organization of individual file folders is shown.

referring diagnosis, method of ascertainment can *all* be recorded directly on this sheet.*

Correct diagnosis and delineation of the genetic nature of a disorder depends on *reliable* information. It is often necessary to substantiate the fact that the proband's maternal first cousin, who is mentally retarded, indeed has Down syndrome as reported by a family member, or whether a critical person in the family, on whom a genetic conclusion rests, shows any signs diagnostic of the disorder in question. The recording of physician's name and address, place and dates of hospitalization, and additional comments on the reverse side of the pedigree form (see Fig. 1b) facilitates the tracing of pertinent medical information.

The Family Record

How does one bring together pedigree information and other selected data of genetic/clinical interest which bear on a particular problem, patient, or family? How does one organize it in a way which will lend itself to easy access and use?

In clinical genetics, information about two or more members of a family often becomes more valuable when considered together. Since the focus of attention is the *family*, it seems logical that pertinent information gathered in the course of a genetic evaluation should be gathered in a *family* rather than a *patient* folder or chart. This is not to minimize the importance of an individual's medical record. The patient folder remains an important and vital document of an individual's medical history. The family record contains specific clinical and laboratory summaries on individuals in a family that are of special importance in the context of the family history. The information is usually obtained from individual patient records. Genetic summaries should likewise appear in the medical record. Thus, the patient and family records are complementary; information contained in each is essential for a thorough genetic and clinical evaluation.

As shown in Figure 2, the family folder may contain the following: family pedigree, pertinent medical records, laboratory results or test summaries, summary of the genetic work-up, written record of the counseling given to individual members of the family, referrals made to other clinics or physicians, any correspondence to and from the patient, family, and physician(s), a record of all clinic and follow-up visits, and other information such as clinical photographs, financial information, or signed consent forms for release of clinical information, for use of clinical photos, and for participation in research protocols. A section set aside for "notes" is particularly useful for recording other types of patient contacts such as telephone conversations, scheduled appointments, home visits, as well as "red flag" notes such as "the proband does not wish anyone in the family contacted".

Research findings also should be entered in the family folder. It is frequently the case that more thorough work-ups and/or specialized tests are performed in

---

*Copies available upon request.

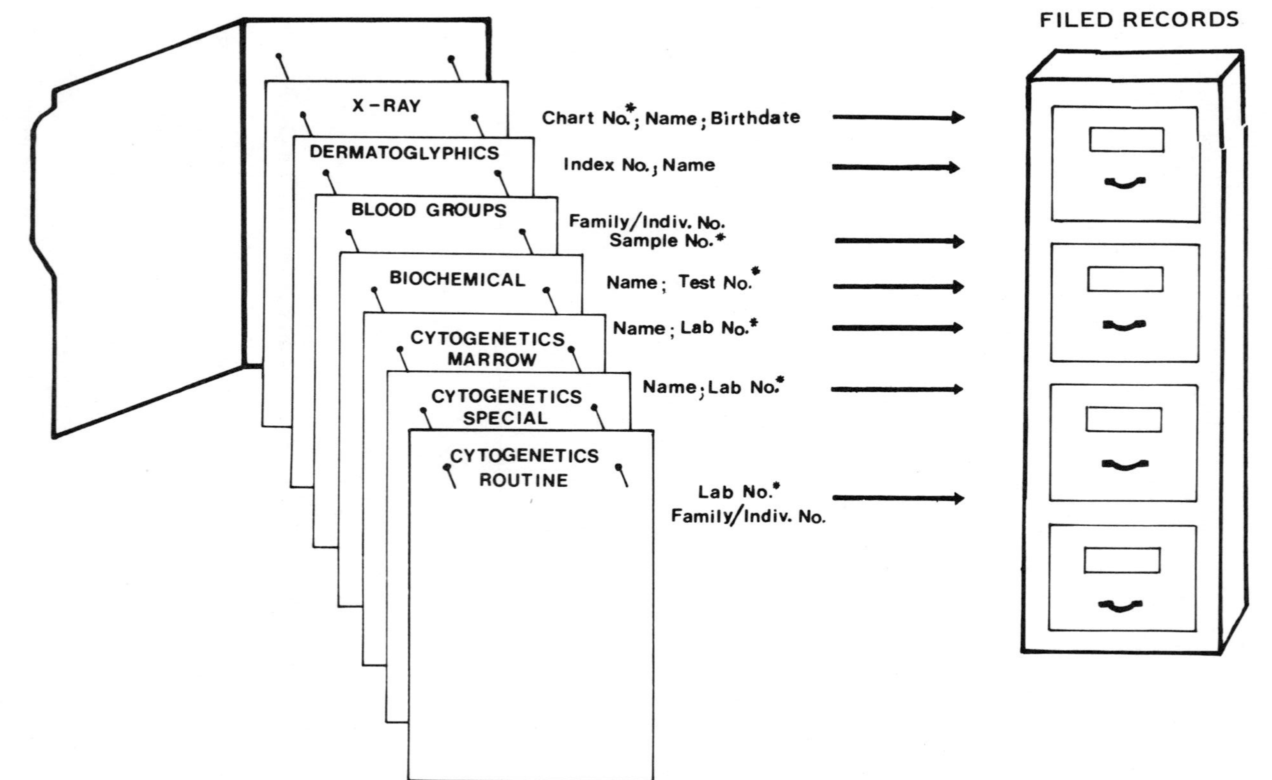

Fig. 3. Cross-indexing within the family folder permits ready access to hard-copy material filed alphabetically or numerically in other record systems. Shown are examples of items on lab summary reports which can service as indices to other files. Asterisks indicate information required to access original laboratory reports and results in our clinical genetics unit.

the course of a research protocol. Considerable costs are involved in generating these data; yet research findings are entered in family records with varying degrees of completeness. All too often they are filed away in individual research laboratory files and find their way to the patient or family folders only when reprints of the published study become available. Routine entry of research summaries in the family folder or at least reference to the availability of such data in another file maximizes the information available to those persons responsible in the future for the care of the patient and family.

Family Folder Record System

A family folder record system is simply *a centralized system of records* (genetic, clinical, and laboratory) *which have been manually linked in family folders.* A central family record, among other things, minimizes duplication of effort, *e.g.,* the recording of information in several places, the retracing of steps previously taken, and the regeneration of data previously obtained. Considerable time and costs are involved in collecting and collating this information initially. To do it twice would cost more than double in effort and funds!

The probability that duplication of efforts will occur in clinical genetic units with one or two professional staff members is minimal. However, in clinical settings in which the "team approach" is practiced, or in a setting in which a number of staff physicians and fellows participate in a rotating fashion, the danger is real that information which is not centrally recorded may be "lost".

Family records are usually filed alphabetically by proband's surname or numerically by family number. A sequential file based on family number (with family members assigned a unique number within that family) has worked especially well for our clinical genetics unit. It avoids the problem of how to file the family folder when several probands or affected individuals (in different sibships and/or with different surnames) are identified in the family. In addition, the numerical system facilitates the identification and tracing of "missing" or "lost" charts.

Elements of a Good Record System

Several more obvious elements of a good record system may be cited. For example, individual file folders should be compartmentalized to facilitate access to specific items of information such as medical, social, and historical information about a particular family member (Fig. 2). Each entry in the folder should be dated, labeled with the individual's family and individual number, cross-indexed with hospital chart number or laboratory number for ease of access to other (laboratory, hospital, health department, etc.) files and their contents (Fig. 3). Information should be recorded legibly and formatted to permit rapid scanning and abstracting, and all file entries should be secured to minimize loss of folder contents.

Perhaps less obvious but nonetheless the most important element of a good

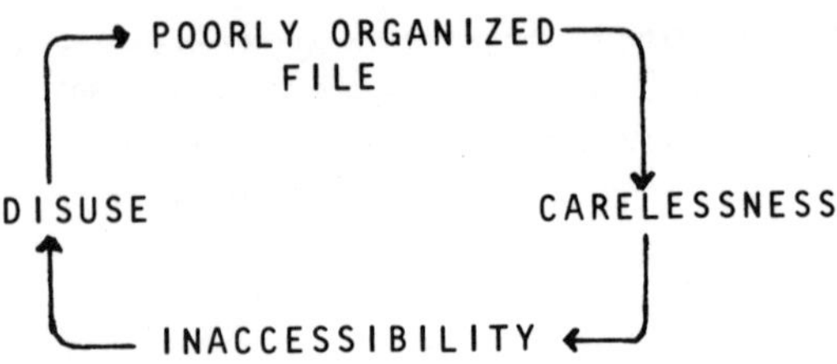

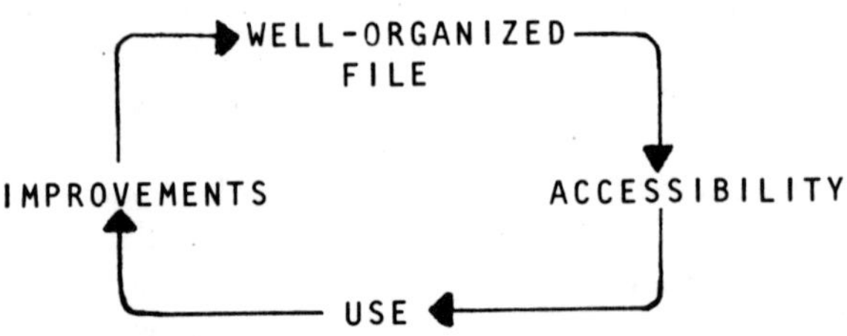

Fig. 4. Most likely flow of events when the central record system is poorly organized (top) and when the file is well organized (bottom).

record system is the *human element.* There is no substitute for conscientious personnel with a positive attitude toward the file and its contents. Persons involved must be committed, compulsive and consistent – *committed* to the concept of a good record system, *compulsive* about how the information is handled, and *consistent* in the recording of information. As Acheson[1] has pointed out, "It is common experience that men and women cannot be expected to perform tasks conscientiously which they consider to be futile. Many of the errors and omissions in medical records arise because the writer knows that due to faulty design and poor file organization the data he is recording will not be accessible when they are required, whether in the service of the invidivual or for research."

As illustrated in Figure 4, a poorly organized file generates a careless attitude in recording of information and handling of file folders. The file becomes less useful and the personnel develop a negative attitude toward the file. Little enthusiasm for the file and its contents prevents corrective action (especially if the task seems formidable) and the cycle continues. A well-organized file, on the other hand, permits ready access to its contents which, in turn, encourages its use. In the process of using the system, problems become apparent and sources of error can be identified and corrected. By using the system, new applications of the stored information may be defined, perhaps requiring modifications of existing methods or procedures. When the cycle of feedback and adjustment begins to operate, a record system which was good initially becomes better.

The Record System and the Delivery of Genetic Services

McKusick[2] and others[3–13] have pointed out the need for some form of a genetic disease register, or genetic data management system, and have indicated various ways in which such a record system may prove useful in the area of clinical genetics. Applications fall into four general categories: (1) patient care, (2) record linkage, (3) research, and (4) prevention.

1. Patient care. One obvious use of a centralized genetic record system is improvement of patient care through prompt and accurate diagnosis. The central file, after all, was generated primarily for this purpose.

In a study involving general practitioners in North Carolina in 1953-54, various aspects of their practices – namely, clinical histories, physical examinations, use of laboratory aids, therapy, preventive medicine, and clinical records – were observed and evaluated.[14] The monograph states, "It was realized that the extent of a physician's clinical record might not necessarily be a valid predictor of his professional skill. Nevertheless, this should provide some indication of the physician's thoroughness and attention to details which add up to good patient care." Physicians in this study were given a score reflecting the extent and quality of their record system. Only 17% of the 87 physicians were considered to have good clinical records. In the final analysis, those physicians in the highest qualitative rank, *i.e.*, those with performances were considered to be outstanding, had

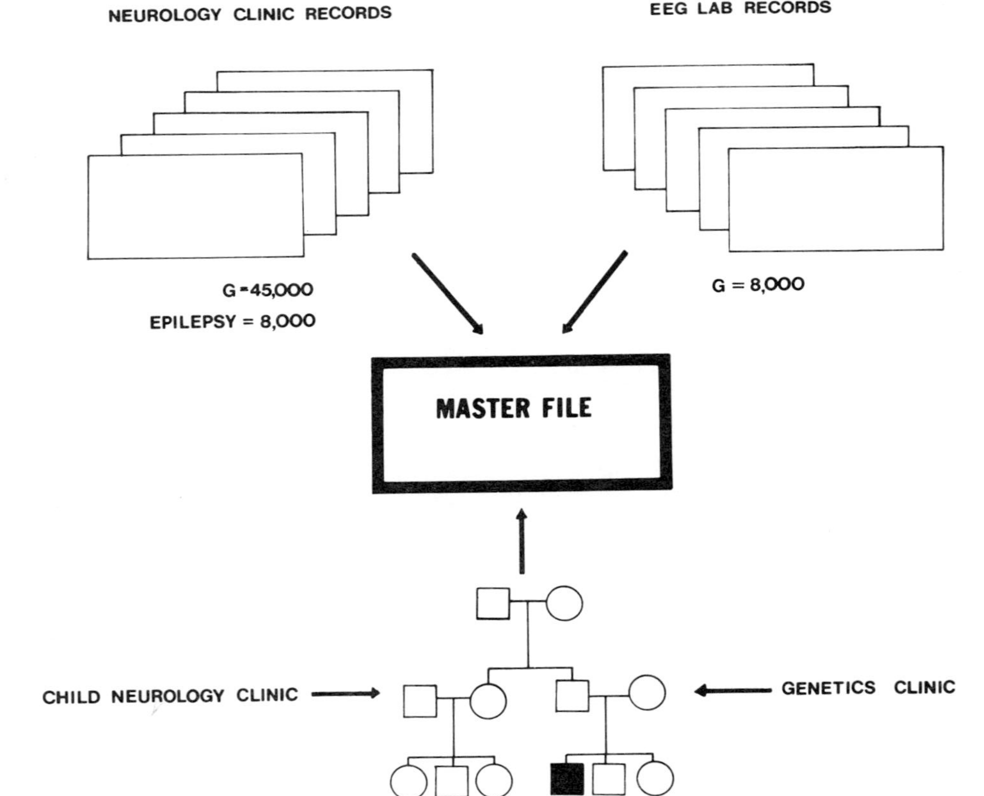

Fig. 5. Record linkage of clinical (top left), laboratory (top right), and genetic center (center bottom) information in a sample of individuals with a seizure disorder. Creation of a master file of *all* individuals (affected and unaffected) identified in the course of the study and searching the master file for "matches" whenever a new family or individual is ascertained is the essence of a record-linking process.

received the highest quantitative scores in the area of clinical records. Thus, a well organized and current record system was shown to be highly correlated with good patient care. It is, most likely, also correlated with good patient care in clinical genetics.

2. Record linkage. Acheson[1] and others[15–21] have written extensively about the methods of linking medical records with records obtained from other sources such a birth registrations, marriage records, etc.; but, as Smith[8] points out "a general medical record linkage system may be too large and too general to serve the specific needs of medical genetics".

Record linkage on a smaller scale, however, may provide unique opportunities for both service and research. An example of how record linkage can be used for both service and research is illustrated in Figure 5. Forty-five thousand records of patients seen since 1938 in the Neurology Clinic (Portland, Oregon) are available. From 1938 to the early 1950's this clinic was the only one of its kind in the Pacific Northwest. Eight thousand of these individuals have a history of a seizure disorder. Approximately 8,000 EEG records dating back to 1938 are also available for record linkage purposes. A third source of information is the body of genetic data generated from family histories taken on epileptic patients (mostly children) seen in either the Genetics Clinic or the Child Neurology Clinic at the Portland Epilepsy Center. Thus, there exists the opportunity to link three bodies of data: clinical, laboratory, and genetic. Individuals among the proband's relatives who were evaluated at an earlier date can be identified from the master file and this information incorporated into genetic analyses of selected epileptic disorders and, in turn, be used to generate and communicate with more precise risk estimates.

Another form of record linkage is linking data *within* the central file. It is often useful to know whether a particular individual is a member of a family previously ascertained as the following example illustrates. The pedigree in Figure 6a was constructed from the limited information provided by the proband's mother (C). To the best of her knowledge this was an isolated case of hemophilia A. She was not aware that four other individuals in this family were also affected (see Fig. 6b), nor did her relatives know that she had an affected son. If the same individual had not conducted both family history interviews, it might not have been ascertained that the two families were indeed one. The description of a rather colorful relative by each of the two interviewees prompted the interviewer to pull the first family record and check for matching names and birthdates. The importance of finding that the four affected sibships were part of the same family lies in the difference in the risk estimate given the mother (C) of the first proband. Her risk of being a carrier, based on the first family history (Fig. 6a), is 0.37, whereas on the basis of the second pedigree (Fig. 6b), her probability of being a carrier is 1.0, or certainty.

Record linking within the centralized genetic record system would assume the availability of accurate pedigree information for diagnosis and assessment of risk; In simplest terms, it involves the creation of a "master file" containing minimal

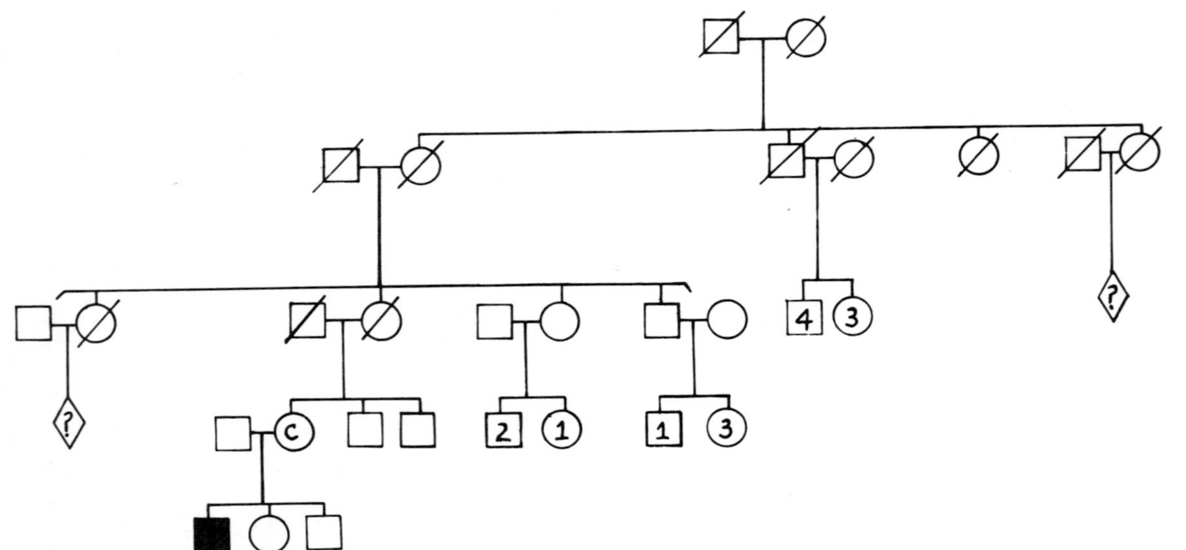

Fig. 6a. Pedigree of a family in which hemophilia A is segregating. This pedigree is constructed from information provided by the proband's (↗) mother (C).

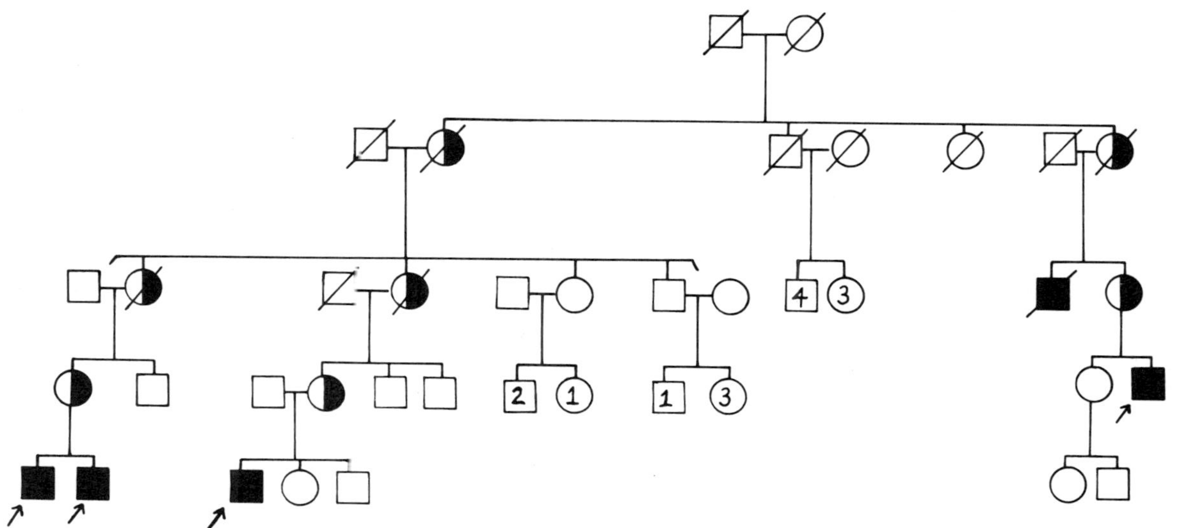

Fig. 6b. Pedigree of a family in which hemophilia A is segregating. This pedigree of the family is constructed from information provided by the proband's mother (C) and her maternal first cousin.

identifying information (name, phonetic coding of the name,[16,17,22] birth date, sex, parents' names) on *all* individuals (affected and unaffected) known to the clinical genetics unit. The size of the master file will depend primarily on the number and extent of the family histories (pedigrees) taken during the genetic evaluation(s). For instance, our genetics unit has 4,500 family records. If on the average, thirty-five individuals per family are identified during the family history interview, our master file will contain some information (even if only name and sex) on over 150,000 individuals. Some of these families are known to be related to other families seen in our Genetics Clinic. For the most part these "matches" have been accidental or coincidental. There is a need to check for "matches" in a systematic way.

Creation of a master file and searching it for "matches" whenever a new family is ascertained in clinic is the essence of internal record linking. Success (in terms of maximizing true "matches") depends on the *quality* of the information available on each individual. Newcombe[15,18] has shown that the surname, first initial, birth date and birthplace of an individual provide a high degree of discrimination between individuals. The more precise the information, the more accurate the record linking process. Thus, special emphasis must be placed on accurate recording of names (including maiden names), addresses, birth and death dates on all family members even if unaffected. If there is limited time available during the clinic visit, consideration might be given to the use of a "self-administered family history form"* or a family history questionnaire[23] which is mailed to the family prior to the clinic visit. Our experience with these mailed intake forms has been a positive one. The mailing of the forms prior to the clinic visit allows the patient to think about his family history, look up requested information, or contact family members who may be more knowledgeable. The family information obtained this way may then be verified at the time of the clinic visit and modifications made. The questionnaire also allows the clinical staff to compile, evaluate and, if necessary, request more information prior to seeing the family in clinic.

3. Research. Providing investigators with a ready source of patient material for research studies of genetic disease is another use of the central record system. In turn, information generated from research activities may prove valuable in diagnosis, patient care, and in providing more precise risk figures for those individuals at risk.

4. Prevention. Genetic evaluation and genetic counseling is directed primarily at individuals who have already demonstrated that they have a relatively higher risk than the population at large either because they are affected or because they have a child who is affected. Counseling in such situations is primarily retrospective counseling in that its focus is prevention of further cases in affected sibships.

---

*Available upon request.

Information gathered in the course of the genetic evaluation of a nuclear family, however, often indicates that other individuals in the extended family are likewise at risk for (a) developing a genetic condition (*e.g.,* a disorder with variable age of onset), (b) developing a serious medical complication of an already diagnosed condition, (c) medical complications due to exposure to drugs or environmental agents, or (d) having a child with a serious abnormality. Many of these individuals are aware of their risk and that diagnosis, treatment, or prevention are available.

Identification of such high risk individuals as those in categories a, b, and c above is preventive medicine in the traditional sense. Another aspect of prevention, albeit not as traditional, is offering genetic counseling to individuals identified as being ar risk for having a child with a serious genetic condition. It has been well documented that prospective counseling could be effective in reducing the proportion of cases of genetic disease in the population, and that single-locus (simple Mendelian) disorders offer the best opportunities for prevention.[7–10, 13]

Preventive medicine is aggressive medicine. An aggressive preventive clinical genetics program requires a sound system for storage, retrieval, and integration of family information. The role of the central record system must be changed from a passive/storage role to that of an active/interactive data management system. Greater emphasis must be placed on developing a routine for locating, testing, and counseling individuals at risk, and keeping the record system up-to-date with changes in family status (*e.g.,* new births, recent deaths, etc.), and migration to and from the geographic area. If the record system is a vital one, individuals at risk could be fully ascertained and monitored during their period of risk. Effectiveness of counseling and preventive measures, such as carrier testing or population and family screening programs, could also be used on both short and long term bases.

We have recently tested our genetic record system to determine whether it could function in a preventive role. Hemophilia A families were selected because of our intent to offer a carrier test to women at risk. Questions for which we sought answers included: How many women are at risk for being carriers? How many of these live in our geographical area? What is the distribution of the degree of risk in this sample of women? How many are of child-bearing age? How many tests are we likely to perform each year? What are our projected manpower needs?

Thirty-nine families with hemophilia A were identified in our central file. Each family folder contained (a) a detailed family history obtained at the initial clinic visit and modified during subsequent contacts with the family or relatives, (b) a list of females at risk for being carriers and (c) a computer printout summary of each woman's risk generated by PEDIG, a computer program which calculates risk using Bayesian conditional probability.[24] These 39 families yielded 440 females (excluding deceased female relatives) at risk for being carriers of 11.3 females per proband.

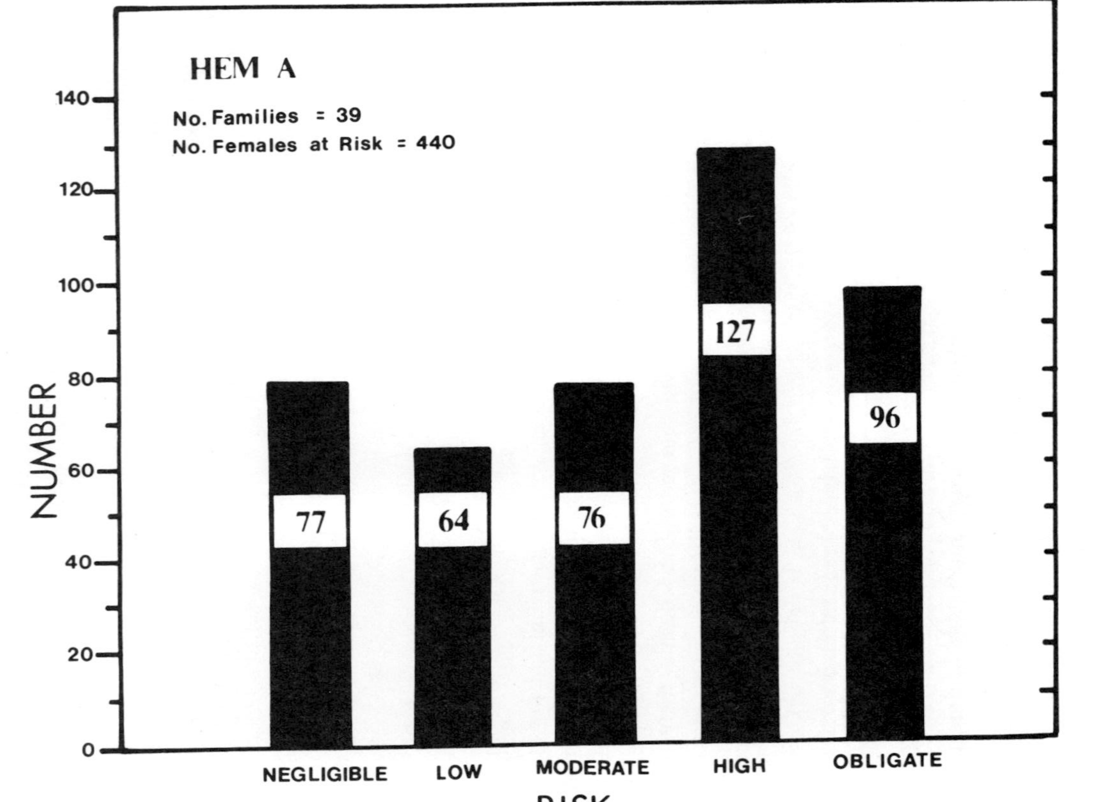

Fig. 7. Distribution by risk group of females at risk for being carriers for hemophilia A. Risks groups: negligible (<1%), low (1-5%), moderate (6-20%), high (20-99%) and obligate (100%).

Figure 7 shows the distribution of risk in this sample of 440 females. Sixty-eight percent or 299 individuals have a risk greater than 6%. If one excludes obligate carriers and those with negligible (<1%) risk, 267 females (61% of the total sample) are most likely to ask for and benefit from carrier testing. The geographical location of 180 of these 267 females was recorded on the pedigree forms; 120 reside in our catchment area. Approximately half of the females in the low to high risk groups are of child-bearing age; a similar percentage was found in our sample of obligate carriers (Fig. 8).

The data cited above were generated solely from information contained in family folders. The information has proved valuable in the standardization of our carrier test (*e.g.*, by identifying obligate carriers from our pool of at-risk females) and in planning the carrier testing program. Now that the program is operative, other questions may be posed and answers sought. How successful is patient contact? How successful is patient contact when the proband or parents of proband are aked to contact specific relatives? How many of these individuals know that they are at risk? How many seek genetic counseling after being informed that they are at risk? How many take advantage of testing procedures such as carrier testing when it is available? What is the cost-benefit ratio of such ascertainment? How do the above correlate with severity of the condition or degree of risk? How do these findings compare with those obtained for other genetic conditions? Answers to these questions can provide data regarding program effectiveness and the relative value of an aggressive preventive approach.

Computerized Record Systems

In this paper reference to computerized data management has been minimal due to the author's belief that the best computerized systems will evolve from existing, well-maintained, manually-kept record keeping systems.

Should the record system be computerized? Each clinical genetics unit will have to answer that for itself on the basis of the status of its present record system, its patient load, the number of supporting laboratories and the volume of data generated, current and projected uses of the stored data and availability of funds.

Computerized record systems offer distinct advantages over manually-linked systems. They are more efficient and because of this they provide one with the opportunity to accomplish more in less time, and to ask more questions of the stored data than one was previously inclined to ask. Once operative, fewer man-hours are required to maintain, correct, and update the system, and the need for manually-kept indexing systems is virtually eliminated.

Machine-assisted record systems, however, are expensive. As Newcombe has pointed out, however, only 10% of the total cost of the British Columbia Health Surveillance Registry involved computer operations. Over 90% of the cost was for preparing the data for the computer including abstracting or coding the data, keypunching, and verifying. These costs do not include the costs of obtaining the data initially.

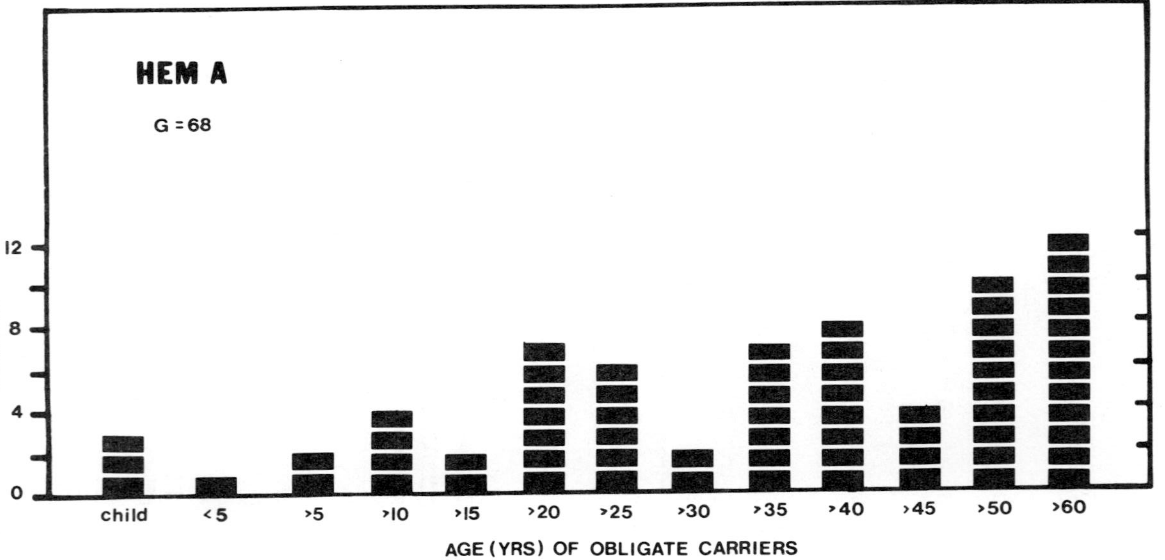

Fig. 8. Distribution by age of obligate carriers of hemophilia A. Approximately one-half of the women are of childbearing age (15-45 years).

Several reports describing computerized record-linking[15–21] genetic data management[25] and cytogenetic register[26,27] systems have appeared in the literature in recent years. Readers interested in initiating such systems may consult these sources for specific information. Many of the reported systems are designed for specific purposes and/or are machine dependent *i.e.*, designed for a particular set of hardware). However, many of their features can be modified for use in existing or proposed genetic and cytogenetic laboratory record systems.

Computerized record systems may be inevitable. If and when that time arrives, will the transition from a manual system be a smooth one? The expense of converting to a machine-assisted system will be formidable if the data are not in an easily abstractable form, or in a form suitable for conventional machine analysis. The message is the same as that of the TV commercial about oil filters. The gas station owner, after describing the cause of the damaged automobile engine, picks up a relatively inexpensive oil filter and states in a rather mater-of-fact tone: "You can pay me now or you can pay me later!"

Summary

What is the present status of your record system?

Scope. Which patients are currently in your central genetics file? Genetic clinic patients only? Patients from specialty clinics such as cystic fibrosis clinic, hemophilia clinic, etc.? Patients referred from in-house consultations? Patients from state or private institutions? What is your present and projected patient load? What are your present and projected needs? Do you foresee an active preventive genetics program feasible in your geographical area? What are the present and projected research interests and needs of the staff?

Content. What information is currently stored in the central genetic file folders? Are the folders patient- or family-oriented? Have you found this arrangement satisfactory? How many copies of file entries, such as the pedigree, must be made in order to assure that every file has a copy? Is the medical, genetic, and laboratory information in individual folders recorded in legible, easily abstractable form? Are the contents of the folders organized in such a way as to facilitate abstracting of information? Are the patient and family records complete? Are file contents securely fastened? What proportion of the pedigrees are in the format shown in Fig. 1a?

Usefulness. Is your present system used for purposes other than storage? How often is information in patient folders used for research purposes? When was the last time a question was asked of the record system? Could the question be answered? Answered easily?

Overall impression. Are you pleased with your present system?

Disposition. Are there plans for improving the present system?

Observe
Record
Tabulate
Communicate

The flight of purpose ne'r is o'rtook
unless the deed go with it.
W. Osler

REFERENCES

1. E.D. Acheson, Medical Record Linkage, Oxford University Press London, 1967.
2. V.A. McKusick, *J. Chronic Disease 22*, 1, 1969.
3. A.D. Merritt, *J. Clin. Comput. 4*, 227, 1975.
4. P.M. Conneally, *J. Clin. Comput. 4*, 231, 1975.
5. A.D. Merritt, K.W. Kang, P.M. Conneally, J.M. Gersting and T. Rigo, *in* Registers for the Detection and Prevention of Genetic Disease, A.E.H. Emery and J.R. Miller (Eds.), Stratton, New York, pp. 31-51, 1976.
6. A.E.H. Emery, D. Elliott, M. Moores and C. Smith, *J. Med. Genet. 11,* 145, 1974.
7. A.E.H. Emery and C. Smith, *Brit. Med. J. 3*, 636, 1970.
8. C.Smith *in* Modern Trends in Human Genetics, Vol. 1, A.E.H. Emery, (Ed.), Appleton-Century-Crofts, New York, pp. 350-369, 1970.
9. C. Smith, S. Holloway and A.E.H. Emery, *J. Med. Genet. 8*, 453, 1971.
10. A.E.H. Emery, M.S. Watt and E.R. Clack, *Clin. Genet. 3* 147, 1972.
11. J.R. Miller, *in* Registers for the Detection and Prevention of Genetic Disease, A.E.H. Emery and J.R. Miller (Eds.), Stratton, New York, pp. 1-7, 1976.
12. W.H.O. Scientific Group, Biological Components of Human Reproduction, Studies of their Variation in Population Groups, *Wld. Hlth. Org. Techn. Rep. Ser. No. 435*, 1969.
13. A.G. Motulsky, G.R. Fraser and J. Felsenstein, *in* Birth Defects: Original Article Series, Vol. VII, No. 5, D. Bergsma (Ed.), Williams and Wilkins Co., Baltimore, for the National Foundation-March of Dimes, pp. 22-32, 1971.
14. O.L. Peterson, L.P. Andrews, R.S. Spain and B.G. Greenberg, *J. Med. Educ., Part 2*, 1, 1956.
15. H.B. Newcombe, *Am. J. Hum. Genet. 19*, 335, 1967.
16. J.M. Kennedy, H.B. Newcombe, E.A. Okazaki and M.E. Smith, List Processing Methods for Organizing Files of Linked Records, Atomic Energy of Canada, Ltd., Chalk River, Ontario, Document AECL-2078, 1964.
17. J.M. Kennedy, H.B. Newcombe, E.A. Okazaki and M.E. Smith, Computer Methods for Family Linkage of Vital and Health Records, Atomic Energy of Canada, Ltd., Chalk River, Ontario, Document AECL-2222, 1965.
18. H.B. Newcombe and J.M. Kennedy, *Commun. Assoc. Computing Machinery 5,* 563, 1962.

19. H.B. Newcombe, J.M. Kennedy, S.J. Axford and A.P. James, *Science 130*, 954, 1959.
20. M.E. Smith, R.R. Schwartz and H.B. Newcombe, Computer Methods for Extracting Sibship Data from Family Groupings of Records, Atomic Energy of Canada, Ltd., Chalk River, Ontario, Document AECL-2530, 1965.
21. B.K. Trimble, *in* Registers for the Detection and Prevention of Genetic Disease, A.E.H. Emery and J.R. Miller (Eds.), Stratton, New York, pp. 87-101, 1976.
22. L. Davidson, *Commun. Assoc. Computing Machinery 5*, 169, 1962.
23. J. Cole, P.M. Conneally, M.E. Hodes and A.D. Merritt, *J. Med. Genet. 15*, 10, 1978.
24. P.M. Conneally and I. Heuch, *Am. J. Hum Genet. 26*, 773, 1974.
25. A.E. H. Emery and J.R. Miller, Registers for the Detection and Prevention of Genetic Disease, Stratton, New York, 1976.
26. G.H. Prescott, M.L. Rivas, L. Shanbeck, D.W. Macfarlane, H.E. Wyandt, W.R. Breg, H. Lubs, R.E. Magenis, R. Summitt, F. Hecht, W. Kinberling and D. Clow, *Am. J. Hum. Genet. 29*, 654, 1977.
27. Human Cytogenetic Registers (1977): A Description of Nine Systems Together with Some Recommendations, Birth Defects: Original Article Series, XIII, 4, The National Foundation, New York, 1977.

GENETIC SERVICES AS HEALTH CARE SERVICES

Vincent M. Riccardi

Introduction

The genetic approach to human disease is an attitude; it reflects a desire to assist patients and their families in avoiding the occurrence or recurrence of genetic or congenital disorders.[1] It also introduces the broadest concept of genetic services: Whoever implements the genetic approach to human disease thereby provides genetic services. Recognition of this broad concept as distinct from individual genetics services (*e.g.*, genetic counseling, cytogenetic analysis) is important as each specific service is formally defined according to particular professional, administrative, legal and financial needs. Then, as limitations and refinements are applied to the individual services, the broader notion of genetic services as part of primary care will not be excessively circumscribed. My concern is that without this distinction, excessively technical definitions of the individual genetic services and providers thereof could remove the natural impact of the primary care clinician, with the net effect of decreasing the availability of genetic health care services rather than expanding them. In order that this exclusion not occur, genetic health care planners must constantly remind themselves of two facts: (1) Each of the genetic services is indeed part of the larger health care responsibility entailed in the genetic approach to human disease. (2) This larger health care responsibility mostly is carried out by non-geneticist clinicians. This presentation will emphasize these facts and deal with genetic services at the level of routine health care.

Overlap of Primary and Speciality Health Care

As indicated above, genetic services may be considered either in broad, generic terms, or in terms of specific tasks. A broad, generic definition of genetic services may be as follows: providing assistance to a patient or family about whom there is concern for a genetic disorder or genetic consequences (*i.e.*, heritability). Specific genetic services represent the particular vantage points by which genetic specialists become involved with a patient or family. These include (1) genetic counseling, (2) clinical diagnosis, (3) laboratory diagnosis (cytogenetic, biochemical, etc.), (4) prenatal diagnosis, (5) genetic screening, (6) therapy/management, and (7) training/education. Although in sum these are the responsibilities

ISBN 0-12-562650-9

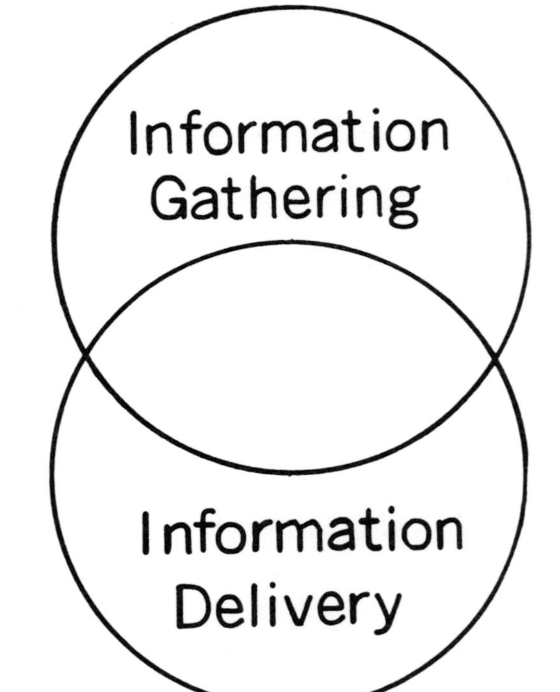

Fig. 1. Preliminary genetic counseling: A product of the overlap of information gathering and delivery efforts. This depiction emphasizes the need for non-geneticist clinicians to have some genetic background and skills. (From V.M. Riccardi, The Genetic Approach to Human Disease, 1977, reprinted with permission from Oxford University Press,)

of geneticists, it would merely confuse the issue to demand that only geneticists provide any of these genetic services. Genetics has been and will continue to be an important aspect of primary care medicine.[1,2] Therefore, we need to ensure that the generic aspects of genetic health care are not overlooked. This is best done by increasing the genetic clinician's overlap and interdigitation with the activities of primary (and secondary) care clinicians.[3–7] This in turn will depend on the development of genetic health care models and programs that recognize multiple levels of providing genetic services.

There are at least three practical consequences to focusing on the multilevel overlap of primary care and specialty genetics: (1) the development of outreach programs to provide genetic back-up on a widespread, routine and frequent basis; (2) the development of operational models of genetic counseling that include non-geneticist clinicians; (3) the development of a mechanism to ensure the earliest recognition or referral of patients who require genetic services. The first of these consequences I have discussed previously,[3,4,8] and it is further considered elsewhere in this volume. Thus, I will proceed directly to the second point on my way to a more elaborate discussion of the third point, which involves the notion of a genetic disposition protocol.

A Genetic Counseling Model

As indicated in Figure 1, my model of genetic counseling has three components: genetic evaluation, definitive genetic counseling and preliminary genetic counseling, defined according to whether there is information gathering only, information delivery only, or both, respectively. The point is that as information is being gathered (*e.g.*, by a primary care obstetrician) information may also be delivered. The resultant preliminary genetic counseling is no less a part of the entire genetic counseling process than is definitive genetic counseling (*i.e.*, that resulting while emphasizing delivery of information). An illustrative scenario would involve an obstetrician taking a family history from a 24 year old woman who is 12 weeks pregnant. Having determined that she has a nephew with the Down syndrome, he explains the need to determine the affected child's karyotype since certain findings (*i.e.*, translocations) may alter her risks and ultimate pregnancy management. As a result of this preliminary counseling the expense and effort of the necessary chromosome analyses are recognized as reasonable and thus are pursued. The proband turns out to have a Robertsonian translocation to explain his Down syndrome. His aunt, the consultand, is then referred to a geneticist for further evaluation and definitive counseling. She is found to be a translocation carrier like her sister, the proband's mother, and amniocentesis is afforded, leading to the intrauterine diagnosis of a chromosome imbalance, whereupon she and her husband elect to terminate the pregnancy. This example demonstrates effectively how the model depicted in Figure 1 both respects the multiple levels of genetic counseling and characterizes the potential interrelationships of geneticists and non-geneticists in providing at least one of the

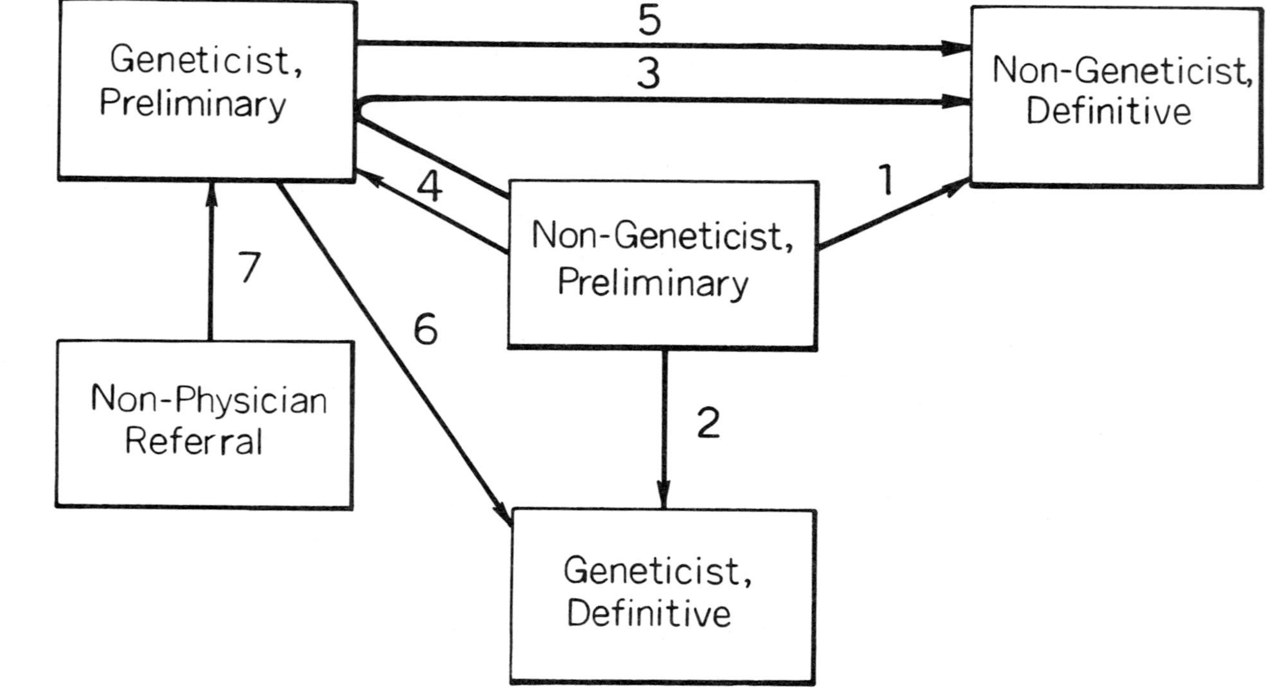

Fig. 2. This diagram indicates that genetic counseling may begin with a non-geneticist physician who also may provide definitive counseling (1) or refer the family to a geneticist who directly provides definitive counseling (2). Minor second-level preliminary counseling (*e.g.*, diagnosis corroboration) may be provided by the geneticist before the non-geneticist does definitive counseling (3). The geneticist may make amajor second-level preliminary counseling contribution (*e.g.*, establishment of a diagnosis, family studies,etc.) (4) before referral (back) to the primary physician for definitive counseling (5). The geneticist may solely be responsible for both preliminary and definitive counseling (6). Occasionally a primary physician is not involved (7). Thus, there are many ways for primary physicians and geneticists to cooperate and mutually contribute to effecting genetic counseling for a family. (From V.M. Riccardi, The Genetic Approach to Human Disease, 1977, reprinted with permission from Oxford University Press.)

specific genetic services. This point is further emphasized in Figure 2, which depicts schematically the fact that both geneticists and non-geneticists may participate in each level of evaluation and counseling.

Genetic Disposition Discharge Protocol

I now wish to focus on the role of non-geneticists in ensuring that as a result of their evaluations, and perhaps preliminary counseling, definitive counseling is afforded the patient or family. There is probably no better circumstance for considering the interdigitation of primary care clinicians with genetic specialists in providing the genetic services than the occasion of hospitalization of a pediatric patient.[9,10] Yet recent discussions of planning for health care needs in hospital settings have virtually ignored this fact[10–13] and, as I will demonstrate below, currently there is very little overlap between pediatricians and geneticists on behalf of hospitalized patients. This probably reflects, at least in part, a failure to respect the mutual responsibilities shared by the geneticists and pediatricians in general. It has been as though there were no genetic responsibilities unless a geneticist was involved and that therefore principles of genetic health care, such as incorporating genetic advisement into the hospital record, have not been implemented. (On the other hand, it would be virtually impossible and unnecessary for a geneticist to consult on every hospitalized pediatric patient.) In order to demonstrate the need for emphasizing the role of pediatricians in providing genetic health care we carried out a chart survey study at Milwaukee Children's Hospital (MCH) in the summer of 1976. We believe the data allow for two conclusions relevant to this discussion of genetic services: (1) Primary (and secondary) care physicians do have daily health care responsibilities that fall within the purview of clinical genetics, particularly preliminary genetic counseling. These practitioners are the ones who make the greatest number of decisions about applying counseling principles as a health care service. (2) Thus, we need to provide an operational mechanism emphasizing the practitioner's role in providing genetic services, such as formalized genetic disposition hospital discharge protocol.

The details of the MCH study are reported in detail elsewhere,[15] but certain elements are recounted here in order to demonstrate that definitions of and plans to implement specific genetic services need to respect the actual and potential roles of primary care practitioners. In a retrospective survey of 38,424 patients spanning 1971-1974, 1,633 patients with either of 10 disorders were identified. (The designated disorders included chromosome abnormalities, hemoglobinopathies, cystic fibrosis, metabolic disorders (*e.g.*, phenylketonuria, adrenogenital syndrome), neurofibromatosis, cleft lip/palate, neural tube defects, congenital heart defects, polycystic kidneys, and multiple anomaly/developmental syndromes.) The charts of 478 such patients were reviewed in detail and scored as to whether genetic counseling was documented to have been (a) "considered", (b) "offered", or (c) "provided". A request for genetic laboratory studies (*e.g.*, karyotype) was not considered on its own to indicate counseling efforts. In 2 cases (0.4%) genetic counseling was offered and in 5 cases (1.1%) it was given, for a total recorded genetic disposition in 1.5% of patients with either of 10 genetic/ congenital disorders. We construe the absence of a discussion about genetic services (whether considered, offered, or provided) to indicate either that there was no counseling effort *or* that the person who dealt with this matter did not recognize the need to make this aspect of health care a part of the patient's hospital record.

I suggest that we can markedly enhance the widespread routine availability of genetic health care and use of genetic services by dealing with the deficiency noted above through the mechanism of a hospital discharge protocol requiring an explicit disposition.[14,15] In this way practitioners would be afforded the chance to routinely initiate the genetic counseling process (evaluation and preliminary counseling) or designate its inappropriateness (which is still a genetic decision). Derivation of an explicit disposition would result from the need to answer two questions for each diagnosis at the time of discharge: (1) Is the disorder genetic? (yes, no, or possibly). (2) Was the patient/family so informed? (yes, no, deferred). Once answers to these questions are derived the additional steps in providing the genetic service of counseling are clear: further evaluation, with or without referral to a clinical geneticist or other specialist, and then definitive counseling, which may involve merely the statement that no further genetic services are required. In any case it is clear that genetic counseling as a genetic service directly involves non-geneticists and that this fact can be capitalized upon for improved availability and utility of genetic services.

Summary

As we begin to consider the accreditation of clinical geneticists and genetic service programs it is critical that organizations such as the American Society of Human Genetics and the (yet unestablished) American College of Clinical Genetics allow for and encourage the provision of genetic services by non-geneticists – not merely by training and education but also by devising, fostering, and implementing health care models that recognize and rely on local primary and secondary care practitioners. The two-stage (preliminary-definitive) genetic counseling model and the hospital discharge genetic disposition protocol described herein are specific examples of how to include both specialists and non-specialists in providing genetic services.

ACKNOWLEDGMENTS

Thanks to Ms. R. Pope for manuscript assistance and to Dr. Arthur Robinson for being himself.

REFERENCES

1. V.M. Riccardi, The Genetic Approach to Human Disease, Oxford University

Press, New York, 1977.

2. M.L. Peterson, *Birth Defects Orig. Art. Ser. 13 (6)*, 171, 1977.
3. V.M. Riccardi, *Am. J. Publ. Hlth. 66*, 268, 1976.
4. V.M. Riccardi, *in* The Prevention of Genetic Disease and Mental Retardation, A. Milunsky (Ed.), W.B. Saunders, Philadelphia, p. 410, 1975.
5. D.L. Rimoin, *Birth Defects Orig. Art. Ser. 6 (1)*, 67, 1970.
6. D.L. Rimoin, *Birth Defects Orig. Art. Ser. 13 (6)*, 105, 1977.
7. Amer. Acad. of Pediatrics Task Force on Genetic Screening, *Pediatrics 58*, 757, 1976.
8. V.M. Riccardi, The Genetic Approach to Human Disease, Oxford University Press, New York pp. 259-266, 1977.
9. N. Day and L.B. Holmes, *Am. J. Hum. Genet. 25*, 237, 1973.
10. J.G. Hall, E.K. Powers, R.T. McIlvaine and V.H. Ean, *Am. J. Med. Genet. 1*, 417, 1978.
11. A.M. Warrington, D.J. Ponesse, M.E. Hunter, D.A. Grant, A.V. Grasset, D.W. Gray, C.D. Hayward, B.F. Long, G.E.C. Morrison and D. Sutherland, *Canad. Med. Assoc. J. 117*, 354, 1977.
12. G.M. Komrower, *Br. Med. J. 2*, 787, 1977.
13. A.F. North Jr., P. Wilkinson and T.K. Oliver, Jr., *Am. J. Dis. Child. 131*, 400, 1977.
14. V.M. Riccardi, The Genetic Approach to Human Disease, Oxford University Press, New York, pp. 4-5, 1977.
15. V.M. Riccardi, A. Cohen and M.T. Chen, *Am. J. Publ. Hlth. 68*, 652, 1978.

STRUCTURE AND ORGANIZATION OF COMMUNITY GENETIC SERVICES*

L.G. Jackson
M.A. Barr
D. Linn

In an attempt to improve the regional provision of genetic services in the eastern Pennsylvania and southern New Jersey area, we established a "center-satellite" system of traveling or community based genetic clinics to serve this population. The original clinic was established in 1968 and the formation of a network system began in 1970. Some of the details of this system have been reported previously[1,2] and, in general, they closely parallel the independently established system of Epstein and his colleagues in California (and Nevada).[3,4] Like the California system, the Pennsylvania-New Jersey network is still growing and evolving as we continue to gain experience in this form of health care delivery. Both systems have experienced growth in referral numbers but have discontinued some clinics for reasons of an individual nature.[4] These have included clinic growth to independence and the assumption of responsibility by a local medical group, as well as the converse experience of declining referrals and lack of local support. In general, experience with this system of community-based genetic programs is one of success both in the delivery of genetic diagnosis and counseling services and in the dissemination of education on the usefulness of genetic services to regional health professionals.[5] The experience has also pointed out some lessons which may be useful to newer programs of this type as well as for improvement of our own or other similar programs. We will briefly describe the establishment of our program, its skeletal structure, and some recent items of interest gleaned from a survey of the past two years of operation.

Establishment of the Satellite Clinics

The first satellite clinic existed as a cooperative monthly clinic to review developmentally disabled children with a pediatric neurologist at a state health department outpatient and inpatient facility. Public awareness of this program and subsequent requests for similar outreach clinics caused us to initiate a planned expansion of this activity in 1970. Preceding and accompanying this expansion

*Supported in part by Grant CE-34 from the National Foundation-March of Dimes.

ISBN 0-12-562650-9

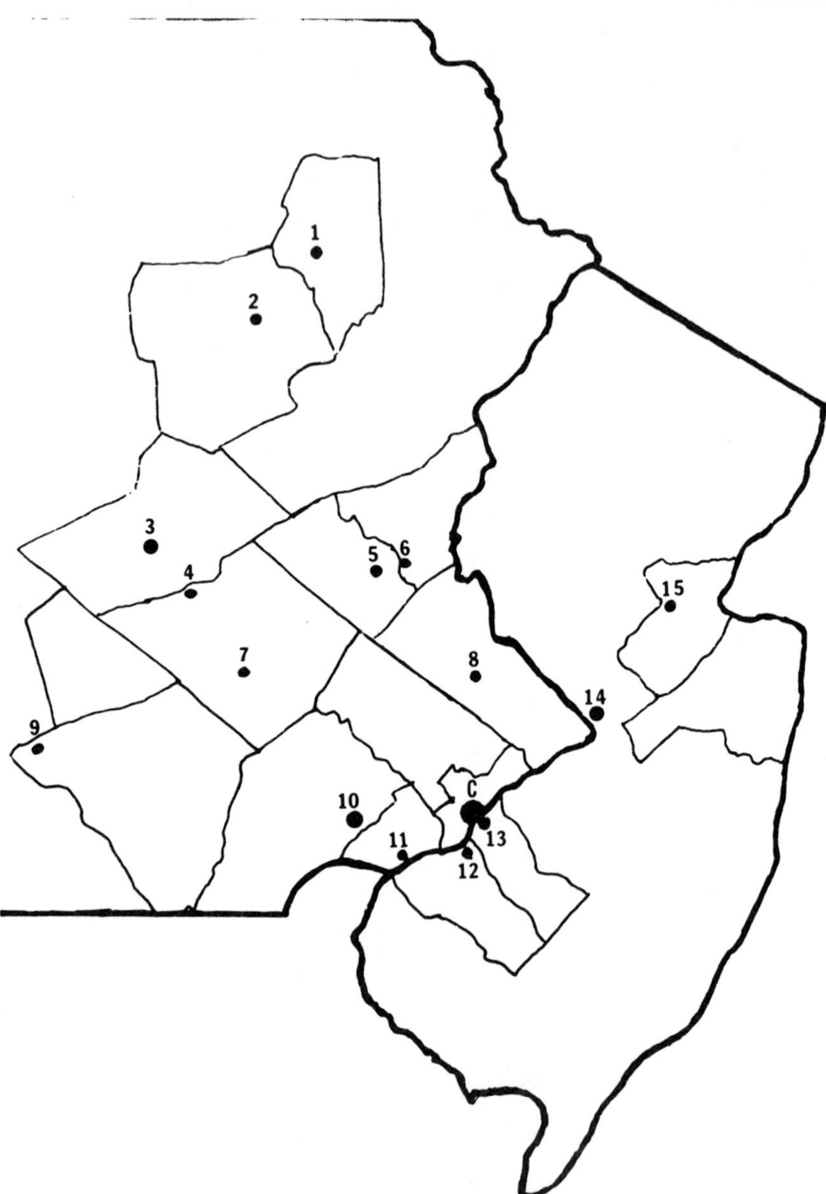

Fig. 1. Outline map of eastern Pennsylvania (left) and New Jersey (right) showing geographic location of Medical Center Genetic Unit (center) and Satellite Genetic Clinics in Pennsylvania: (1) Scranton, (2) Wilkes-Barre, (3) Pottsville, (4) Hamburg, (5) Allentown, (6) Bethlehem, (7) Reading, (8) Doylestown-Penndel, (9) Elizabethtown, (10) West Chester, and (11) Chester; and in New Jersey: (12) Westville Grove, (13) Camden, (14) Trenton, and (15) New Brunswick (now operated by the Rutgers Medical School).

was an ongoing program of public (lay and medical) education through speaking engagements, hospital seminars, parent group (retarded citizens associations, Mental Health-Mental Retardation parent groups, handicapped children) meetings, and professional symposia (M.D., R.N., special education, physical medicine, etc.). Although the need for services exists within such groups, it is not organized or focused, and specific delineation of genetic services which may be made available, as well as the mechanics of their availability, are important items for discussion. It is also important to include the local medical community in the planning of satellite clinical activities so that they will develop an interest in the success of the program and avoid the feeling that the activity has been introduced outside their sphere of interest and influence.

After initial education, a cooperative approach to a local medical facility was made, usually with the area representative of the National Foundation-March of Dimes. The program has grown and exists largely under National Foundation-March of Dimes sponsorship and local executives are usually familiar with the existing medical community. Discussions with the local group would then lead to an organizational format, location of the clinic within an existing local medical facility, and creation of local publicity for the medical community (professional staff or county medical organization) and the lay community (hospital public relations office and National Foundation-March of Dimes chapter office). New clinics were generally established singly and at reasonably spaced intervals more by demand than by plan.

Structure of the Center-Satellite Program

The satellite genetic clinics are distributed on a county basis in Eastern Pennsylvania and South-Central New Jersey (Fig. 1), in local health care facilities (usually the outpatient clinic area of a hospital). However, we also use a county health department clinic, a school for mentally retarded children, and a Mental Health-Mental Retardation Clinic. Each clinic is scheduled for one-half day of time, or 3-5 hours of patient contact time. Each is within a two hour driving distance of the genetic center in Philadelphia and, where possible, the clinics are scheduled so that two will occur on the same day in a close geographic area. This minimizes the travel time per clinic but commits the staff to a long day and sometimes forces haste in the morning clinic if interviews take longer than anticipated.

The local medical facility essentially provides only a waiting room, space for interviewing and counseling patients, and an examining room. Usually the basic medical tools are available, such as examining equipment, syringes, needles, etc. In addition, we also carry with us the usual equipment that you would find in a physician's bag – containers for special test samples, some material for developmental evaluation of children, a variety of forms that we use in our own center and photographic equipment, which is important. We make a conscious effort to have a photographic record of each of the patients we see because all are ultimately discussed in our regular conference at the medical center to get other consultant's diagnostic opinions, and the visual record is invaluable in facilitating these discussions. Each one of the clinics provides us with a local contact for referrals – usually a nurse from the medical facility. Initially this varied from clinic to clinic. We recently completed a nurse training program specifically addressed to this. We trained one or more nurses from each of the satellite clinics. The course consisted of 40 hours of formal classroom work, including the basic fundamentals of genetics and genetic counseling, and how to handle laboratory samples for metabolic screening, chromosome studies, and fluids for amniotic fluid cell culture, thus making it possible for the nurse to to serve not only as the local contact for appointments but also to answer questions from both physicians and lay-people about the appropriateness of genetic counseling for their problem, and complete follow-up calls to patients and medical facilities in the area. In addition, she is a single local contact person for physicians who want to send samples for testing in advance of the patient's appointment.

The clinics frequently have other local personnel in attendance, including house staff or the patient's physician. Occasionally a social worker or a member of the health agency referring the patient will accompany them.

Our center always provides two staff members who travel to each of the satellite clinics: a physician-geneticist and a non-physician genetic counselor. More than one physician or genetic associate may attend depending upon the clinic load. In addition, there are usually fellows, residents, or students who are spending elective time in the medical center genetic unit and travel with us. This provides them with a unique educational opportunity. The patients are seen more frequently as whole family units than they are in the medical center and there is less formality and a more relaxed atmosphere in these counseling sessions.

Clinics are scheduled on a monthly or bi-monthly basis, depending on the case load, and the number of families served varies from 6-10 in a clinic day in the "active" satellites. Historical interview, physical examination for medical evaluation, diagnosis, and genetic counseling are then carried out exactly as they would be in the medical center, with return visits for completion of counseling, reinforcement, or simple medical follow-up scheduled as we would in our own facility. Even diagnostic amniocentesis is carried out with ease in clinics where the staff is capable of the procedure. Only the laboratory activity is missing from the satellite centers.

Utilization of Satellite Genetic Clinics

As with Epstein's experience,[4] our active clinics serve about 16 families per 100,000 population per year. However, there is considerable variability in that figure so we undertook a survey of other factors involved in clinic utilization in an attempt to discover measurable differences between the center and satellite clinics. The survey involved only the Pennsylvania clinics, for reasons of sponsorship and state planning, and concerns an area which includes 24% of the annual

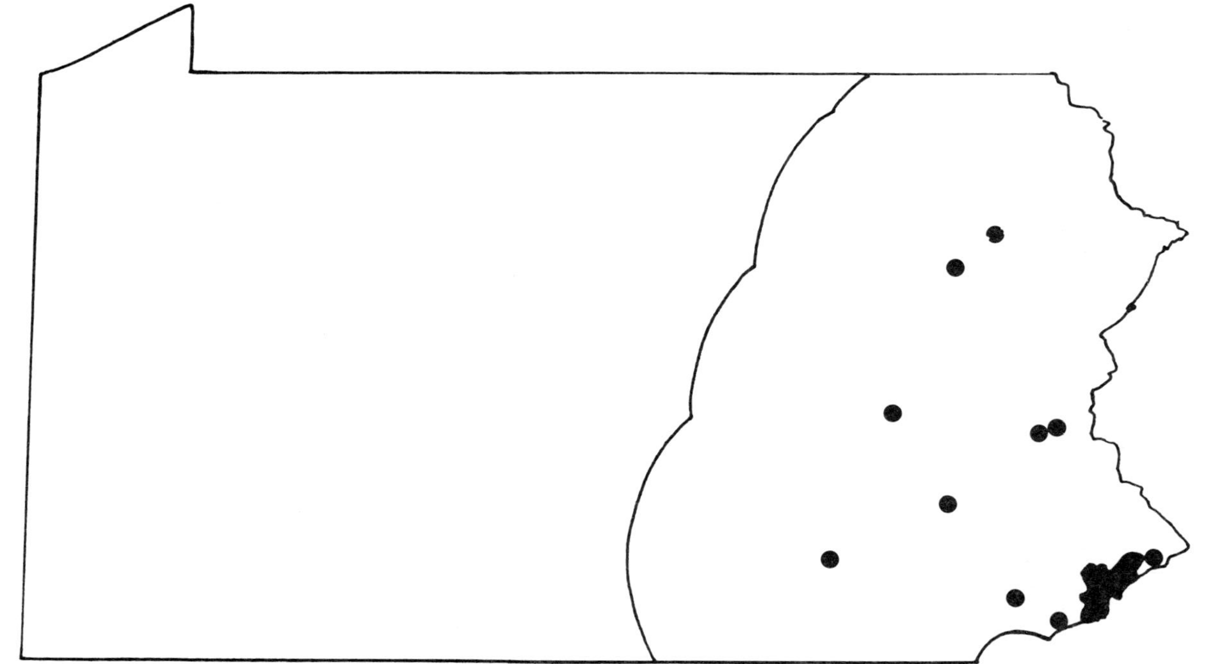

Fig. 2. Outline map of Pennsylvania showing the area that is within 50 miles of the satellite genetic clinic (radii). This area, which includes 24% of Pennsylvania's annual births, is therefore within one hour of genetic services affiliated with our medical center.

births of the Commonwealth of Pennsylvania (Fig. 2). The survey was conducted by analysis of all referrals to either a satellite or center genetic clinic for genetic counseling, as opposed to specific diagnostic testing or evaluation, from July 1975 to June 1977. Clinic records were analyzed, patients were questioned, and counselors were questioned. The sample included 250 patient families from the medical center clinic and 465 from the satellite clinics. The population surveyed is primarily middle class with 90% white clients in the medical center and 98% at the satellites (Table 1). This is in contrast to the area population distribution and strongly suggests a need to develop more effective means to reach the non-white and non-middle class populations of all areas served.

TABLE 1

Summary of Survey Population

Total Patients Surveyed			
250 Center	20% Self	49% Couple	22% Proband
465 Satellite	20% Self	23% Couple	51% Proband

All Patients from Commonwealth of Pennsylvania
Center 90% White
Satellite 98% White

Comparison of diagnostic categories as seen at the satellite and center clinics reveals good correlation (Table 2). This suggests that the satellite clinic referrals are as appropriate as those to the genetic center and that a significant case load of real genetic problems exists in the satellite areas. Inspection of the sources of referral (Table 3) shows only a difference in pediatrician-obstetrician referrals in the two areas. Our medical center has a developmental disability clinic in the pediatric department where a substantial amount of genetic counseling is done, which is reflected in the decreased number of center referrals to a separate genetic clinic. In addition, the center has an active obstetrical staff dealing in problems of reproduction and high-risk pregnancy, accounting for an increased percentage of obstetrician referrals. Finally, Table 4 examines usage of the clinics by two patient groups and again there is good correlation between groups, with the majority of families referred for diagnosis of genetic cause for their problem or for estimating the genetic risk for recurrence of the problem.

If the satellite clinics are doing an appropriate job of serving area patients with genetic problems there should be no significant difference between patient groups in the time between recognition of the condition and obtaining genetic services. services. Table 5 examines this and suggests that any difference in the time taken to obtain genetic counseling services is minimal. Of course, the correlation between groups may also mean that similar degrees of unawareness of the utility of genetic services may exist in both areas. To take a look at that possi-

TABLE 2

Diagnostic Category of Patients Seen at Center and Satellite Clinic by Percent

Diagnostic Categories	Center	Satellite
Cytogenetics	14%	24%
Single gene	18%	19%
Polygenic	14%	11%
Mental retardation	10%	12%
Multiple congenital anomalies	7%	7%
Single congenital anomaly	4%	10%
Reproductive failures	10%	6%
Amniocentesis	10%	5%
Other	13%	6%
Total	100%	100%

TABLE 3

Referral Source, by Percent, for Patients at Center and Satellite Clinics

Referral Source	Center	Satellite
Pediatrician	13%	28%
Obstetrician	58%	32%
Family practice	4%	7%
Nurse	–	.6%
Self	5%	6%
Specialist	11%	5%
Health agency	9%	16%

TABLE 4

Usage of Genetic Services

Usage	Center	Satellite
Diagnostic	34%	42%
Risk	59%	44%
Supportive	5%	11%
Risk Confirmatory	2%	3%

TABLE 5

Time Delay (Patient)

	Center	Satellite
1. No delay	65%	63%
2. Delay in recognition of signs or symptoms, patient or physician	4%	9%
3. Delay following recognition and seeking medical intervention	3%	2%
4. Unavailability, inaccessibility or unawareness	28%	26%

bility, the items listed in Table 6 were studied. This attempts to see if the opportunity for genetic counseling intervention was recognized promptly and, if so, seized. The table shows that there is some increased lack of recognition of the need for genetic counseling in the satellite areas, as opposed to the urban area. About 50% more patients were correctly recognized as having a genetic condition, but were not referred for counseling or counseled by the primary physician. It is interesting that once counseling is suggested, the referral is apparently made appropriately and the family is not left without resource. It must be remembered in both of these questions that we are only examining those families who actually come to one of the clinics. The reasons why families with genetic problems do not appear at clinics can only be examined through statistics from various other health records and undoubtedly there is still a significant unserved group.

Finally, there is the question of impact of genetic services on the population they serve. Several complex methods of assessing the effects or outcome of genetic counseling have been described but these are more extensive than our program permitted. We attempted a simple estimate of impact by assessing change in the client's reproductive behavior. In a majority of instances this outcome was clear, as decisions for continuation of pregnancy, termination, prenatal diagnosis, etc., were made within the survey period. In others, our interpretation is based on direct questions and clients' answers although time has not permitted them to demonstrate fidelity to their answers. In some, as with those who declined reproduction in the face of a high risk, time may allow them to change their decision either with new procedures which will allow modification of the risk, or because of changed attitudes toward risk. In any event, the responses show several interesting trends (Table 7). A large percentage of clients who seek counseling have a magnified perception of their risk which can be moderated by counseling. This invariably provides reassurance and relief and usually allows family planning where none was considered or continuation of a pregnancy fraught with anxiety and uncertainty. Another sizable segment is using prenatal diagnosis or other risk modifying techniques to proceed with reproductive plans in the face of high risk. There is no doubt that this segment of the population will continue to increase. Finally, it is noteworthy that few who come for counseling will ignore high risks and proceed without modification of reproductive plans. At least those who get to genetic counseling appear to utilize it.

Summary

We have described one example of regionalization of clinical genetic services through the establishment of community based satellite genetic clinics maintained by a cooperative effort between a medical school based genetic center and local medical facilities. These satellite community genetic clinics are organized in a similar fashion to genetic clinics elsewhere except for certain technological resources which are not directly at hand to deliver services. The clinics

TABLE 6

Opportunity for Genetic Counseling (Physician)

	Center	Satellite
1. No opportunity, condition not recognized as genetic	8%	9%
2. Condition recognized but no counseling given or suggested	16%	24%
3. Counseling suggested but no referral or direction to service	0%	1%
4. Counseling delivered accurately or referral instituted	76%	67%

TABLE 7

Impact of Genetic Service

	Center	Satellite
1. Low risk – no change in reproductive behavior	19%	22%
2. Low risk –reassurance and positive reproductive change	41%	34%
3. High risk – no change in reproductive behavior	6%	8%
4. High risk – negative reproductive change – no reproduction (adoption?)	3%	3%
5. High risk – positive reproductive change – use of prenatal diagnosis, AID	15%	24%
6. Unknown	16%	9%

depend on quality resources, especially in personnel to act as local contacts, referral sources, and advocates for the service. With appropriate cooperation the clinics deliver the same quality genetic services available in large medical centers and, in addition, offer unique opportunities for education and service to a new population.

REFERENCES

1. L.G. Jackson, L.A. Peris, F.S. Cowchock, G.C. Carpenter and M.A. Barr, *Am. Soc. Hum. Genet (Abs.)*, 44a, 1974.
2. L.G. Jackson and M.A. Barr, *in* Genetic Counseling, H.A. Lubs and F. de la Cruz (Eds.), Raven Press, New York, pp. 83-91, 1977.
3. C.J. Epstein, R.P. Erickson, B.D. Hall and M.S. Golbus, *Am. J. Hum. Genet. 27*, 322-332, 1975.
4. C.J. Epstein, Regionalization of genetic services, see elsewhere this volume.
5. V.M. Riccardi, *in* The Prevention of Genetic Disease and Mental Retardation, W.B. Saunders Co., Philadelphia, 1975.

EVOLUTION OF A CENTER-SATELLITE SYSTEM FOR GENETIC COUNSELING

Charles J. Epstein

The distribution and delivery of medical and health care are matters of paramount public concern at the present, and genetic counseling – despite its relative newness as a medical service – has not escaped scrutiny. With the passage of the National Genetic Diseases Act of 1976 (P.L. 94-278), the federal government formally expressed an interest, still to be realized, in improving the availability and quality of genetic services. For many reasons the mechanisms for accomplishing these goals have not as yet been implemented or even decided upon, and it is important, therefore, to consider a variety of approaches before any specific system is adopted. In this article, I shall describe a satellite system for genetic counseling which has developed over a period of nine years and which, perhaps more significantly, is still evolving and adapting to changing circumstances. Other satellite clinic systems have been developed and are described elsewhere.[1–6]

The genetics clinic at the University of California, San Francisco (UCSF) was started 10 years ago as a conventional University Hospital referral clinic, and it still continues to operate essentially in that manner. However, a year after the USCF clinic began, the first satellite clinic was started in Ross, a suburban community about 16 miles away from San Francisco. During the following nine years, a total of 14 clinics was established (Fig. 1), covering at one time an area of 120,600 square miles (113,800 in California, 73% of the state's land area; the remainder in Nevada) and a population (in 1974) of 9,150,000. At the present time the number of satellite clinics in operation has, for reasons to be discussed below, been reduced to 9 (Fig. 1). Although the area served has decreased by only 15%, to 103,000 square miles, the population has been reduced by a third to about 6,000,000.

The growth of this center-satellite system was controlled partly by chance and partly by design. The element of chance was contributed principally by the

---

*This work was supported in part by grants from the National Foundation-March of Dimes, the National Institutes of Health (GM-19527), and the Maternal and Child Health Service (Project No. 455). The author is an Investigator of the Howard Hughes Medical Institute.

ISBN 0-12-562650-9

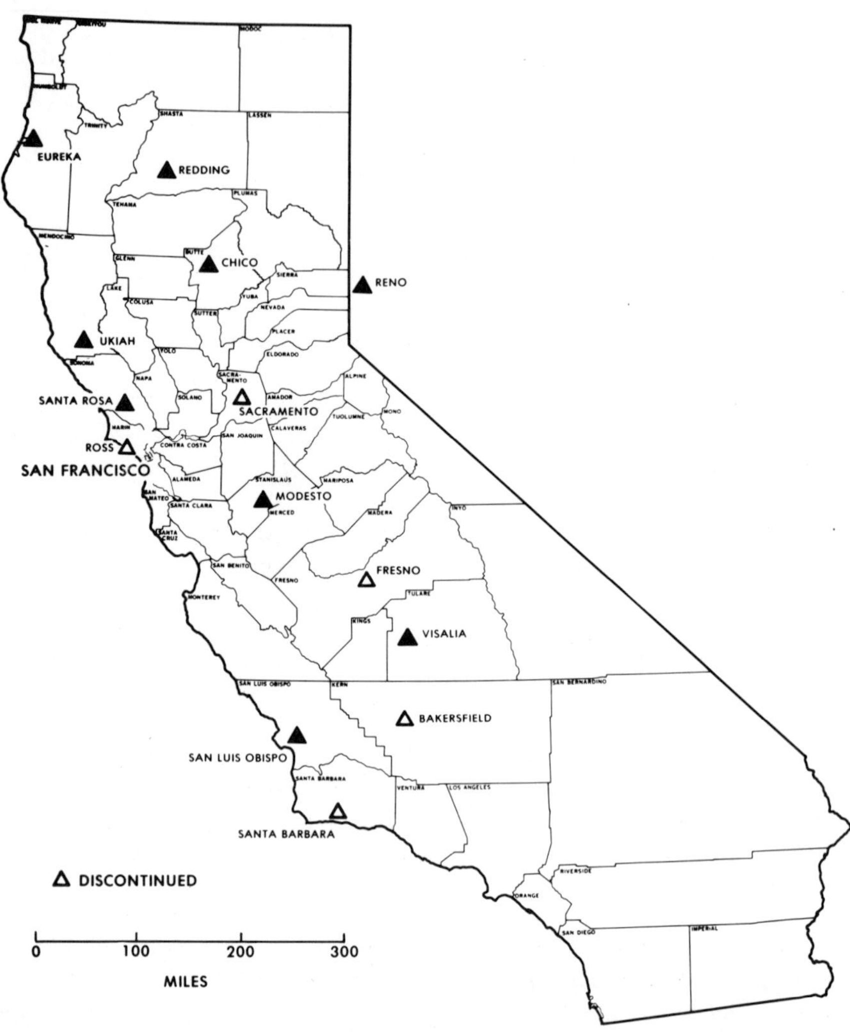

Fig. 1. Locations of existing and discontinued satellite genetic counseling clinics of University of California, San Francisco, as of November 1977.

combination of local expression of interest in having a satellite clinic established in the community and our willingness to establish one. It is for this reason that clinics were established in cities such as Santa Barbara and Bakersfield which are as distant as 340 miles from San Francisco and within 100 miles of Los Angeles with its profusion of medical genetic units. The element of design was represented by our desire to have clinics located in major population areas which were not receiving any significant amount of service and were receptive to the idea of having a clinic located there. The more recent clinics in Eureka, Santa Rosa, Ukiah, and Reno fall within this category.

The methods for establishing and operating clinics have been extensively discussed in an earlier report[7] and will not be described in detail here. In brief, each satellite clinic meets once every two or three months at a community medical facility such as a county public health clinic, a regional center for the mentally retarded, or a hospital. The UCSF medical genetics group is always represented by a staff medical geneticist, usually by one or more postdoctoral fellows, and sometimes by a nonphysician genetic counselor. The local community is represented by public health nurses who do preclinic information gathering and postclinic follow-up, and in some instances by physicians with related interests, or by nonphysician geneticists. Specialized laboratory studies such as chomosome analysis and amino acid chromatography are performed at USCF, but other studies are done locally whenever possible. The general "flavor" of each clinic is a function of local factors and of the particular USCF medical geneticist (there are now five) who is in charge, and no two clinics operate in precisely the same manner.

Since no reliable measures of the effectiveness and quality of genetic counseling yet exist, there is no appropriate way to evaluate the counseling carried out at the central UCSF clinic. Nevertheless, it is possible, as in the initial report,[7] to present some subjective impressions. Overall, there appears to be little difference in diagnostic acuity, risk calculation, and initial counseling between the central and the satellite clinics. This uniformity is insured by the close communication among all of the medical geneticists and postdoctoral fellows in the group. However, since it is often carried out by persons without specialized training and experience in genetic counseling, the initial information gathering tends to be more variable in the satellite clinics, but it is still generally quite satisfactory. The same is also true of follow-up services. Because of the distances involved and the greater number of people involved in the counseling on a part-time basis in the satellite clinics, the rapport between the medical geneticists and the other counselors is often not as close as in the central clinic. On the other hand, the satellite clinics, by virtue of a combination of factors including proximity to the patient's or family's home, lack of the university hospital and clinic aura, the presence of fewer people in the general vicinity, the appreciation of the fact that the medical geneticist has traveled some distance from San Francisco to the local clinic, and the generally more pleasant and relaxed surroundings, are often more conducive to the establishment of a warm and comfortable relationship between

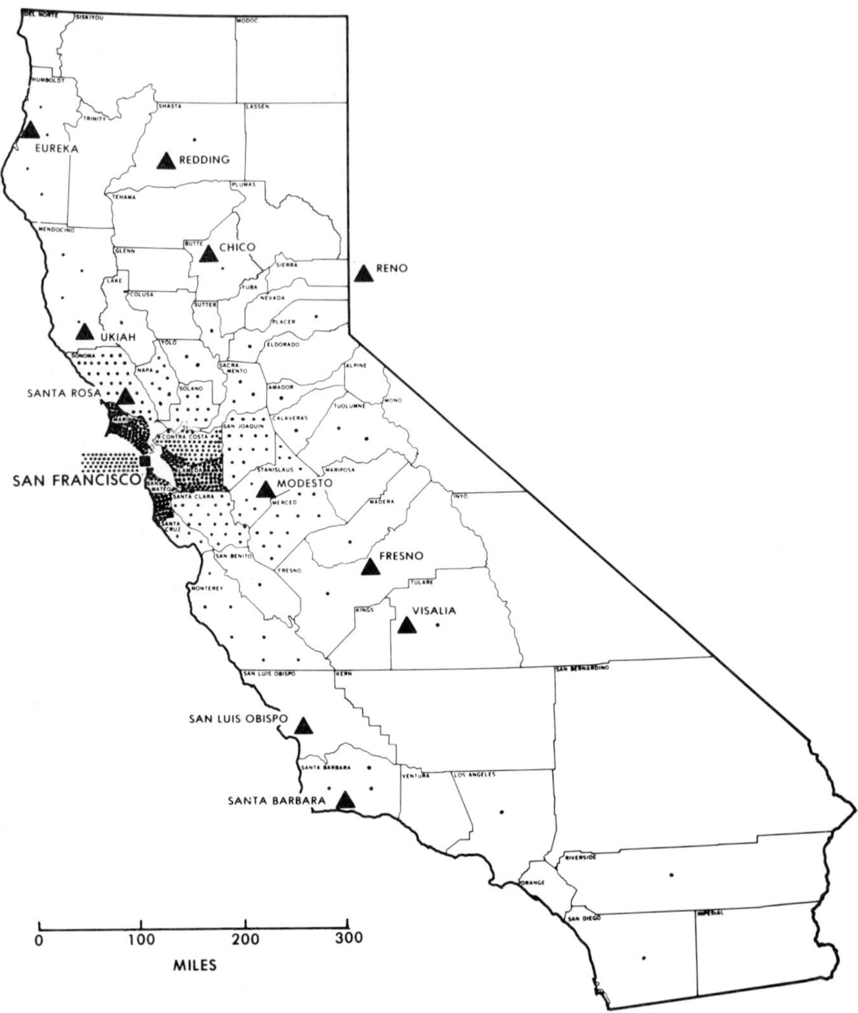

Fig. 2. Families seen in the central San Francisco genetic counseling clinic in 1976, by county of residence. Each dot indicates an individual family.

clients and counselors. Furthermore, the families seen in the satellite clinics often come from less affluent social groups and represent ethnic groups such as Mexican-American, not as often seen at the USCF central clinic. Nevertheless, it is our overall impression that counseling in the central and satellite clinics, while differing in many details, is generally similar and equivalent in quality.

It is, of course, much easier to compare the central and satellite clinics in terms of the numbers of families or patients seen and the geographic areas represented. In the earlier report[7] it was demonstrated that the establishment of a satellite clinic in a specific area led to our seeing many times the number of families from the area than had previously been seen in the central clinic. This has clearly been the case with the newer clinics as well. Furthermore, when the distributions of families seen at UCSF and in the satellite clinics are compared, it is clear that they are complementary. The UCSF clinic primarily serves San Francisco itself and the surrounding area within a radius of about 100-150 miles (Fig. 2). The satellite clinics, on the other hand, while overlapping to some extent at the periphery of the central clinic region, primarily reach the population living between 100 and 300 miles from San Francisco (Fig. 3).

While absolute numbers give an idea of how many families are seen and where they come from, they do not provide a very good estimate of how effective the satellite clinics are in reaching and providing services to the population. Thus, while certain counties are represented by one or only a very few families, these figures become much more significant when considered in relationship to the actual populations of the regions. The data applicable to our central and satellite clinics for 1976 have been calculated in terms of families per 100,000 population per year and the results are shown in Table 1. For the central UCSF clinic, the rates of clinic utilization for the counties close to San Francisco range from 5 to 17.5, with the rates for the city of San Francisco itself and the immediately adjacent Marin, Conta Costa, and Alameda counties being 10.9, 17.5, 6.9, and 6.6, respectively. These are counties which are not heavily served by the genetics clinic at Stanford. By comparison, when the counties in which satellite clinics are located are analyzed, the rates for clinic utilization ranges from 6.4 to 33.4. Four counties, Mendocino, Shasta, Tulare, and Washoe in Nevada, have rates of greater than 20. Furthermore, there is a spreading effect so that adjoining counties also reach high rates of utilization. For example, Tehama county, between the Redding and Visalia clinics, has a rate of 19; Kings County, equidistant from Fresno and Visalia, has a rate of 16.2.

It appears, therefore, that the satellite clinics are more effective in reaching the surrounding population than is the central UCSF clinic itself. The mean rate of utilization for the counties which themselves have satellite clinics is 16.3, while that for San Francisco and its adjacent three counties is 8.7, a ratio of 1.9:1. The explanations for this difference are fairly obvious. Patient referrals to the UCSF clinic occur by conventional means, with a mixture of physician, agency, and self referrals. All of these sources also apply to the satellite clinics as well, but there are three important differences. One is the large amount of case finding by the

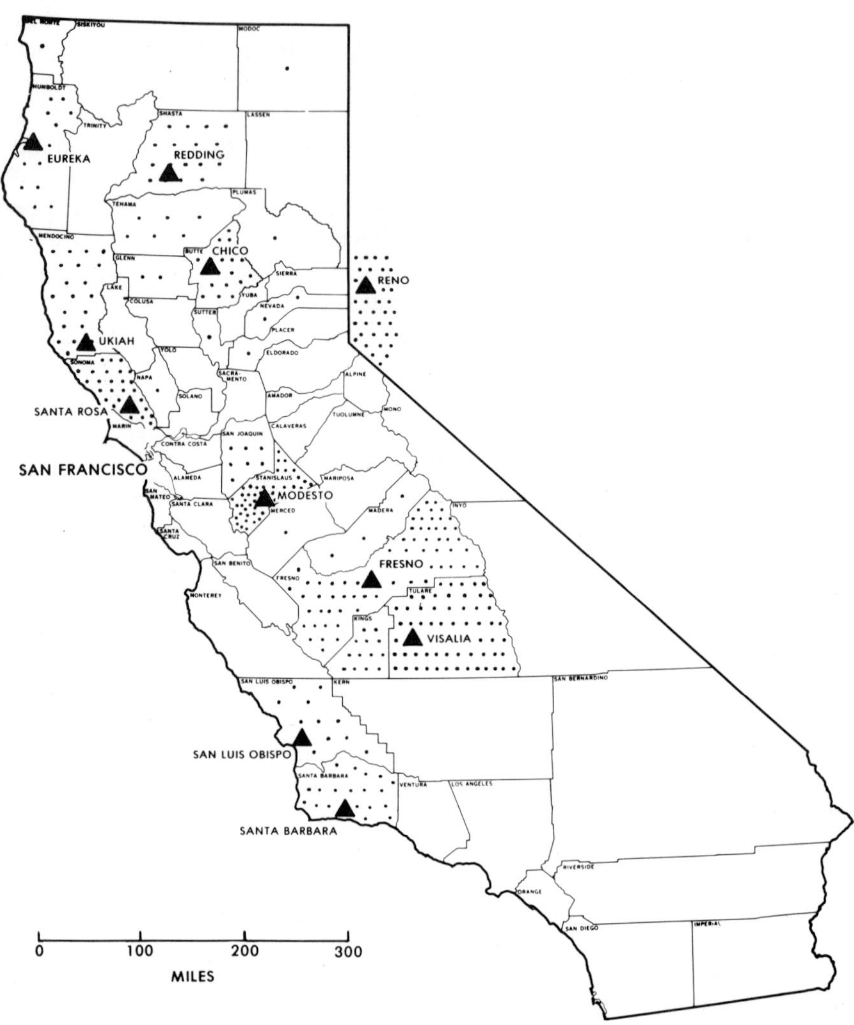

Fig. 3. Families seen in satellite genetic counseling clinics in 1976, by county of residence. Each dot indicates an individual family.

public health nurses associated with the satellite clinics. Because of their involvement in a variety of programs relating to mental retardation, physical and developmental disabilities, and family planning, the public health nurses, particularly in less urban areas, are in a unique position to ascertain families for whom genetic counseling would be appropriate. And, once ascertained, the personal involvement of these nurses with the satellite clinic makes referral immediate and direct. The second difference relates to the nature of physician referrals. In smaller communities, the bulk of specialized services, such as pediatrics and the evaluation of retarded and disabled children, are provided by a relatively small number of physicians. Once these physicians become convinced of the usefulness of genetic counseling, they are likely to be more consistent in making referrals than are physicians in the urban San Francisco area who are less likely to have had contact with the UCSF clinic. A third difference relates to publicity. Most satellite clinics were initiated and continue to operate with the financial support of the National Foundation-March of Dimes. As part of their public information programs, the local National Foundation chapters have done much to publicize the clinics and their services and thereby to stimulate referrals of all types. There may still be other differences between UCSF and satellite referrals, but the net effect is the same; in areas with satellite clinics, in which there are aggressive case finding, referral, and public information, genetic counseling services are more heavily utilized than they are in the central university hospital clinic.

Coupled with, but not ncecessarily dependent upon, the increase in the number of satellite clinics has been an increase in the number of families seen for genetic counseling each year. In the 5 years between July 1, 1968 and June 30, 1973, 803 patients were seen in San Francisco and 295 in one of the satellite clinics. In the calendar year 1973, 216 families (264 patients) were seen in San Francisco and 185 (210 patients) in one of 12 satellite clinics (5 of which were established in 1973). A two-fold increase in both UCSF and satellite clinic referrals occurred between 1973 and 1976, and in 1976, 412 families were seen in San Francisco and 370 in one of the 10 satellite clinics. Despite this growth over the past four years, the proportion of total cases seen in the satellite clinics has remained tively constant, with 46.1% and 47.3% of families being counseled in a satellite clinic in 1973 and 1976, respectively. These figures do not include the very large number of patients seen in San Francisco for prenatal diagnosis who are counseled in a separate clinic.

Although a total of 14 satellite clinics were at one time operated by the UCSF medical genetics group, this number has now been reduced to 9 (Fig. 1). With a view to what can be learned about the establishment of satellite clinics, it is instructive to consider the factors which led to discontinuation of these clinics. An overriding factor was time. No clinic was discontinued solely because there was not enough medical geneticist time available to run it. However, it did not require very much more in the nature of adverse factors to lead to a decision to discontinue a clinic.

The Ross clinic was the first to be established and, for sentimental reasons, the

TABLE 1

Families Seen for Genetic Counseling in 1976

County of Origin	Population in 1974	USCF Clinic		Satellite Clinics	
		Total	Per 100,000	Total	Per 100,000
Alameda	1,087,300	72	6.6		
Amador	14,700	1	6.8		
Butte*	114,100	1	0.9	14	12.3
Calaveras	15,500	1	6.5		
Contra Costa	578,300	40	6.9		
Del Norte	15,300			1	6.5
Fresno*	439,500	1	0.2	66	15.0
Glenn	18,600			2	10.8
Humboldt*	104,900	4	3.8	17	16.2
Kings	68,000			11	16.2
Lake	24,200	1	4.1		
Los Angeles	6,955,500	1	0.01		
Madera	45,100	1	2.2	3	6.7
Marin	211,500	37	17.5		
Mendocino*	56,900	4	7.0	19	33.4
Merced	115,100	11	9.6	1	0.9
Modoc	8,200			1	12.2
Monterey	261,600	7	2.7		
Napa	86,900	8	9.2	1	1.2
Nevada	31,900			2	6.3
Placer	87,900	2	2.3	1	1.1
Plumas	13,600			1	7.4
Riverside	514,200	1	0.2		
Sacramento	682,600	3	0.4		
San Benito	19,200	1	5.2		
San Diego	1,527,700	1	0.07		
San Francisco	679,200	74	10.9		

TABLE 1 (Continued)

Families Seen for Genetic Counseling in 1976

County of Origin	Population in 1974	USCF Clinic		Satellite Clinics	
		Total	Per 100,000	Total	Per 100,000
San Joaquin	298,500	15	5.0	7	2.4
San Luis Obispo*	122,000			12	9.8
San Mateo	568,900	39	6.9		
Santa Barbara*	279,200	3	1.1	17	6.4
Santa Clara	1,169,400	19	1.6		
Santa Cruz	145,000	3	2.1		
Shasta*	86,200	1	1.2	19	22.0
Solano	181,200	9	5.0		
Sonoma*	238,500	26	10.9	30	12.6
Stanislaus*	207,800	9	4.3	31	14.9
Sutter	45,200	1	2.2	1	2.2
Tehama	31,600			6	19.0
Tulare*	202,600	1	0.5	65	32.1
Tuolumne	25,400	2	7.9		
Washoe (Nevada)*	121,068			31	25.6
Yolo	98,600	2	2.2		
Other and Unknown		10		1	
Total		412	782	370	
% of Total		52.7%		47.3%	

*County with satellite clinic

most difficult to stop. The factors leading to its cessation were the desire to devote more time to the nearby Santa Rosa clinic which was rapidly growing in referrals, the proximity of Ross to San Francisco, and a general decline in census because direct referrals to UCSF were being made because of the shorter lag time between referral and counseling. The Santa Rosa clinic, which is still within convenient driving distance of San Francisco, about 1 to 1½ hours, has not suffered similarly although about equal numbers of families from Sonoma county are seen at UCSF and in Santa Rosa (Table 1). A low rate of referral, coupled with *great* distance from San Francisco, was responsible for discontinuation of the Santa Barbara clinic, the last clinic to be discontinued. While the distance *per se* was not critical, since Santa Barbara and San Luis Obispo were seen in tandem, the low referral rate was. While all of the reasons for the poor utilization of the Santa Barbara clinic will never be known, there is one which, operative from the start, and while recognized, was not acted upon when the decision to start the clinic was made. Each major medical center has its own area of influence. Despite the presence of other major university and non-university medical centers in Northern and Central California, most communities, even as far south as San Luis Obispo, feel that they belong, in whole or in part, to the UCSF orbit. Santa Barbara definitely does not and looks to the Los Angeles institutions for consultation. The Santa Barbara medical community never appeared willing to accept a satellite clinic coming from the North rather than the South and, as a result, enthusiasm was never more than lukewarm. In addition, it is quite likely that many families were being referred directly to medical genetics units in the Los Angeles area.

The Bakersfield clinic was discontinued because of its great distance, our inability to provide as much medical geneticist time as the local collaborators desired, and our feeling that it ought to be affiliated with a Los Angeles area group. The Sacramento clinic, which was run jointly with the University of California, Davis Medical School, was discontinued because of lack of appropriate local support. The Fresno clinic has also been discontinued quite recently because it is no longer needed, for a reason which is very important to discuss.

The satellite clinic system was developed because we felt that wide-scale provision of genetic counseling was desirable and knew of no other way to provide these services in a large geographical area with a very spread-out population. However, the availability of a medical geneticist from San Francisco every two or three months is still not the same as having a specialist present in the area all of the time. By a series of fortuitous events, including establishment by UCSF of a regional postgraduate medical program, the precedent of a successful genetic counseling clinic, and the presence of a trained medical geneticist in the area, it became possible to establish a full-time community hospital based genetic counseling clinic in Fresno (Fig. 4). This clinic, which has been operative for only a year, saw a total of 283 patients between September 1, 1976 and August 31, 1977 – four times the number seen in the USCF-Fresno satellite clinic during the preceding year. Blood samples are still sent to UCSF for cytogenetic evaluation,

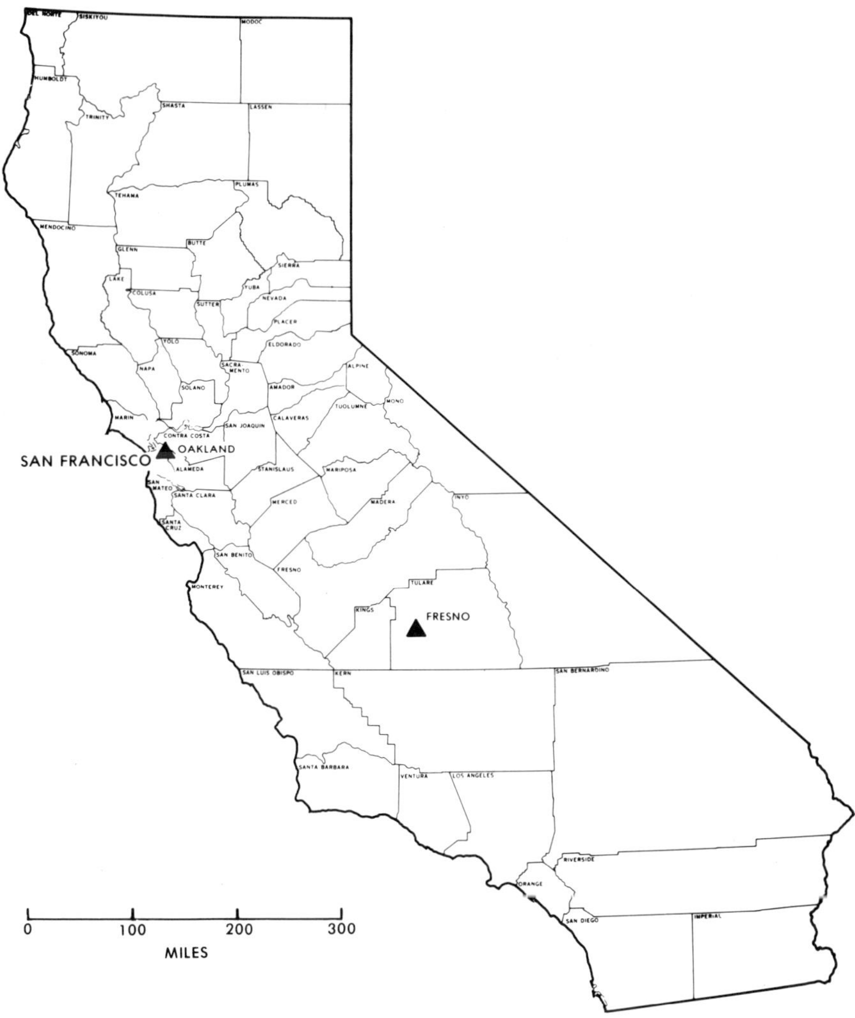

Fig. 4. Locations of independent genetic counseling centers affiliated with the University of California, San Francisco.

and frequent consultation by phone, and occasionally in person, with the UCSF medical genetics group takes place. Thus, what was originally a satellite clinic has evolved into a full time, independent but still affiliated community based genetic counseling clinic. This is a form of evolution which we consider to be highly desirable and would encourage whenever possible.

A similar type of full time, independent but affiliated counseling unit has also been established in Oakland (Fig. 4), within 10 miles of the UCSF clinic. The Oakland clinic, again community hospital based, has its own cytogenetic capabilities and is now developing capabilities for prenatal diagnosis. To maintain close liaison, the members of the Oakland clinic actively participate in the activities of the central UCSF clinic. Although 134 patients were seen and 172 karyotypes performed during the 14 month period between August 1, 1976 and September 30, 1977, there has not been any decrease in the number of families seen and karyotypes performed in San Francisco during the same period of time. The immediate inference is that the availability of resources leads to a marked and rapid increase in their utilization and in the number of families served.

For those less populous areas in which the establishment of independent genetic counseling clinics is unlikely, improvement in the quality of the services in the existing clinics is still desirable. As was mentioned earlier, there is a major difference between the UCSF and many (not all) fo the satellite clinics with regard to preclinic information gathering and postclinic follow-up services. This difference stems from the greater training and experience possessed by the nonphysician genetic counselors at UCSF as compared with that of the public health nurses and others who fill similar roles in the satellite clinics. Recently the California Legislature passed a law, SB 873, which provides for the funding, on a two year trial basis, of eight nonphysician genetic counselors in non-urban areas. It is my hope that several of these counselors, who must by law be supervised by a medical geneticist and will be individuals with a masters degree in genetic counseling or with equivalent training and experience, will be directly affiliated with one or more of the existing satellite clinics. They will then be in a position to directly influence the quality of the service, both by their own activities and by educating the other professionals who work with the satellite clinics. There is, of course, a danger that the nonphysician counselors might be placed in the undesirable position of having to provide genetic counseling in an independent manner, but it is hoped that, with judicious planning and implementation, this can be avoided.

In the earlier report on the UCSF center-satellite system a detailed financial analysis was presented.[7] The satellite clinics have been operated without cost to the consulting families, and the major expenses for the operation of these clinics have been borne by the National Foundation-March of Dimes in the form of a single comprehensive service grant. How long such support can or will continue is unknown, but outside support from private, state, or federal sources is essential for continued maintenance of the program. Otherwise it will be come necessary to charge fees which would be likely to act as a serious deterrent to many in seeking genetic counseling and would, because of the significant business aspects which would be necessitated, make the satellite mechanism much less attractive to the providers.

Summary

The continued evolution of the UCSF center-satellite system for the delivery of genetic counseling services has been discussed. Since its inception with one satellite clinic in 1968, this system has progressed through the establishment of 14 satellite clinics and has, for the moment, stabilized with 9 satellites throughout northern and central California and northwestern Nevada. While the quality of counseling provided is considered to be comparable with the central and satellite clinics, the rate of clinic utilization is about two-fold greater in the areas served by satellite clinics than in San Francisco and its surrounding counties. The work of the satellite and central clinics is now being complemented by that of other genetic counseling units, including two which are community based and independent but still affiliated with UCSF. Financial support for nonphysician genetic counselors by the state should lead to an improvement in the nonmedical aspects of the counseling process, and outside financial support will continue to be necessary for optimal operation.

REFERENCES

1. C.L. Clow, F.C. Fraser, C. Laberge and C.R. Scriver, *Prog. Med. Genet. 9*, 159, 1973.
2. V.M. Riccardi, *Amer. J. Pub. Health 66*, 268, 1976.
3. K.R. Reid, N. Sakati, L.L. Pritchard, L.J. Schneiderman, O.W. Jones and B.K. Dixson, *West. J. Med. 124*, 6, 1976.
4. L.G. Jackson and M.A. Barr, *in* Genetic Counseling, H.A. Lubs and F. de la Cruz (Eds.), Raven Press, New York, p. 83, 1977.
5. L.B. Schechter, N.F. Bartnoff and S.F. Wang, *Amer. J. Hum. Genet. 29*, 94A, 1977.
6. R.E. Stevenson, *Amer. J. Hum. Genet. 29,* 104A, 1977.
7. C.J. Epstein, R.P. Erickson, B.H. Hall and M.S. Golbus, *Amer. J. Hum. Genet. 27*, 322, 1975.

A COMMUNITY APPROACH TO PRENATAL DIAGNOSIS

Godfrey P. Oakley, Jr.
Karlene Brantley
Andrew T.L. Chen
Paul M.Fernhoff
Marshall F. Goldberg
Jean H. Priest
Suzanne Trusler

THE PROBLEM

The President's Committee on Mental Retardation has set as a national goal the reduction of the incidence of mental retardation by 50% by the year 2000. Clarke and Clarke[1] have recently reviewed the likelihood of reaching this goal. They note that 25% of mental retardation is characterized as severe and 75% as mild. They conclude that prospects of reducing the incidence by 50% is good for the causes of severe mental retardation, but it is not likely for the causes of mild mental retardation.

The incidence of severe mental retardation can be reduced through two general approaches – those due to social changes and those due to specific attempts to lower mental retardation by genetic counseling, prenatal diagnosis, and the treatment of metabolic defects. Down syndrome is the most common cause of severe mental retardation, accounting for approximately 30% of severe mental retardation.[2] With social changes, the decreasing percentage of births to older women has made a substantial impact on this disease, and much of that impact has occurred over the past 15 years. In 1960, 10.7% of all births in the United States were to women 35 and older.[3] In 1973, the percentage had dropped to 5.1%. Between 1960 and 1973 the estimated frequency of Down syndrome changed from 1/833 births or about 1.2 per thousand, to 1/1,123 births or 0.9 per thousand. In 1960, 45% of the infants with Down syndrome were born to these older women, while in 1973 it was only 28%. Recent data indicate that the proportion of births to women 35 and older has plateaued.[4] Thus, this demographic change has had an influence on the incidence of Down syndrome, but it is unlikely that it will have much additional impact. General improvement in health and medical care seem unlikely to have much impact on this problem either. We must then look at what specific activities or programs are feasible. We

ISBN 0-12-562650-9

look here at fetal chromosomal diagnosis.

The mere availability of preventive or ameliorative services does not mean they will be used.[1] It is necessary to find a way for those in need of the service to have access to it. Prenatal chromosomal diagnosis, for example, is a case in point. It is theoretically available but those at high risk, for some reason, were not using the service. We wanted to look at this issue and try to increase access to prenatal chromosomal diagnosis. Our purpose in this paper is to describe our efforts and some of the results.

There are several groups at high risk for having a fetus with Down syndrome. In general, these groups can be divided into those with a positive family history of Down syndrome or translocation Down syndrome carrier state, and those with advanced maternal age. In the former group the *a priori* risk for a fetus with a chromosomal disorder ranges from 1% to 100%, while in the latter the risk ranges from 0.5% to 5%. There is, however, quite a notable difference in the number of women in each group. No one knows for certain the number in the former group, but it is unlikely to be larger than 10,000 a year in this country. More than 10 times this number are known to be at increased risk due to maternal age. In 1975 in the United States, there were 143,000 births to women 35 and older.[5]

We suspected that there was also a difference in the availability of prenatal diagnosis for the two groups. It seemed that families with a Down syndrome child would be more likely to find out that they were at increased recurrence risk and that prenatal chromosomal diagnosis was available. On the other hand, we felt that the probability of older women being informed about the test was lower. A survey done in 1976 by the President's Committee on Mental Retardation[6] had indicated that only 10,000 prenatal chromosomal diagnoses were done in that year, indicating an under usage of the service. With the preceeding assumptions in mind, we took a community approach to increase the availability of prenatal diagnosis for older pregnant women.

THE PLAN

There are several steps that must be taken to implement such a program. First, one must establish a goal. Our goal was that all women in the seven-county metropolitan Atlanta area, 37 and older, would make a timely, informed decision for or against prenatal chromosomal diagnosis. Then one must identify the program elements. One needs availability of high-quality laboratory services through the cooperation and collaboration of various laboratories in the community. An estimate of the capacity of these laboratories will indicate how to focus the program. One does not want to generate more samples than can be handled.

There must also be support from the medical community – particularly the physicians who practice obstetrics – and the public health sector. There must be lay support as well. When the number of specimens that can be handled is established and the cooperation of the laboratories, physicians, and the lay community is obtained, one can plan and implement the program.

The program must have several components: (1) identification of high-risk groups, (2) counseling regarding the availability, benefits, and dangers of prenatal diagnosis, (3) access to amniocentesis, and (4) post-amniocentesis counseling.

The seven-county metropolitan Atlanta area was selected as a target population and has approximately 25,000 births a year. Nine hundred of these births are to women 35 and older, and 137 are to women 40 and older. A laboratory doing chromosomal analysis of amniotic fluid and other studies had been set up at Emory University in the Department of Pediatrics, Division of Medical Genetics, in 1972. An additional laboratory was established at the Center for Disease Control (CDC) in late 1975. It was agreed that CDC would handle, without charge, the analysis of amniotic fluids from women in the seven-county area who would be 40 or older at delivery. The Emory University Laboratory would accept all other prenatal diagnoses on a fee for service basis.

The target group identification would obviously be a function of the persons doing obstetrics. We anticipated that some obstetricians would want to do the counseling and amniocentesis and that others would want to refer to a center. Center counseling facilities appeared to be a possible rate-limiting function, so we offered to support and teach those physicians who wanted to do the counseling, particularly of older pregnant women. We presented a seminar on prenatal diagnosis at the obstetric staff meeting of each hospital in the seven-county metropolitan Atlanta area. These seminars were presented between January and May 1976. Table 1 shows the handout we used at these seminars. We made a deliberate attempt to simplify this handout by highlighting those indications that a practitioner might be expected to see. We also gave the telephone numbers of each laboratory so that they would be available for consultations and patient scheduling. Appendix I is a "Questions and Answers" pamphlet we developed for the physician to have available for his patients. We then wrote a detailed informed consent, including a quiz (Appendix II, a and b) which was used for CDC specimens. We believe that patients who can pass this quiz are informed about the most pertinent points concerning prenatal chromosomal diagnosis. However, it was necessary to have a different informed consent form for use at Emory University (Appendix III). Appendix IV shows our amniocentesis intake form. We have encouraged physicians to call either of the laboratories when they have identified a women who wants the service. We make these materials available by mailing them to physicians. The CDC mailing also includes a syringe for transport of amniotic fluid and a heparinized tube for a sample of the woman's blood.

THE RESULTS

We can look first at the women 40 and older. In 1975, before the community effort was initiated, 10/138, or 7.2%, had fetal chromosomal diagnosis (Table 2). In the first six months of 1976, the percentage rose to 10.3% and in the last six

TABLE 1

Present Indications for Prenatal Diagnosis

1. Maternal age 37 and over
2. Previous child with trisomic Down syndrome or other trisomy
3. A parent known to carry a chromosomal abnormality
4. Previous child with anencephaly or myelomeningocele
5. Families at risk for an X-linked recessive disorder, or at risk for an autosomal recessive disorder known to be detectable *in utero*.

TABLE 2

Percentage of Older Gravidas in Metropolitan Atlanta Having Fetal Chromosomal Diagnosis, 1975-1977

Ages	1975	Jan.-June 1976	July-Dec. 1976	Jan.-June 1977
35-36	10/464	8/242	9/242	26/242
	2.2%	3.3%	3.7%	10.7%
37-39	8/298	15/153	26/153	32/153
	2.7%	9.8%	17.0%	20.9%
⩾40	10/138	8/78	22/78	18/78
	7.2%	10.3%	28.2%	23.1%

TABLE 3

Fetal Chromosomal Diagnosis: Metropolitan Atlanta, 1976

Number of Amniocenteses and Number of Fetal Chromosomal Diagnoses

	Center Amniocentesis		Non-center	
	Physician No. 1	Physician No. 2	Amniocentesis	Total
Number patients tapped	72	15	47	134
1st tap and culture successful	67 (93%)	13 (87%)	35 (74%)	115 (86%)
2nd tap and culture successful	1 (1%)	2 (13%)	8 (17%)	11 (8%)
Number of patients with fetal chromosomal diagnosis	68 (94%)	15 (100%)	43 (91%)	126 (94%)

months it was 28.2%; in other words, it had tripled. In the first six months of 1977, it was 23.1%. In this 18-month period, we detected two fetuses with trisomy 21 Down syndrome and one trisomy 13. Each of these women elected abortion. In the 37 to 39 years old group, the percentage of women having the test has risen from 2.7% or 8/298 in 1975, to 9.8% in the first 6 months of 1976, to 17.0% in the last six months of 1976, and was 20.9% in 1977. In the 37-39 age group, between January 1976 and June 1977, there was one fetus diagnosed as trisomy 18. The pregnancy ended with a spontaneous abortion. For women 35 and 36, there was a slight increase to 3.7% in the last six months of 1976, compared to 2.2% in 1975. In 1977, 10.7% of women 35 and 36 had the procedure.

In a communty rather than a genetic center approach, there is the possibility that safety and reliability could suffer. In 1976, 126/134, or 94%, of women who underwent amniocentesis for prenatal chromosomal diagnosis had a diagnosis, 86% requiring only one amniocentesis (last column, Table 3). In the first half of 1977, 98% of women had a diagnosis, 87% requiring only one amniocentesis (last column, Table 4). These figures are comparable to the NICHD national amniocentesis study.[7]

In our experience, the most common reason for a second amniocentesis was the initial failure to obtain fluid the first time. Two obstetricians who are closely affiliated with the Emory University Division of Medical Genetics (Center Amniocentesis), needed to repeat amniocentesis less often than the remaining physicians in the community (Non-center Amniocentesis – Table 3 and Table 4. In 1976, the percentage of patients who had an amniocentesis and received a fetal karyotype report was slightly less for the Non-center group, but the percentages for the two groups in the first part of 1977 were similar.

DISCUSSION

It was our intention that the physicians' educational program would promote an increased access to fetal chromosomal diagnosis for women in the risk group ⩾ 37 years, while protecting the laboratories and other clinical genetic services from being overwhelmed by specimens and consultations from the lower risk group, women 35 to 36. This inundation was a real possibility, as there are more births to women 35 and 36 than there are to those ⩾ 37. The data in Table 2 show that in the last six months of 1976, compared to the first six months, there was logarithmic increase in use by women in the two older age groups, while the use was essentially unchanged in the 35 to 36 year group. These data suggest that the educational seminars were effective. Use of the procedure by women 40 and older plateaued in the 25% range suggesting that only about 25% of older women will have the procedure. The percentage of women 37 to 39 has approached this level even though there is a fee for the analysis, indicating that cost has apparently not prevented access to the amniocentesis in this community.

What are the problems, and what needs to be done? We have had some

TABLE 4

Fetal Chromosomal Diagnosis, Metropolitan Atlanta, January-June 1977:
Number of Amniocenteses and Number of Fetal Chromosomal Diagnoses

	Center Amniocentesis		Non-center	
	Physician No. 1	Physician No. 2	Amniocentesis	Total
Number of patients tapped	43	36	31	110
1st tap and culture successful	38 (88%)	34 (94%)	24 (77%)	96 (87%)
2nd tap and culture successful	5 (12%)	1 (3%)	6 (19%)	12 (11%)
Number of patients with fetal chromosomal diagnosis	43 (100%)	35 (97%)	30 (97%)	108 (98%)

problems communicating with physicians. Assuring that specimens would be scheduled has been difficult. Some specimens have arrived unannounced or after regular laboratory hours and not transported properly. Specimens have been transported in unorthodox containers such as urine jars. Both laboratories would prefer that the fluid be transported in the disposable syringe in which it is obtained. This reduces the chance of bacterial contamination of the fluid, and has been a safe way to transport fluid. It does not mean, however, that no problems will arise from using syringes, because one manufacturer did use a sealant that was toxic to the amniotic fluid cells.[8]

What needs to be done? It is obvious that even when cost of analysis is free and when a substantial effort is made, only about 25% of those in the highest maternal age risk group (age 40 and older) have the procedure. We do not know about the remaining 75%. Perhaps many did make timely decisions about fetal chromosomal diagnosis and decided not to have it. If so, then we have reached our goal to have every older pregnant woman make an informed, timely decision about fetal chromosomal diagnosis. A study of those women who did not have fetal chromosomal diagnosis is needed before we can know how close we have come to achieving our goal.

We believe those individuals planning programs similar to ours need to anticipate, over the first 18 months of operation, that a maximum of 25% of the highest risk target group will ask for fetal chromosomal diagnosis.[1] This estimate should help in planning for service needs. We, for example, are working with the State of Georgia to establish a statewide effort and are using 25% as an estimate for determining the provision of services.

SUMMARY

We have tried to approach fetal chromosomal diagnosis for older women from a community, population viewpoint. The community we selected was the seven-county metropolitan Atlanta area. We provided laboratory services and conducted an educational program to teach community obstetricians about indications for and availability of prenatal chromosomal diagnosis. We have seen an increase in the proportion of women having the test in our target group of women age 37 and over. Still, only about one-fourth have it. We believe those planning similar programs need to anticipate, over the first 18 months of operation, that a maximum of 25% of the target group will ask for fetal chromosomal diagnosis. This estimate should help in planning for service needs. There are many unanswered questions about why women either do or do not have prenatal chromosomal diagnosis. We must seek answers to these questions and design sensitive program elements to maximize the number of timely, informed decisions about prenatal chromosomal diagnosis among older gravidae.

REFERENCES

1. A.D.B. Clarke and A.M. Clarke, *Am. J. Ment. Defic. 81*, 523, 1977.
2. N. Goodman and J. Tizard, *Brit. Med. J. 1*, 216, 1961.
3. Center for Disease Control, Congenital Malformations Surveillance Report, July 1974-June 1975, issued December 1975.
4. National Center for Health Statistics, Monthly Vital Statistics Report, Vol. 26, No. 12 Supplement, March 29, 1978.
5. National Center for Health Statistics, Monthly Vital Statistics Report, Vol. 25, No. 10 Supplement, December 30, 1976.
6. C.B. Jacobson, Amniocentesis Update: 1976, Proceedings of the International Summit on Prevention of Mental Retardation from Biomedical Causes, December 1977 (in press).
7. The NICHD National Registry for Amniocentesis Study Group, *J.A.M.A. 236*, 1471, 1976.
8. K. Garver, S.L. Marchese and E.G. Boas, *N. Engl. J. Med. 295*, 286, 1976.

APPENDIX I

QUESTIONS and ANSWERS
AMNIOCENTESIS AND FETAL GENETIC DIAGNOSIS IN ATLANTA

U.S. Department of Health, Education, and Welfare
Public Health Service
Center for Disease Control

What is Informed Consent?

Before agreeing to amniocentesis and fetal genetic diagnosis, (one or both) parents will be asked to sign a statement that they understand and have thought about what they have read here and have been told by their physicians.

What are Chromosomes?

Chromosomes are structures made up of genes; they carry hereditary traits. All normal cells in the body (except egg and sperm cells) have 46 chromosomes.

What is Amniocentesis?

Amniocentesis is a medical procedure in which an obstetrician uses a thin hollow needle to withdraw from the uterus (womb) a small amount of amniotic fluid, usually a little less than 1 ounce (20 ml.). The amniotic fluid comes from the sac surrounding the developing fetus. Cells in amniotic fluid are shed from the fetus. The procedure takes only a few minutes, and the patient then goes home.

What is Sonography?

Sonography or ultrasound is a test in which sound waves are used to tell certain things about the pregnancy, such as the position and size of the fetus, if twins are present, and where the placenta is located. There is no known danger to the mother or fetus from the test. A physician may request sonography before performing an amniocentesis.

What is Fetal Chromosomal Diagnosis?

Fetal chromosomal diagnosis is a test to find out if the cells from the amniotic fluid have normal chromosomes. This test can identify fetuses with chromosomal abnormalities, the most common of which is Down syndrome (mongolism). The best time to do an amniocentesis for fetal chromosomal diagnosis is in the 15th week after a woman's last menstrual period.

How is Fetal Chromosomal Diagnosis Done?

After an amniocentesis, the amniotic fluid is sent to a laboratory where the cells are grown and the chromosomes studied. Results are obtained in about 1 month. About 10% of amniocenteses are repeated either because fluid was not obtained or the cells in the fluid did not grow in the laboratory.

Can Amniocentesis Harm the Mother or Her Fetus?

Although amniocentesis has been performed many times and is an accepted medical procedure, there can be no guarantee that the test will do no harm. Bleeding, infection, or damage to internal organs may occur, but these serious complications usually develop infrequently, no more than 1 time in 200 (0.5%). A miscarriage can occur during any pregnancy, usually during the early weeks. Even after the 3rd month of pregnancy, 3 or 4 out of every 100 pregnancies still end with a miscarriage. Amniocentesis does not increase the chance of a miscarriage.

Who Should Consider Having Fetal Chromosomal Diagnosis?

1. Any pregnant woman who will be 37 years or older when she delivers.
2. Any pregnant woman who already has a child with a chromosomal abnormality, such as Down syndrome (mongolism).
3. Any pregnant woman who knows that she or her mate carry a chromosomal abnormality.

How Often is a Fetal Chromosomal Abnormality Found?

One or two out of every 100 pregnant women between the ages of 37 and 40 will have an abnormal fetal chromosomal result. About 4 of every 100 pregnant women over 40 will have an abnormal fetal chromosomal result.

Women who have had a child with Down syndrome (mongolism) and who are younger than 37 have 1 or 2 chances in every 100 of having an abnormal fetal chromosomal result if neither they nor their husbands carry a chromosomal abnormality. If either parent carries a chromosomal abnormality, the chances of the woman having a chromosomally abnormal child are increased.

Does a Normal Chromosomal Result Guarantee That the Baby Will be Normal?

NO! This test identifies only those fetuses with chromosomal abnormalities. Most infants who are born with retardation or some other type of birth defect have normal chromosomes, and the defects therefore cannot be detected with this test.

Will the Chromosomal Result Always Be Correct?

Results are usually correct, but not always. In a twin pregnancy, for example, each fetus is surrounded by its own amniotic fluid, so the fluid from any one amniocentesis will show the chromosomes of only one twin. In some instances the effects upon the fetus of certain chromosomal abnormalities are not clear. In such cases, the decision of whether to continue the pregnancy can be difficult.

If a Fetal Chromosomal Abnormality is Found, Must a Woman Have an Abortion?

NO! But the possibility of abortion should be carefully thought about before the amniocentesis.

Is an Abortion Done After the First 3 Months Dangerous?

No medical procedure, even delivering a baby, is entirely safe. Abortion done in the 4th to 6th month of pregnancy usually requires overnight hospitalization and is more risky than an abortion done during the first 3 months. Still, the risk is quite low – about equal to the risk of having a baby. Since fetal chromosomal diagnosis may take up to a month to complete, the earliest an abortion can be done is during the 4th-5th month of pregnancy. Usually by this time a pregnant woman will have felt the fetus move.

Can Fetal Chromosomal Diagnosis Detect Other Diseases?

Not directly. Fetal chromosomal diagnosis can be used when it is important to know the sex of the fetus. In certain types of hemophilia and in muscular dystrophy, the inheritance is "sex-linked". This means that a male fetus has a 50% chance of having the disease, but females are not affected. Since these diseases cannot be tested directly from the amniotic fluid, the parents may decide to use fetal chromosomal diagnosis to determine the sex of the fetus so that only daughters will be born.

Can Amniocentesis Detect Other Birth Defects?

Yes. Amniocentesis can detect types of severe defects of the head (anencephaly) and spina bifida (open spine). If a fetus has either of these defects, there is too much protein material, called alpha-fetoprotein, in the amniotic fluid. If a woman or her mate has an open spinal defect or if either of them has had a child with one of these defects, she should consider having amniocentesis for the alpha-fetoprotein test.

Amniocentesis can test certain rare "metabolic" diseases. These are usually inherited diseases which often produce severe mental or physical retardation. They are caused by a missing or abnormal enzyme (protein). If parents think they might pass on a genetic disease to their children, they can discuss this possibility and amniocentesis with a genetic counselor.

How Can I Have Fetal Chromosomal Diagnosis Done in the Atlanta Area?

If you are pregnant and will be 37 years of age or older when you deliver, or if you already have a child with a chromosomal disorder, such as Down syndrome (mongolism), or if you or your mate carry a chromosomal abnormality, talk to your doctor. Your physician will discuss the procedure and will arrange for you to have all of the proper tests.

What is the Cost of Fetal Chromosomal Diagnosis in Atlanta?

The physician doing the amniocentesis will set the cost. If sonography is requested, this fee is separate. If you are a resident of Clayton, Cobb, DeKalb, Douglas, Fulton, Gwinnett, or Rockdale counties, and will be 40 or older when you deliver, the Center for Disease Control (CDC), as part of a pilot study, can perform the laboratory analysis without charge. At present, the Division of

Medical Genetics, Emory University, School of Medicine, has a laboratory fee for fetal chromosomal diagnosis. Medical insurance policies and public assistance programs may pay all or a part of these fees.

Note: These appendices have been modified slightly for use in this volume.

APPENDIX IIa
PROGRAM FOR PRENATAL CHROMOSOMAL DIAGNOSIS IN HIGH-RISK PREGNANT WOMEN

PART 1. INFORMED CONSENT

I understand that the Center for Disease Control (CDC), in cooperation with the Georgia Department of Human Resources and the Atlanta Obstetrical and Gynecological Society, is evaluating a community-based program for chromosomal diagnosis of fetuses of pregnant women who expect to be 40 or older at delivery. I have agreed to take part in the program because I have an increased risk of having a baby with a chromosomal abnormality and want to know what the chromosomal constitution of my fetus is. I understand that as a part of this program, I may be asked questions concerning my experience and opinions about amniocentesis. I have been told that I will not be identified by name when program results are published and that no personal information will be voluntarily released by CDC. If important facts about my personal health should be learned during the program, I have asked that they be given to my physician. I realize that **I AM FREE TO WITHDRAW MY PARTICIPATION IN THIS PROGRAM AT ANY TIME.**

As part of this program, I have requested Dr.________________ to obtain a sample of amniotic fluid from my uterus (womb) and send it to CDC for analysis (study). I understand that the fluid will be drawn by a procedure called "transabdominal amniocentesis" which involves inserting a needle into my uterus (womb) through my abdominal and uterine walls. If a local anesthetic (medicine to reduce pain) is used before inserting the needle, I understand that there is a small chance that I might have an adverse reaction to this medicine. **I HAVE NEVER HAD ANY ADVERSE REACTION FROM A LOCAL ANESTHETIC.**

The following points have been explained to me and I understand and accept them:

1. At present, amniocentesis is the only known method for diagnosing chromosomal abnormalities in a fetus.
2. The "transabdominal amniocentesis" procedure has been used many times and is an accepted medical practice. No one, however, can guarantee that it is harmless. The fetus might be struck with a needle, or I might have a miscarriage, infection, pain, or internal damage after the procedure. Such complications due to amniocentesis are believed to occur no more often than one time in 200 (0.5 percent). The chance for miscarriage in this pregnancy, whether or not I have an amniocentesis, is 3-4 percent.
3. There is about 1 chance in 10 that the amniocentesis will have to be repeated, either because the attempt to obtain fluid was unsuccessful or the laboratory analysis was unsuccessful.
4. Tests results are not guaranteed to be 100% accurate, although they are usually correct.

5. If tests results show my baby's chromosomal pattern is normal, my baby might still be mentally retarded or have a birth defect caused by factors which this test will not reveal.
6. If test results show any chromosomal abnormalities, the findings will be explained to me and I will be given the chance to decide whether to continue my pregnancy or to have an abortion.
7. If I am carrying more than one fetus (twins, triplets, etc.), the test results could be misleading. For example, if one twin were normal and the other abnormal and the fluid was taken from the normal one, there would be no indication that I was carrying an abnormal child.
8. The test results will not be available for several weeks.
9. Amniocentesis and chromosomal analysis are available from other sources in the Atlanta area, and I am free to use those services.

Date ______________________ Signed ______________________
(Patient)

Date ______________________ Signed ______________________
(Physician)

APPENDIX IIb

PART II. INFORMED CONSENT

Please write out the words true or false in response to the statements below:

1. Down syndrome (mongolism) is a condition caused by a chromosomal abnormality. Children with Down syndrome usually have physical defects and are mentally retarded.

   ____

2. The chance of having a baby with Down syndrome rises with mother's age. After age 40, a woman has a 1 in 100 chance of having a child with Down syndrome.

   ____

3. Amniocentesis involves inserting a needle through the pregnant woman's abdominal and uterine walls. It is considered to be a safe procedure but occasionally (less than 1 percent of the time) can cause an adverse effect.

   ____

4. The amniocentesis procedure may need to be repeated either if the doctor cannot obtain amniotic fluid or if the cells from the amniotic fluid do not grow or are not usable.

   ____

5. Even if the test results are normal, my baby still might have a birth defect or be mentally retarded, since usually these abnormalities are caused by factors which this test cannot determine.

   ____

6. Under unusual circumstances, the result of the test may be unclear or may present a chromosomal pattern for which, at the present time, only limited information is known. This information and its possible effects will be explained to me, and I will decide whether to continue my pregnancy or terminate it (have an abortion).

   ____

APPENDIX III

INFORMED CONSENT FOR ANTENATAL DIAGNOSIS

We, the undersigned, have requested of Dr. ______________________________
and Dr. ______________________________ that an attempt be made to perform a biochemical or chromosome analysis of our unborn child. We understand that the cells required as a basis for such an analysis are obtained in amniotic fluid by a transabdominal amniocentesis procedure which involves penetration of the mother's abdominal and uterine walls by hypodermic needle.

The following points have been explained to us, and we understand and accept them:

1. That although transabdominal amniocentesis is a proven technique which has been used extensively, and hazard to the mother or fetus is considered to be extremely small, it cannot be guaranteed that the procedure will not cause damage to the mother or the fetus or initiate premature labor, possibly resulting in spontaneous abortion.
2. That any particular attempt to obtain amniotic fluid by transabdominal amniocentesis may be unsuccessful.
3. That any attempt to obtain a viable cell culture from the cells of any particular sample of amniotic fluid may be unsuccessful or the chromosome preparations may be of poor quality and unusable.
4. That although the likelihood of a misinterpretation of the chromosome karyotypes in this case is considered to be extremely small, a complete and correct diagnosis of the condition of the fetus based on the karyotypes obtained cannot be guaranteed.

The results obtained from these procedures may benefit us by confirming the diagnosis of a suspected genetic disease and by giving the sex of the unborn child. Additional studies of cultured cell morphology and biochemistry or virus studies may be performed to provide information needed for interpreting the results of diagnostic amniocentesis or for determining causes of birth defects. There is no guarantee that these additional laboratory studies will provide information useful for this particular pregnancy.

In full recognition of these possible hazards and limitations of the techniques and interpretations involved in the biochemical or chromosome analysis of our unborn child, we elect to have the analysis attempted.

We have read the foregoing information and fully understand it.

Signed: Mother ____________________ Date ____________________

Father ____________________

Please sign and return as soon as possible after a decision is made to have amniocentesis.

APPENDIX IV

AMNIOCENTESIS INTAKE REPORT

AMNIOCENTESIS INTAKE REPORT

FOR STAFF USE ONLY

IDENTIFYING NO. ____________

CDC ________ EMORY ________

DEPARTMENT OF HEALTH, EDUCATION, AND WELFARE
PUBLIC HEALTH SERVICE
CENTER FOR DISEASE CONTROL
BUREAU OF EPIDEMIOLOGY
BUREAU OF LABORATORIES
ATLANTA, GEORGIA 30333

Patient's Name (First, Maiden, Last)	**Date of Birth** ☐☐ Month ☐☐ Day ☐☐ Year	**Race**	**Marital Status** ☐ S ☐ M ☐ W ☐ D ☐ Sep

Address (Number and Street)	**City**	**State**	**Zip Code**	**County**

Home Phone	**Work Phone** (Circle one: husband's, wife's)	**If married, Husband's Name** (First, Middle, Last)

PRESENT PREGNANCY:

LMP: ____________ EDC: ____________

Has the patient had any problems or complications during this pregnancy? ☐ Yes ☐ No ☐ Don't know **IF YES**, what problem(s)? ____________

What medications has the patient taken since the pregnancy began? (Please include non prescription and prescription drugs especially hormones to retain pregnancy, birth control pills and antibiotics.) ____________

PREVIOUS PREGNANCIES:	TOTAL NUMBER	BORN ALIVE	STILLBIRTH OR SPONTANEOUS ABORTIONS	THERAPEUTIC ABORTIONS	NUMBER OF MULTIPLE PREGNANCIES (Twins, etc.)

If stillbirths or spontaneous abortions, check trimester of pregnancy in which the 3 most recent ones occurred.

	TRIMESTER FIRST	SECOND	THIRD
1.	☐	☐	☐
2.	☐	☐	☐
3.	☐	☐	☐

PAST MEDICAL AND FAMILY HISTORY:

Patient's Blood Type: ☐ A ☐ B ☐ AB ☐ O

Rh Type: ☐ Positive ☐ Negative

If Rh Negative, check husband or mate's Rh type: ☐ Positive ☐ Negative ☐ Don't know

Has patient had **DIABETES MELLITUS?** ☐ Yes ☐ No ☐ Don't know

Has the patient or members of her family (or her husband's or mate's family) ever had?

	Yes	No	Don't know	**IF YES,** relationship to fetus:
DOWN'S SYNDROME (mongolism)	☐	☐	☐	
ANENCEPHALY or SPINA BIFIDA (open spine)	☐	☐	☐	
HYDROCEPHALY	☐	☐	☐	
HEMOPHILIA	☐	☐	☐	
MULTIPLE PREGNANCIES (Twins, etc.)	☐	☐	☐	

AMNIOCENTESIS INDICATION: ☐ ADVANCED MATERNAL AGE ☐ PREVIOUS DOWN'S SYNDROME ☐ OTHER

IF OTHER, please specify: ____________________

ULTRASOUND TO BE DONE ☐ Yes ☐ No ☐ Don't know **IF YES,** Where? ____________ Date: ________

Physician performing amniocentesis:	When (date)?	Where will amniocentesis be performed?

Who will transport specimen to the laboratory ?	What is the estimated time of arrival of the specimen to laboratory?

Physician's Signature	Date	Address	Telephone

LARGE SCALE PRENATAL CYTOGENETIC DIAGNOSIS IN NEW YORK CITY*

Rene I. Jahiel

INTRODUCTION

The New York City Prenatal Cytogenetic Screening Program (PCSP), which will start operating in the Fall of 1978, was undertaken in order to make high quality prenatal diagnosis available and accessible to all pregnant women residing in New York City (NYC) who are at high risk of bearing a fetus with chromosomal abnormalities or neural tube defects (NTD). The categories of women eligible for PSCP are shown in Table 1.

Planning for this project began in 1974, under the impetus of a group of scientists in a task force of the N.Y. Scientists' Committee for Public Information (SCPI). A two-fold problem was addressed. First, public and private services in NYC were operating at nearly full capacity in 1974, yet they were serving less than 3% of the pregnant women 35 or older residing in NYC.[1] Therefore, a massive increase in the capacity of services was needed. Secondly, the task force was aware that such massive expansion might be accompanied by dangerous side effects if all the services involved in prenatal cytogenetic diagnosis were not adequately controlled: tragedies might result from avoidable errors of diagnosis, from inadequate counseling of pregnant women, or from complications of amniocentesis performed by obstetricians inexperienced or untrained in that procedure. Therefore, quality control during the phase of expansion of services was essential.

In 1976, the task force completed its report, in which three options for the expansion of services in NYC were discussed.[2] According to one option, which was favored by the vast majority of the task force's scientists, the expanded

*I wish to acknowledge the support given in the early stages of the project by a grant of the Greater New York Chapter of the National Foundation-March of Dimes to SCPI (Dr. Jahiel) in 1975-76, and by the Maternal and Child Health Services, Health Resources Administration, U.S. Department of Health, Education and Welfare to the N.Y.U. Medical Center (Dr. Selma Snyderman), in 1976-77, and the support given in the implementation of the project by the New York State Department of Health, the New York City Department of Health, and the New York City Health Systems Agency.

ISBN 0-12-562650-9

TABLE 1

NYC Women Eligible for the Prenatal Cytogenetic Screening Program

Indication for	Category
Chromosome studies	Age 35 or older at EDC Previous birth of a child with a chromosomal abnormality When one of the mates has a chromosomal abnormality Family history of X-linked disease
AFP determination	Elevated maternal serum AFP Previous birth of a child with NTD

TABLE 2

Pregnancies Lasting 16 Weeks or More in NYC Women 35 and Older in 1976 (By Single Year of Maternal Age)*

Age	Live births	Spontaneous abortions 16 weeks and over	Induced abortions 16 weeks and over	Total
35	1,741	28	56	1,825
36	1,439	23	50	1,512
37	1,099	25	37	1,161
38	884	23	33	940
39	640	15	28	683
40	439	15	20	474
41	303	6	24	333
42	193	6	21	220
43	125	3	11	139
44	64	1	8	73
⩾45	76	4	11	91
Total	7,003	149	299	7,451

*New York City residents only. Data from the New York City Department of Health.

services would be provided by a central laboratory, under public health auspices, in which some 4,000 specimens of amniotic fluid could be tested yearly, and by decentralized medical facilities, under public or private auspices, in which counseling, ultrasonography, and amniocentesis would take place. This division of work is illustrated in Fig. 1. The laboratory would be under direct control of the public health agency responsible for the program. The participating facilities would have to abide by quality standards for counseling, sonography, amniocentesis, and follow-up services specified in agreements between the facilities and the agency in order to utilize the laboratory. Therefore, the agency responsible for the program would exercise quality control directly over laboratory services and indirectly over the other services. Cost control would be facilitated by the economies of scale that are feasible in a large central laboratory.

Later in 1976, the New York State (NYS) Department of Health approved this option and, in 1977, it provided funding to develop it into the present program. The NYC Department of Health provided space for the central laboratory. NYC's PCSP is sponsored jointly by the NYS and NYC Departments of Health and operated by a not-for-profit corporation, the Medical and Health Research Association of New York (MHRA), under contract with the NYS Department of Health. The MHRA will administer the central laboratory, provide public and professional education and make and enforce the agreements with participating facilities. The participating facilities will be medical facilities (chiefly hospitals), which meet the program's requirements for quality of counseling, sonography, amniocentesis, and follow-up services. The program will be open to all pregnant women in the categories listed in Table 1 who reside in NYC. All obstetricians may refer such women to the program through one of the participating facilities. Each participating facility will designate a genetic service for counseling of women with abnormal or equivocal findings. Policy and technical committees will advise the PCSP's management committe, so as to provide input from consumers and from scientific or technical experts. The relations among these administrative components are shown in Fig. 2.

NYC's PCSP has four principal characteristics:

1. It will bring about rapid expansion of services until there is, regionally, the capacity to provide prenatal diagnosis of chromosomal abnormalities or NTD to all NYC women in the high risk categories listed in Table 1.

2. The laboratory is very large in comparison with the usual prenatal cytogenetic laboratories. Indeed, the term "megalab" has sometimes been applied to it. Such large size presents challenges for ensuring the smooth operation of the laboratory, as well as opportunities for cost and quality control.

3. Measures to uphold the quality of the entire set of services involved in prenatal diagnosis of chromosomal abnormalities and NTD are built into the program.

4. The program is not directive. Its object is to help women to make their own informed decision about whether to have amniocentesis or not and, when prenatal

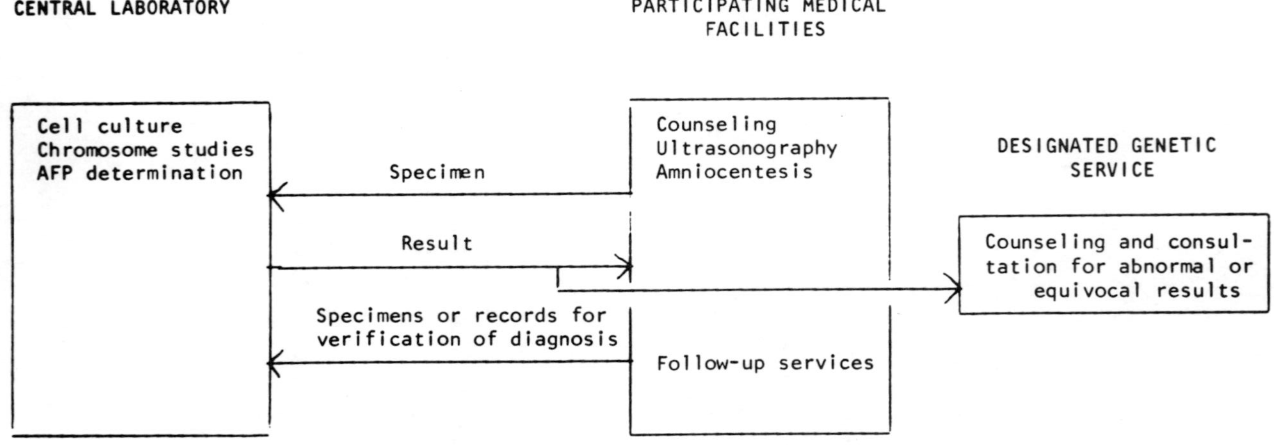

Fig. 1. Division of work among major components of program.

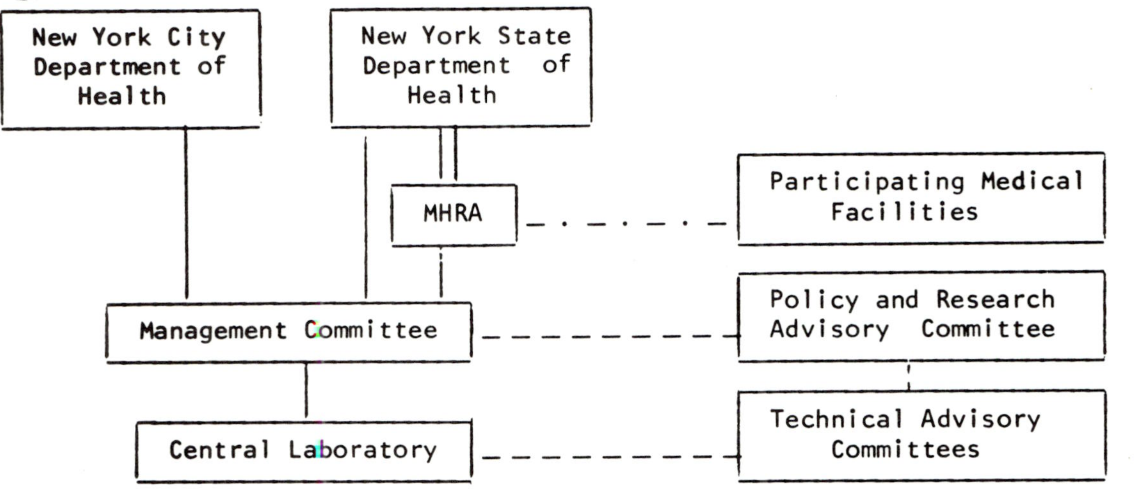

Fig. 2. Relationships among administrative components of the program. The management committee is the executive body of the program, which is responsible to the NYS and NYC Departments of Health and to the MHRA. It is presently composed of the project directors from the NYS and NYC Departments of Health, the Assistant Commissioner of Laboratories for NYC, the project's laboratory director, the executive director of MHRA, and the writer of the proposal (Dr. Jahiel).

TABLE 3

Pregnancies Lasting 16 or More Weeks in NYC Women 35 and Older, by Maternal Age Group, Based on 1976 Data.*

Age group	Live births	Spontaneous abortion 16 weeks and over	Induced abortion 16 weeks and over	Fetal death over 28 weeks*	Total
35 and over	7,003	149	299	170	7,621
36 and over	5,262	121	243	128	5,754
37 and over	3,823	98	193	93	4,207
38 and over	2,724	73	156	66	3,019
39 and over	1,840	50	123	45	2,058
40 and over	1,200	35	95	29	1,359
41 and over	761	20	75	18	874
42 and over	458	14	51	11	534
43 and over	265	8	30	6	309
44 and over	140	5	19	3	167
$\geqslant 45$	76	4	11	2	93

*New York City residents only. Data from the New York City Department of Health.

diagnosis of a fetal anomaly is made, whether to carry the pregnancy to term or terminate it. The program is to help women receive the services needed in any of these eventualities.

In this article, the quantitative aspects of these four characteristics will be presented in relation to the planning and implementation of the program. Although the laboratory will also do alpha-fetoprotein determinations in amniotic fluids and grow cultures that will be referred to other laboratories for metabolic studies, this article will cover only the program's functions in the prenatal diagnosis of chromosomal abnormalities.

RATIONALE FOR PROJECTED EXPANSION OF SERVICES IN NYC

Projection of the Population Eligible for Fetal Chromosome Studies

Of the various groups of women with indications for fetal chromosome studies listed in Table 1, the largest, by far, consists of women 35 or older at the estimated date of confinement (EDC). The number of women 35 and older residing in NYC who had live births or who had spontaneous or induced abortion after the 15th week of pregnancy was retrieved from the 1976 Birth Certificate Tapes of the NYC Department of Health by single year of maternal age (Table 2). The cut-off time of 16 weeks was chosen because this is the optimum time for amniocentesis performed for chromosomal diagnosis. From these data and from the number of stillbirths, the number of pregnant women in each year of age or older was calculated (Table 3). The consensus of the cytogenetics advisory committee of the program was that the number of women with indications for fetal chromosome studies other than advanced maternal age is under 500 a year in NYC. Therefore, the total numbers of women who would have been eligible for the program in 1976 because of increased risk of fetal chromosomal abnormalities if the minimum ages for eligibility had been 35, 36, or 37 are estimated to be about 8,000, 6,200, or 4,700, respectively.

The size of the population with indications for fetal chromosome studies will be affected in the future by several factors. There was a decrease in the number of live births from women 35 and older in the 1960s, followed by stabilization at a level of about 7,000 per year in recent years (Table 4). As the women born in the baby boom of the 1940s and 1950s reach the age of 35 during the next 15 years, a rise in live births from women 35 and older might be expected. Furthermore, the program and its public and professional education campaigns may have two side effects. Public education may make some women over 35 more concerned over the risk of fetal chromosomal abnormalities. This may lead to fewer pregnancies or more abortions in this group of women. On the other hand, knowledge that fetal chromosomes may be monitored during pregnancy may lead some women over 35, who would otherwise practice contraception or have induced abortion, to carry pregnancies to term, provided that prenatal diagnosis shows no chromosomal abnormalities of the fetus. Since there were 7,112 women

TABLE 4

Number of Live Births in New York City*

	Age of Mother	
	All ages	35 and older
1967	145,802	13,130
1971	131,920	9,584
1973	110,639	7,717
1974	110,642	7,493
1975	109,418	7,635
1976	109,995	7,585

*Data from the New York City Department of Health. The figures are for all births occurring in NYC. In 1976, about 92.5% of those were births from NYC residents.

TABLE 5

Amniocentesis for Women 35 or Older Residing in NYC

Year	No. AFCS*	No. live births	No. AFCS/ No. live births	No. AFCS/No. pregnancies lasting 16 weeks or longer
1974	221	6,912	0.032	
1976	1,055***	7,003	0.151	0.138**

*AFCS women with amniotic fluid chromosome studies.

**1,055/7,621 (denominator from Table 3).

***This figure does not include the estimated 300 women who had their amniotic fluid chromosome studies in laboratories that did not participate in our study.

35 or older residing in NYC who had induced abortions in 1976 (data from the NYC Department of Health Birth Certificate Tapes), and a much greater number who practiced contraception, a decision by a small proportion of this population to have prenatal cytogenetic diagnosis would significantly increase the number of those eligible for the program. Taking all these factors into consideration, it is likely that the number of women eligible for the program because of advanced maternal age will increase in the next decade.

Projections for Increased Capacity of Services in NYC

In order to estimate the need for increased capacity of laboratory services for the monitoring of fetal chromosomes, we found how many pregnant women 35 or older who were NYC residents had amniotic fluid chromosome studies in laboratories in NYC in 1974 and 1976. These studies were done in collaboration with Dr. Holger Hansen and with the cooperation of the directors of the laboratories. We examined the records of all laboratories in NYC which had received more than 50 specimens of amniotic fluid for chromosome studies per year in 1974. In 1976, one institution did not participate and collection of data from two other laboratories is still under way, so that the number of patients who had chromosome studies of amniotic fluid cells in these three laboratories were estimated from oral communication with the staff of these institutions, rather than from examination of records. The results are shown in Table 5. In 1975, the number of women residing in NYC who had amniotic fluid chromosome studies was about 3% of the number of live births. By 1976, it had risen to about 15% of the number of live births or 13.8% of the number of pregnancies lasting 16 weeks or more. In 1976, a New Jersey commercial laboratory, MetPath, became an important outlet for prenatal diagnosis of NYC women. We estimate that the number of NYC residents who had amniotic fluid chromosome studies at MetPath could not have exceeded 250 in 1976, and that the number who had these studies done in other laboratories not included in our survey was less than 50. Therefore, we estimate that not more than 1,355 women 35 or older residing in NYC had amniotic fluid chromosome studies in 1976. This would be 17.8% of the 7,621 women who had pregnancies lasting 16 weeks or longer.

Communication with the laboratory directors or their genetic counselors showed that by 1977 all the laboratories were working at full capacity. Several laboratories reported that they could not meet all the demand. Different mechanisms were used to cope with this situation, including referral to other laboratories outside NYC, refusal to accept out-of-town patients, raising the age limit for accepting specimens to 36, 37, or even 38 at EDC, or stressing the laboratory by accepting more specimens than the laboratory could handle comfortably. Furthermore, the laboratory directors saw, in general, no ready source of funds for significant further expansion. Many laboratories had had their work supported in part in earlier years by research grants and, as the test had moved from the realm of research into that of service, research funds were decreasing as a source of support.

TABLE 6

Projected Growth of Capacity for Prenatal Diagnosis of Chromosomal Abnormalities in NYC

Year	Projected Capacity*		
	Present laboratories	NYC Central Laboratory	Total
1976	1,355	–	1,355
1977	1,750	–	1,750
1978	2,000	750	2,750
1979	2,000	2,500	4,500
1980	2,000	4,000	6,000
1981	2,000	5,000	7,000

*Number women who could be served by the laboratories (NYC residents only).

In view of these findings, projections of growth of laboratory capacity for amniotic fluid chromosome studies in NYC were made in which it was assumed that the currently active laboratories would continue to operate at or near their present capacity, except for some continued growth of MetPath, and that the program's central laboratory would start functioning in 1978 and expand gradually to a yearly capacity to serve 4,000 women by 1980, and, if demand warrants, 5,000 women by 1981 (Table 6). According to these projections, NYC would have the capacity to provide amniotic fluid chromosome studies to 7,000 women by 1981.

Projected Utilization of NYC's PCSP

There is no way, now, of making a reliable estimate of the number of women who will have amniotic fluid chromosome studies on the basis of past experience, since public and professional attitudes towards amniocentesis and prenatal diagnosis are evolving rapidly. Public education programs in other cities have led to utilization of services by over 30% of pregnant women 35 or older.[3] Because of changing attitudes and of the public and professional education organized by NYC's PCSP, we are assuming for long-term planning that 80% of the population of pregnant women 35 and older in NYC who have not already decided to have an abortion would want to have amniotic fluid chromosome studies. If we use as an estimate of that population, the 7,621 women estimated to have had a pregnancy lasting 16 weeks or longer in NYC in 1976, 50% of that population would be about 3,800, and 80% would be about 6,100. The latter figure would amount to the capacity projected for the combined laboratory resources in NYC by 1980-81.

Number of Live Births of Infants with an Abnormal Number of Chromosomes (Exclusive of Mosaics) Expected in the Population Eligible for the Program, With and Without Prenatal Diagnosis

The risk of a Down syndrome live birth is known by single year of maternal age from several studies.[4] The potential number of Down syndrome live births from NYC residents 35 or older, in the absence of prenatal diagnosis, is shown by single year of maternal age in Table 7, and by age groups in Table 8. The number of Down syndrome live births from NYC residents 35 or older in the absence of prenatal diagnosis would, on the basis of the live birth data for 1976, be expected to be about 42. Projections of the number of Down syndrome live births from these women that would be prevented by the program, and of those for which the family would be prepared by prenatal services following the diagnosis, depend upon assumptions concerning utilization of prenatal diagnosis and parental decisions following the finding of a fetus with Down syndrome. For instance, if 80% of women 35 or older at EDC decide to have amniocentesis (with the same rate at all maternal ages above 34), if the test failure rate is negligible, and if 90% of women who have a fetus with Down syndrome decide to have an abortion, one

TABLE 7

Live Births and Expected Number of Down Syndrome Births Per Year of Age, In New York City

Age of mother	No. live births (in 1976)*	Expected prevalence of Down syndrome at birth (per 1,000 live births)**	Expected No. of Down syndrome births
35	1,741	2.63	4.58
36	1,439	3.39	4.88
37	1,099	4.37	4.80
38	884	5.64	4.99
39	640	7.27	4.65
40	439	9.38	4.12
41	303	12.11	3.67
42	193	15.64	3.02
43	125	20.20	2.53
44	64	26.08	1.67
45	39	33.70	1.31
46	17	43.54	0.74
47	14	56.26	0.79
48	6	(80.00)	0.48

*From the New York City Health Department's Birth Certificate tapes.

**From Ernest B. Hook. Differences between rates of trisomy 21 (Down syndrome) and other chromosomal abnormalities diagnosed in live births and in cells cultured after second-trimester amniocentesis – suggested explanations and implications for genetic counseling and program planning. *In* Bergsma, D. and Summitt, R.L. (Eds), Proceedings of the 1977 Birth Defects Conference, Original Article Series, Alan R. Liss, Inc., New York, 1978, Table 4. The figures are for expected prevalences calculated from the New York State and the Swedish data. (See reference 7.)

TABLE 8

Live Births and Expected Down Syndrome Births Per Age Interval, In New York City*

Age of mother	Cumulative expected number of live births per (year of age + older women)	Cumulative expected number of Down syndrome births per (year of age + older women)
⩾ 35	7,003	43.23
⩾ 36	5,262	37.65
⩾ 37	3,823	32.77
⩾ 38	2,724	27.97
⩾ 39	1,840	22.98
⩾ 40	1,200	18.33
⩾ 41	761	14.21
⩾ 42	458	10.54
⩾ 43	265	7.52
⩾ 44	140	4.99
⩾ 45	76	3.32

*Derived from the data shown in Table 7.

would expect that 30 Down syndrome live births would be prevented and that, in about 3 instances, the women would decide to carry a pregnancy with a Down syndrome fetus to term and prepare for the birth of the affected infant.

In six studies of chromosome number in newborns,[5] altogether there were 72 newborns with trisomy 21, and 102 with other abnormalities of chromosome number (exclusive of mosaics); *i.e.*, the total number of cases with an abnormal chromosome number (exclusive of mosaics) was 2.42 times the number of Down syndrome cases. Multiplying the number of Down syndrome live births from NYC residents 35 or older, in the absence of prenatal diagnosis, by 2.42 yields an estimated 102 cases of live births with an abnormal number of chromosomes, exclusive of mosaics, in the same population. If 80% of that population has amniocentesis and the test failure and error rates are negligible, one would expect that the program would have detected prenatally 82 fetuses with an abnormal number of chromosomes (exclusive of mosaics) that would have progressed to live birth in the absence of prenatal diagnosis. These projections are based on a number of assumptions which may introduce some errors: for instance, the assumption that the number of cases with abnormal chromosomes is 2.42 times the number of cases with Down syndrome, at birth, was derived from studies in which all maternal ages were included and may not hold as well when the population is restricted to women 35 or older. Therefore, the projections above are only rough approximations.

Prevalence of Fetuses With an Abnormal Number of Chromosomes (Exclusive of Mosaics) as Determined in Studies of Amniotic Fluid Cultures Following Second Trimester Amniocentesis

Chromosome studies of cultures of amniotic fluid collected by amniocentesis (prenatal studies) have shown a considerably higher prevalence of trisomy 21 than in studies of prevalence at birth (postnatal studies).[6] Unfortunately, maternal age was aggregated in these studies into groups of women aged 35-39, 40-44, and 45 or older. This makes comparisons by single year of maternal age impossible at this time. Several explanations have been advanced for the differences in prevalence between prenatal and postnatal studies,[7] such as unrepresentative distribution of women by age within the group 35-39 years old who had amniocentesis (since the proportion of women who have amniocentesis increases markedly between the ages of 35 and 39), selection of amniocentesis studies with unusually high prevalence of abnormal findings for publication, and increased mortality of Down syndrome fetuses, as compared with fetuses without chromosomal number anomalies in the second half of pregnancy. To eliminate the effect of unrepresentative age distribution in the 35-39 year old group and of selective publication, estimation of an approximate factor to relate pre- and postnatal prevalences of Down syndrome will be based on the prenatal prevalence in women aged 40-44 reported in the NICHD and Canadian studies and summarized by Hook,[7] and on the postnatal prevalence data in women aged 40-44 summarized in Table 7 of this paper. There were 12 cases of trisomy 21 among 428 women

40-44 with successful cultures; *i.e.,* a prenatal rate of 2.8%. From Table 7, the number of Down syndrome live births expected in the NYC resident population of women 40-44 at the time of EDC (in the absence of prenatal diagnosis) is 15.01 out of 1,124 women; *i.e.,* a postnatal rate of 1.34%. From these estimated rates, and from the estimated 42 live births of Down syndrome infants that would have occurred in the population eligible for the program in the absence of prenatal diagnosis, we can project that there would be 88 cases of fetal trisomy 21 in that population at the 16th week of pregnancy (*i.e.,* the optimal time for performing amniocenteses.

In second trimester amniotic fluid cultures, the diagnosis of trisomy 21 was about twice as frequent as that of all other abnormalities of chromosome number, exclusive of mosaics.[6] Therefore, we may project that there would be 88 x 1.5 = 132 fetuses with abnormal chromosomes in the 7,621 NYC residents 35 or older at EDC, at the 16th to 20th week of pregnancy (Table 3).

If the NYC central laboratory does laboratory chromosome studies on a sample of 4,000 women representative of that population, and if the test failure rate is negligible, the laboratory would be expected to have 132 x 4,000/7,621 x 52 = 1.33 cases with an abnormal number of chromosomes per week, on the average. If other chromosomal abnormalities, such as mosaics, structural abnormalities, etc., are added to that figure, the NYC central laboratory may expect a rate of 1.5 to 2 cases with clinically significant chromosomal abnormalities per week.

The estimates made in this section have involved several assumptions, and are very rough. They are the best that can be made with the data at our disposal. This points to the need for more refined studies of the prevalence of chromosomal abnormalities prenatally by single year of maternal age, and for careful definition of the age and duration of pregnancy of the women utilizing the program.

THE LABORATORY COMPONENT OF THE PROGRAM

The Laboratory

The NYC central laboratory has an area of 3,500 square feet in the NYC Department of Health Building at 1st Avenue and 26th Street in Manhattan. The area for cell culture and chromosome studies comprises 2,300 square feet. Preparation of media, processing of amniotic fluid, cell culture procedures, microscopic examination of cultures, and harvesting of cells will take place in four cell culture modules. Each module is about 100 square feet and contains a laminar flow hood, a bench, storage space, a CO_2 incubator, an inverted microscope, a

*42 x 2.8/1.34 = 88. This estimate must be used with caution. The data from which the prenatal rates were derived was obtained from a small number of cases. Furthermore, several assumptions were made. For instance, the ratio of prenatal to postnatal prevalences in women 35 or older was assumed to be the same as in the population subgroup that is 40 to 44 years old.

TABLE 9

Estimates of Technician Time for Processing of Amniotic Fluid

Activity	Working Time (Hours)*		
	1 Specimen	3 Specimens Simultaneously	5 Specimens Simultaneously
Initial work-up of specimen. This comprises recording relevant information, centrifugation, sending supernate to AFP laboratory, distribution of cells into 4 flasks with growth medium and starting incubation.	1	1½	2
Observation and feeding of cultures. This involves an average of 6 observations per culture and of 4 feedings, and addition of a metaphase-arresting agent when the cultures are ready for harvest.	2	3½	6
From harvesting of cells to preparation of slides. This involves removal of cells from culture flask, concentration of cells, treatment with hypotonic solution, fixation and preparation, and staining of slides.	3	3½	4
Microscopic study of slides. This involves microscopic examination of 2-3 slides per specimen, locating and marking 20-30 well spread metaphases, enumerating their chromosomes and photographing some or all of the selected metaphases.**	3	9	15
Development and printing of films.	2	3	4
Karyotype preparation. This includes cutting of chromosomes from photographs, karyotyping and mounting 3-4 representative metaphases.	2	6	10
Total number of hours for complete work-up of specimen(s)	13	26½	41
Total number of hours per specimen	13	8.8	8.2

*"Slack" time, such as during incubation or other waiting periods of more than 15 minutes is not included in the "Working" time.

**There are two possibilities at this step: either the chromosomes are counted during the microscopic examination of the cells and only 3-4 are photographed or about 20 cells are photographed and chromosomes are counted on the photographs.

table centrifuge, and a water bath. There are two constant temperature rooms, 10 x 15 feet each, one of which is at 4°C and the other at 37°C. There is a 600 square feet area for the preparation of cells for microscopic examination, inclusive of all staining procedures, and for general purpose. Microscopic examination of slides, photomicrography, and cutting up and mounting of karyotypes are done in an 800 square feet area with 8 research microscopes and an enclosed space with a fluorescent microscope. Each microscope is equipped for photography. There are two dark rooms, about 50 square feet each, within a room 200 square feet.

The remainder of the laboratory consists of a 400 square feet room for AFP determination and for storage, and 800 square feet divided into a small library-conference room, and office space for the laboratory director, associate director, and secretarial staff. The entire building is air conditioned and air to the laboratory is filtered. In addition to the 3,500 square feet of laboratory space, the program has an area about 600 square feet in the same building which is used by the record keeping staff, genetic counselors, and health educator attached to the program under the supervision of the laboratory director.

Laboratory Personnel and Division of Work

The productivity of technicians may be increased in at least two ways by division of labor: (1) by starting the processing of several specimens together, and (2) by "specialization" of certain technicians. The time needed to perform the various laboratory procedures was estimated with the help of Ms. Andrea Scheidt. A comparison of technician time required for amniotic fluid chromosome studies when specimens are processed singly, in groups of three, or in groups of five is shown in Table 9. Productivity (*i.e.*, the number of specimens processed per unit of technician time) is increased by more than a third when specimens are processed simultaneously. However, even if several specimens are started on the same day, their cultures may not grow at the same rate, and they are not likely to be ready for harvesting on the same day.

This problem may be alleviated in a large laboratory by specialization of several technicians. Thus, one technician could process harvested cells through staining, another would develop, fix, and enlarge the photomicrographs, and a third would prepare media and solutions. The cytogenetics technician would perform all the other procedures (initial processing of the amniotic fluid, seeding, feeding and observation of cultures, harvesting of cells, microscopic studies of metaphases, taking photomicrographs, karyotyping and mounting of karyotype), under the supervision of the laboratory directors and with the help of assistants. The staining and photography technicians would process specimens worked up by several cytogenetics technicians, thereby increasing the number of specimens that can be processed in the same batch.

Estimates of the number of technical workers needed in laboratories handling different numbers of amniotic fluids a year are shown in Table 10, along with a brief description of the division of work. A marked increase in productivity takes place in laboratories with 624 specimens and a continuing, but less dramatic,

TABLE 10

Example of Division of Work in Relation to Volume of Present Cytogenetic Diagnostic Work

Specimens per year	208	624	1,040	4,160
Specimens per week	4	12	20	80
Specimens/wk/cytog. technician	2	4	5	5.75
No. cytogenetics technicians	2	2	4	14
No. staining technicians		1	1	2
No. photography technicians			1	2
No. medium preparation technicians				1
No. assistants				1
Total no. technicians per laboratory	2*	3**	6***	20****
No. technicians per 80 specimen week	40	27	24	22

It is assumed that the work week of each technician has 35 hours, that a time equivalent to about 4 hours a week is used up in vacations, holidays and sick leave and that about 2-3 hours a week are taken up by meetings, conferences or unexpected occurrences. This leaves 28-29 hours a week for laboratory procedures time (inclusive of slack time periods of less than 15 minutes that occur during a procedure).

*Each technician does all the procedures for the culture and cytogenetic study of the specimens. Preparation of media and glassware preparation are divided among the 2 technicians. Amniotic fluid supernates are sent to other laboratories for AFP determination.

**Each cytogenetic technician works with 4 cultures that they start simultaneously and they do the observations or feeding of cultures, microscopic examination, chromosome counts, photomicrography and karyotype preparation. The staining technician does the processing of cells following harvest and staining of slides (3 batches per week), developing and printing of photomicrographs, as well as the preparation of media and glassware. One of the 4 technicians does AFP determination on the AF supernates once a week, or the supernates are sent to another laboratory.

***The cytogenetics technicians have the same tasks as outlined in footnote 2, except that they get help for karyotype preparation from the other technicians. The staining technician does the processing of cells following harvest and staining of slides (3 batches per week) and the preparation of media and glassware, and helps with the karyotype preparation. The photography technician does the developing and printing of photomicrographs (3 times a week) and helps with preparation of karyotypes. AFP determinations are done in another laboratory or are done in this laboratory by one of the technicians, once a week.

****The cytogenetics technicians have the same tasks as in footnote 3. The staining technicians are responsible for processing of cells following harvest, and staining of slides (4 to 5 batches a week), and for helping with karyotype preparation. The photography technicians are responsible for developing and printing and for helping with karyotype preparation. The media preparation technician has responsibility for preparation and quality testing of all media and that technician may also carry on some cytogenetic work as needed. The assistant helps the cytogenetics technician as needed, and has responsibility for glassware. One of the technicians does AFP determination once a week.

improvement occurs as the size of the laboratory increases further.

Economies of Scale and Other Effects of Laboratory Size on Cost

Table 10 shows that considerable economies of scale might be achieved in large laboratories by increasing technician productivity. Other economies of scale would result from reductions in the unit cost of equipment when several units are bought together, and of supplies when large quantities are ordered. Further economies might be made in large laboratories by preparing the media in the laboratory.

On the other hand, a large centralized laboratory might increase certain costs, as compared to smaller, decentralized laboratories. For instance, in a centralized laboratory, a driver and a car would be needed for the transport of specimens to the laboratory.

The effect of size on certain costs is difficult to evaluate. For instance, in a large centralized laboratory serving low- as well as middle-income individuals, a clerk for the handling of Medicaid and other third party payments may be justified. The salary and social benefits of such a clerk wouldincrease the budget of the laboratory. In the instance of decentralized laboratories attached to medical centers, the medical center would employ personnel for the collection of all third party payments to the center, including those for the laboratory procedures. It is not clear, in the absence of empirical studies relating to such a laboratory, which of the two alternatives is most cost effective. Only a fraction of the laboratory director's time and salary would be devoted to supervising operation of a small laboratory, while two full-time professionals, including a laboratory director would be needed for a laboratory handling 4,000 or more specimens a year. Without empirical studies, it is difficult to know which would be the most effective use of professionals and laboratory directors.

Projected Operating Costs of the Central Laboratory

The projected operating cost of the NYC central laboratory is shown in Table 11. A volume of 4,000 specimens per year, and 1977 prices and salaries are assumed. It should be clear that this budget includes not only laboratoy activities, but also counseling, public and professional education, and certain statistical and data-retrieving activities, since all these activities are under the administration of the laboratory.

The professional personnel comprises a laboratory director and an associate laboratory director (both cytogeneticists), and a health educator. The technical staff of 20 is broken down as shown in Table 10, although some rearrangement of tasks may well occur following experience in running the laboratory. The managerial and clerical staff comprises a supervisor with training in data retrieval and computerization of records, a clerk for billing and collection of third party payments, and two secretaries. The consultant funds are set aside for contingencies requiring expert advice on technical or legal problems. Liability insurance

TABLE 11

Projected Cost of Operating Centralized Laboratory*

Expense Category**	Projected Cost	
	Per year	Per specimen
Personnel: professional (3)	$ 90,000	
technical (20)	260,000	
management & clerical (4)	52,000	
driver (1)	10,000	
Fringe benefits (rate: 26%)	107,120	
Consultants	5,000	
Liability insurance	15,000	
Quality control program	25,000	
Supplies	110,000	
Equipment (pro-rated)***	25,000	
Maintenance & repair	5,000	
Others	20,000	
Total direct costs	$ 724,120	$ 181.0
Indirect costs (approx.)	70.000	
Total laboratory costs	$ 794,120	$ 198.5
Genetic counselors (6)	$ 90,000	
Fringe benefits (rate:26%)	23,400	
Indirect costs (approx.)	11,400	
Total counseling costs	$ 124,800	$ 31.2

*Assumptions: operating rate: 4,000 cases/year; 1977 prices and salaries.

**Numbers in parenthesis after personnel category are number of persons per expense category.

***Assumed life time: 10 years.

was included instead of malpractice insurance, upon legal advice that the former type of insurance was more appropriate for this laboratory. The funds for the quality control program are to be applied to external as well as internal monitoring of quality of the laboratory work. The supplies have been computed at $25 worth of supplies per specimen, plus an additional $10,000 for Xeroxing, office, and other needs. The equipment has been computed on the basis of an initial investment of $250,000 pro-rated over a life-time of two years. Actually, because of marked economies of scale in buying equipment, especially microscopes, it appears that the initial equipment cost will be closer to $200,000. The estimated $5,000 in maintenance and repairs applies to all activities under the administration of the laboratory director. The items under "other expenses" comprise telephone, mailing, some computer expenses, books and journals, car rental, traveling, and expenses for supplies for public and professional education. The expenses for genetic counselors are computed on the basis of one genetic counselor for every 666 patients a year. The indirect costs are for administration of the program by MHRA.

The total projected cost per specimen for the laboratory would be just under $200. Several points must be made in comparing this figure to the cost per specimen in other laboratories, besides the remarks made earlier about economies of scale. First, since the NYC Department of Health provides the space and basic utilities (excluding telephone) free to the program (in fact, giving it a NYC subsidy in addition to NYS financing), the estimate does not include rent and utilities, which might add considerably to indirect costs in other laboratories. Secondly, the cost per specimen comprises the cost of the public and professional education program, and of statistics and data retrieving activities, which are not laboratory activities *per se*.

Further economies may be made in the future. The program's health educator may be phased out as the public and professions become well informed about prenatal diagnosis, and any remaining health educational tasks may be fulfilled by the NYC Department of Health. The managerial and clerical staff might be decreased. When prenatal diagnosis is better understood by the population at risk, more patients may be counseled by fewer genetic counselors. The efficiency of cytogenetics techniques is likely to increase, possibly in conjunction with partial automatization of some steps in the procedure.

Functional Organization of the Central Laboratory

The central laboratory has centralized as well as decentralized features, as shown in Table 12. There are three levels of organization, referred to in the Table as the laboratory, the cell culture module, and the cytogenetics technician. The items listed in the Table as being integrated at the laboratory level are centralized in order to improve quality control, cost control, or both.

Space for cell culture and certain equipment (*i.e.*, laminar flow hood, CO_2 incubator, etc.) is decentralized at the cell culture module level. The cytogenetics technicians will be divided into four groups of 3 or 4 technicians each. Each group

TABLE 12

Functional Organization of the Central Laboratory

Unit of organization	No. specimens in culture at any given time	Items integrated under unit or organization
Laboratory	240	– Overall administration under laboratory director – Laboratory procedure and record keeping system – Monitoring and control of quality – Preparation and pre-testing of media and solutions – Buying of equipment and supplies – Common storage facilities – Sharing of "specialized" technicians – Sharing of information among modules
Cell culture module	60	– Common use of space and equipment in module (with restriction that only one person can use the module at any time.
Cytogenetics technician	15 – 20	– Own set of 5 or 6 specimens per week – Own time for using cell culture module – Own boxes for CO_2 and large incubators – Own batches of media, solutions and reagents – Two technicians share one photomicroscope – Own film cassette

will use one cell culture module. One of the reasons for decentralization at the cell culture module level is to facilitate administration of the laboratory. Another reason is to prevent certain rare, catastrophic events, such as equipment failure, contamination associated with a room or an item of equipment, from affecting the entire laboratory. Since the presence of more than one technician at the same time in the module would increase the hazards of contamination or of mixing of specimens, only one technician can work at any time in the module. It is estimated that each technician will spend less than two hours a day in the module. The technicians will use the module according to a set schedule.

Most of the laboratory procedures will be decentralized at the level of the cytogenetics technician, as shown in Table 12. Each technician will carry all steps of cell cultivation independently from other technicians, with separate materials and in separate incubator boxes. Each amniotic fluid specimen will be divided, and part will be cultured in the incubator room and part in the CO_2 incubator in the cell culture module. The technicians will begin using new batches of media or solutions at different times, so that a problem which has escaped the central pretesting procedure may be picked up by some technicians before it has had a chance to affect all of them.

In view of these precautions, it is expected that the risk that a major hazard will affect a large number of cultures at any time is extremely low. However, since such a risk cannot be entirely excluded, the central laboratory will have agreements with at least two large laboratories in New York which will serve as back-up facilities if needed. These agreements will be reciprocal.

Another hazard is the risk of mislabeling a specimen or misentering a result in the record. To guard against such a hazard, each specimen, or any culture, slide, or other item derived from that specimen, will be identified by both laboratory number and patient's name. All the procedures on that specimen will be done by the cytogenetics technician who does the initial work-up of the specimen, except for those steps which are done by the specialized technicians. The cytogenetics technician responsible for that specimen will share one research microscope; however, each technician will have an individual cassette for photomicrography, which will be removed from the microscope after each period of use by the technician.

Quality of the Laboratory Work

Guidelines for amniotic fluid cell culture and chromosome studies have been written by the Cytogenetics Advisory Committee of NYC's PCSP.[8] These guidelines cover the following items:

- establishment of laboratory and validation of its reliability;
- requirements for procedures of amniotic cell culture and chromosome studies (inclusive of the optimum amount of amniotic fluid for starting cultures, the number of containers to be set as primary cultures, the minimum number of mitoses that shall be counted, analyzed under the micro-

scope and karyotyped by photograph, requirements for either Q or G banding and availability of other banding procedures, and requirements for a laminar flow hood, and for periodic monitoring of amniotic fluid cell cultures for mycoplasma);

- minimum culture analysis success rate standards, standards for promptness of reporting results, and procedures that the laboratory must follow when it fails to meet these standards;
- nature of follow-up data needed to verify all cytogenetics laboratory results;
- nature of records that must be kept by the laboratory and maintenance of these records;
- precautions for protecting confidentiality of information about patients;
- referral information needed by the laboratory and specimen intake procedure;
- procedure for reporting of results;
- participation of central laboratory in NYS Chromosome Registry;
- indications for parental peripheral blood chromosome analysis;
- determination of need for repeat amniocentesis; and
- establishment of a panel of cytogeneticists for consultation regarding laboratory problems at the request of the laboratory director.

The laboratory director will decide whether to use flask or dish cultures, what media and other solutions to use, whether to karyotype individual colonies *in situ* or cells harvested from an entire flask, what criteria to use for a diagnosis of mosaicism, when to request parental peripheral blood for chromosome studies or repeat amniotic fluid cultures, what banding procedures to use routinely and what array of banding procedures to have available in the laboratory, and other procedures within the framework set by the guidelines. The Cytogenetics Advisory Committee, in concert with the laboratory director, will review the guidelines periodically and revise them in response to scientific and technical advances and to the experience of the laboratory.

Monitoring the Quality of the Laboratory Work

The laboratory work will be monitored in at least three ways. First, the laboratory will be subject to the inspection and proficiency testing procedures of the NYS Department of Health. Secondly, the laboratory will be inspected at least yearly by a special committee with NYS as well as out-of-state members, as described in the guidelines of the Cytogenetics Advisory Committee.[8] Finally, there will be internal monitoring.

Measures of accuracy of the diagnosis, test success rate, and promptness in making and reporting the diagnosis, which are outlined in Table 13, will be used to derive an objective evaluation of the quality of the laboratory's output. The central laboratory's aim is to meet at least the best standards that have been achieved in any diagnostic cytogenetic laboratory and to keep up with improvements in standards as they occur. Since techniques and standards have improved

TABLE 13

Measures of Quality of Laboratory Work

Item measured	Quantifiable features
Accuracy of diagnosis	Sex diagnosis error rate: No. of pregnancies in which prenatal diagnosis of sex was different from sex found after birth or abortion/No. of pregnancies with prenatal diagnosis and follow-up report of sex determination after birth or abortion.
	False negative rate: No. of pregnancies in which a normal fetal karyotype was reported by prenatal diagnosis and an abnormal karyotype was found after birth or abortion/No. pregnancies in which prenatal diagnostic studies were made and chromosomal abnormalities of the offspring were found in follow-up studies after birth or abortion.
	False positive rate: No. pregnancies in which an abnormal fetal karyotype was reported by prenatal diagnosis and no evidence of abnormal karyotype was found in follow-up studies after birth or abortion/No. of pregnancies in which prenatal diagnostic studies were made and there was no evidence of abnormal karyotype in follow-up studies after birth or abortion.
Success of fetal chromosome studies	Overall failure rate: No. pregnancies in which no fetal karyotype was obtained with any of the amniotic fluid specimens submitted from that pregnancy/No. of pregnancies from which amniotic fluid specimens were submitted.
	Initial failure rate: No. of pregnancies in which no fetal karyotype was obtained with the first amniotic fluid specimens submitted from that pregnancy/No. of pregnancies from which amniotic fluid specimens were submitted.
Promptness of diagnosis	Days from seeding to first successful harvesting.
	Days from seeding to last successful harvesting of cells used for karyotyping.
	Days from seeding to transmission of information to physician or genetic service in charge of patient.

rapidly in this field in the last few years, a brief discussion of each outcome measure of quality is given below.

Accuracy of Diagnosis

Every fetal chromosome study includes sex chromosome identification, and verification of sex is usually available within 5 months of the diagnosis, either at birth or after abortion. Therefore, data needed to derive the sex diagnosis error rate will be collected relatively fast. There were 5 erroneous sex diagnoses in the NICHD collaborative study of amniotic fluid cell chromosomes from 1,014 patients,[9] and 2 in the Canadian collaborative study which involved 1,020 patients.[10] A sex diagnosis error rate of less than 2 per thousand appears reasonable as an initial aim for the central laboratory.

It takes much longer to accumulate enough data to have reliable rates of false positive and false negative errors, as defined in Table 13, since the vast majority of cases examined have a normal fetal chromosome complement. The NICHD study had a false negative rate of 2/6, which is extremely high. The Canadian study had no false negatives in a series in which there were 8 cases with an abnormal number of chromosomes (7 of which were verified). By analogy with the sex diagnosis error rate, the central laboratory might aim for false negative and false positive error rates of less than 2 per thousand.

In order to check accuracy of diagnosis, it is necessary to have good follow-up studies. The PCSP's participating medical facilities will be required, in their agreement with MHRA, to provide clinical summaries on newborns, pathologic reports on stillborns and abortuses, and specimens appropriate for chromosome studies from all newborns with suspected chromosomal abnormalities, and from fetal fluids or tissues obtained at induced abortion, in order to verify the prenatal diagnosis.

Test Failure Rate

The survey of NYC laboratories performed in collaboration with Dr. Hansen, which is in progress, has already shown considerable variation in culture analysis failure rate from a low under 3% to a high over 20%. The failure rate has two components. The first is the failure rate per specimen received in the laboratory. This may be subdivided further into the initial failure rate and the failure rate for the second specimen submitted from the same pregnancy. The second component is the rate at which the laboratory was unable to obtain a second specimen of amniotic fluid following initial culture analysis failure. The former component depends upon the quality of the laboratory procedures and of the care with which amniotic fluid was collected at amniocentesis and transported to the laboratory. The latter component depends upon the patient and physician attitudes, the time of pregnancy when the specimen was submitted to the laboratory, and the time when the second specimen was requested.

The test failure rate is a relatively crude index. It should be broken down into those with a known cause (*i.e.*, a contaminant, temperature control failure in incubator, etc.), and those without one. With respect to the latter, the culture failure rate should be related to the number of cells seeded per culture.

A reasonable goal for the laboratory, at present, would be a failure rate of 2% with specification of factors associated with each failure as described above.

Promptness of Diagnosis

This is an important criterion of quality, since a delayed diagnosis might prevent a woman from exercising her option to have an abortion, or lead her to have one late in pregnancy with increased risks. Furthermore, a delayed diagnosis increases the psychological stress caused by uncertainty about the outcome of the test.

The time interval between the date of the tap and the date when the diagnosis is communicated to the patient may be subdivided into several segments: (1) time interval to the first successful harvesting; (2) time to complete all the harvesting needed because of the requirements to examine cells from at least two containers; (3) time to karyotype; (4) time to report diagnosis to patient's physician or to the genetic service (which may be further broken down into time for reports of preliminary and final diagnosis); and (5) time until the patient is informed.

In the survey of NYC laboratories under progress with Dr. Hanson, preliminary results show that successful harvesting of cultures from two or more containers took place within three weeks after seeding in from 55% to 78% of instances in different laboratories in 1976. This interval appears to have been prolonged because most of the NYC laboratories were overloaded during much of 1976. A relation between overloading and delay in diagnosis has been documented.[11] Therefore, it is reasonable to expect that, without overloading, the central laboratory should be able to achieve successful harvesting from at least two containers in less than 3 weeks in 95% of the cases or more. In general, the interval from harvesting to karyotyping and communicating of information to physician or genetic service should not take more than 2 to 3 working days.

OTHER SERVICE COMPONENTS OF THE PROGRAM

Among the other service components of the program, public and professional education, and the transportation of specimens are under the administration of the laboratory director, and counseling, ultrasonography, amniocentesis and follow-up services are under the administration of participating medical facilities which are committed, under agreements with MHRA, to uphold specified standards of quality of services.

The integration of the various service components of the program will be as follows. Physicians who provide prenatal care will refer patients who are eligible for the program to one of the participating medical facilities. At the medical facility, the patient will receive counseling by a genetic counselor. Such counseling shall be informative but not directive. If the patient decides to have amniocentesis, the referring physician and the patient will select an obstetrician who fulfills the program's requirement for performing second trimester amniocentesis at that facility, in accordance with the agreement between the medical facility and the MHRA. This obstetrician may be the referring physician (if qualified) or another physician. The counselor, who acts as coordinator of the various services, will make the appointments for sonography and amniocentesis. Also at this time, a genetic service will be designated so that it may be used for consultation and counseling of the patient if there is an abnormal or equivocal result in prenatal diagnosis. After amniocentesis is performed (usually in the same facility where the patient was counseled), the specimen of amniotic fluid will be transported to the central laboratory by the program's driver, along with the information that accompanies the specimen.

If the results of the laboratory tests are normal, they will be reported by the laboratory to the referring physician and to the patient. If there is need for a second tap, the laboratory will promptly notify both the referring physician and the counselor, and an appointment made for a repeat tap. If the results are abnormal or equivocal, the laboratory director will notify the referring physician and the designated genetic service as well as the counselor. Either the referring physician or the counselor will inform the patient of the need for a genetic consultation, and will set an appointment with the genetic service. The consultation with the genetic service will be attended by the patient and the counselor and, in many instances, by the referring physician and the director of the central laboratory. The results of the test will be explained to the patient, and further counseling will be given to enable her to reach an informed decision about her next step. If she makes the decision to carry the pregnancy to term, the counselor and referring physician will help her to obtain the services of social workers, parent organizations, mental retardation service centers, and others, as needed, to prepare the family for the birth of the affected infant. If her decision is to terminate the pregnancy, the counselor and referring physician will help her to have an induced abortion quickly and without financial barriers. The counselor will also assist the laboratory in obtaining records or specimens to verify the diagnosis following birth or abortion.

The monitoring and control of quality presents different problems for each component of this program. Table 14 lists measures or indices of quality which may be used for monitoring and it shows the agencies which have to cooperate in such monitoring.

Public and Professional Education

The targets for public education are the approximately 8,000 pregnant women residing in NYC who have an indication for monitoring of fetal chromosomes, as well as all women of reproductive age, since they may eventually have pregnancies after the age of 35. The public education strategy is also concerned with individuals who influence women at risk, such as husbands, physicians, etc. With respect to the professional education program, all obstetricians, midwives, family physicians, public health nurses, and clinic administrators must be well informed about the program, since they may be involved in the referral of patients. Public and professional education will be the responsibility of the health educator, under the laboratory director. Two quantifiable features related to the effectiveness of public and professional education are the number of women in the eligible population who have early prenatal care (*i.e.*, before the 16th week of pregnancy) and who have individual counseling by a trained genetic counselor. These features are affected by economic and other constraints, but other things being equal, they should reflect the quality of the public and professional education programs.

Counseling Before Amniocentesis

The aim is to help women to make an informed decision about whether to have amniocentesis or not. Counseling shall usually be done by genetic counselors who are employees of the program, but who are also responsible to the obstetrician who gives prenatal care to the patient and to the facility where amniocentesis is performed. Counseling done by an obstetrician who has the qualifications and the time to do it shall be subject to the same requirements as that by a genetic counselor.

Guidelines for counseling have been written by the Genetic Counseling Advisory Committee of the program.[12] These guidelines cover the following items:

- qualifications for counseling prior to amniocentesis;
- components and timing of counseling;
- optimum patient load for amniocentesis counselors;
- information elicited from patient, inclusive of genetic pedigree;
- material sent to patient before interview;
- counseling of patient (including review of reason for referral, explanation of the biologic basis of chromosomal abnormalities of the syndromes associated with these abnormalities, discussion of risk status of the fetus, comprising both prenatal and postnatal prevalence data, explanation of the procedures of ultrasonography and amniocentesis and of their risks, explanation of the conditions that the test can detect and of those that it cannot detect, and of the causes of errors in the laboratory tests and their frequency;
- informing the patients about how they will be notified of the results and about the possibility that a repeat procedure may be needed.

The quality of counseling will be monitored in part by ehecking a sample of charts for compliance of the counseling with the program's guidelines. Furthermore, a questionnaire may be used to assess retrospectively the satisfaction of patients with the decision they made concerning prenatal diagnosis and with the counseling that assisted them in reaching it.

Ultrasonography

Ultrasonography helps to locate the placenta, to establish the duration of

TABLE 14

Approaches to Monitoring the Quality of Service Components of the Program Other than the Laboratory

Component	Quantifiable feature related to quality of service	Source of Data*
Public and professional education:	1. Number of women in the target population who have prenatal care early in pregnancy (*i.e.*, before 17th week).	2
	2. Number of women in the target population who have counseling by a trained genetic counselor.	2,4
Counseling:	1. Examination of sample of counseling records for extent of compliance with standards for: a. history and pedigree; b. assessment of patient's understanding of the tests and conditions that may be detected; c. assessment of psychological, psychosocial, or economic problems.	4
	2. Frequency of satisfaction with counseling, as revealed in follow-up questionnaire to sample of patients.	5
Ultrasonography:	1. Results of periodic testing of apparatus.	6
	2. Proficiency testing of personnel.	6
	3. Rate of missing diagnosis of twin pregnancy.	4
Amniocentesis:	Profile of obstetrician or of medical facility based on:	
	1. Rate of utilization of genetic counselor for pre-amniocentesis counseling.	4,1
	2. Mean error in weeks in estimating the duration of pregnancy, obtained by comparison with estimate made by ultrasonography.	4,1
	3. Mean number of insertions of needle through uterine wall per tap and/or rate of amniocentesis in which needle was inserted more than twice.	4,1

TABLE 14 (Continued)

Approaches to Monitoring the Quality of Service Components of the Program Other than the Laboratory

Component	Quantifiable feature related to quality of service	Source of data*
Amniocentesis (continued):	4. Rate of dry taps.	4,1
	5. Rate of bloody taps.	1
	6. Rate of spontaneous abortions within 3 weeks of amniocentesis.	4,5
	7. Rate of major maternal complications (*i.e.*, bleeding, infection).	4,5
Follow-up services:	1. Women who have a fetus with chromosomal abnormalities or NTD and decide to have an abortion.	
	a. number of such women who are able to obtain an abortion;	4,5
	b. time interval between decision to have abortion and performance of abortion.	4,5
	2. Women who have a fetus with chromosomal abnormalities or NTD and decide to keep the pregnancy going.	
	a. number of such women who have counseling and are referred to services to prepare for birth of the infant.	4,5
	b. time interval between decisions to keep the pregnancy going and appointment following referrals.	4,5
	3. All women who have a fetus with chromosomal abnormalities or NTD.	
	a. frequency of satisfaction with follow-up services as revealed by questionnaire, one year later.	5

*1 – Records of centralized laboratory and of other laboratories serving NYC population,
2 – Birth certificate, fetal deaths and abortion records of NYC Department of Health,
3 – N.Y. State chromosome registry at the Birth Defects Institute,
4 – Records of participating medical centers,
5 – Special follow-up studies or questionnaires,
6 – Special inspection or proficiency testing program.

pregnancy, and to detect twins. Therefore, not using it would increase the risks of having a bloody tap, misjudging the duration of pregnancy, and missing twin pregnancies. On the other hand, follow-up studies of fetuses exposed to ultrasound *in utero* have been reported up to one year after birth only, and the possibility that some ill effects might become manifest several years after birth, which appears to be very remote, cannot be excluded. For this reason, several obstetricians have been reluctant to use ultrasound routinely before amniocentesis. However, most obstetricians who do amniocentesis in NYC appear to use it routinely. Therefore, it is likely that ultrasonography will be used extensively prior to amniocentesis in the program. The apparatus should be inspected and calibrated every 3 to 4 months. Proficiency testing of the personnel operating it and interpreting the results should also be done periodically, possibly through a peer review mechanism. Over a long period of time, the rate of missing a diagnosis of twin pregnancies, which should be extremely low, may be used as an additional test of the accuracy of the procedure.

Amniocentesis

Amniocentesis will be performed in participating medical facilities by qualified obstetricians who are responsible to the facilities, and to whom patients will have been referred by the physicians in charge of the patients' prenatal care.

Guidelines for amniocentesis have been written by the Obstetrics Advisory Committee of the Program.[13] These guidelines cover the following items:

- optimal time for procedure of amniocentesis;
- requirements for facilities where amniocentesis is done;
- qualification of obstetricians for performance of amniocentesis in the program;
- performance of the procedure of amniocentesis;
- Rh sensitization; and
- informed consent.

The performance of an obstetrician, as well as that of the group of obstetricians who do amniocentesis at a facility may be assessed at intervals by the profile outlined in Table 14. The facility's agreement with MHRA will provide assurances that the facility will make available information for such profiles to the PCSP.

Transportation of Specimen

Transportation of the specimen is the responsibility of the program, which will provide a car and a driver, and which will assure that the specimens are transported promptly and are not exposed to deleterious temperatures or other hazards.

Services Following Finding of a Chromosomal Abnormality

Following the finding of a chromosomal abnormality, the patient will be

TABLE 15

Approaches to Monitoring the Outcomes of the Program

Outcomes	Sources of data*
Percentage of women eligible for the program who have counseling, by single year of age or other indications.	2,4
Percentage of women eligible for the program who have prenatal fetal chromosome studies or amniotic AFP studies, by a single year of age or other indications.	1,2,3
Number of instances of chromosomal abnormalities and neural tube defects detected.	1,3
Number of women who have induced abortion because of the finding of an abnormal fetus, and calculated number of live births of infants with Down syndrome, other chromosomal abnormalities or NTD prevented.	1,2,3,4
Number of women who "prepare" for the birth of an infant with chromosomal abnormalities, or NTD detected by prenatal diagnosis	1,2,3,4

*1 – Records of centralized laboratory and of other laboratories serving NYC population.

2 – Birth certificate, fetal deaths and abortion records of NYC Department of Health.

3 – New York State chromosome registry at the Birth Defects Institute.

4 – Records of participating medical centers.

referred to the designated genetic service. There, the significance of the finding will be explained by the staff of the genetic service and by the counselor who had seen the patient before amniocentesis, and the options that the patient has will be explained to her. There should be particularly close cooperation at this stage between the counselor, the referring physician and the genetic service. The counseling will not be directive, and the patient will be assured of help whether she decides to continue or to terminate the pregnancy.

When the patient chooses to carry the pregnancy to term, the counselor and referring physician will help the patient to obtain services that would prepare her and her family for the birth of an affected infant. The services may comprise meetings with parents of similarly affected children or with agencies that provide services for such children, help from a psychologist or other professional in dealing with the emotional reaction to the situation, or social services concerning economic or other relevant problems. Gradually, the responsibility for coordinating the services will shift to an agency specialized in providing services for such affected infants and their families. The program will keep a record of the number of women who have such services, and of the time interval between their decisions to seek them and their appointment following referral (Table 14). Any instance in which a woman who wants such services and is unable to get them, or experiences delay in getting them will be investigated and corrective measures taken.

When the patient chooses to have an abortion, the referring physician will usually make the arrangements. The counselor will be available to help at the discretion of the patient or physician. The agreements with the participating medical facilities should insure that no delay or financial obstacle in the performance of the abortion occurs, and that abortion will be available either at that facility or at a back-up facility which was designated for such purpose at the time of the agreement between MHRA and the facility, and which has endorsed that agreement. The program will keep a record of the number of women who obtain an abortion and of the time interval between the woman's decision to have an abortion and its performance (Table 14). It will investigate instances in which there was delay or inability to obtain an abortion, and take appropriate corrective measures.

MONITORING THE OUTCOMES OF THE PROGRAM

The direct outcomes of the program and the sources of data which can be used to monitor them are shown in Table 15. The program attempts to maximize only the first outcome listed in Table 15, *i.e.*, the number of eligible women who have counseling, since the intent of the program is to give the women at risk an opportunity to make informed decisions concerning prenatal diagnosis, but not to influence these decisions. However, in order to assess the impact of the program, it is necessary to monitor the other four outcomes listed in Table 15.

In addition to its direct outcomes, the program may also have several significant side effects. The public education program may induce pregnant women 35 and older to have earlier prenatal care than they would have otherwise. This is expected to improve prevention or management of complications of pregnancy other than chromosomal abnormalities of the fetus. The public education program may also lead to changes in the number of live births from women 35 or older as discussed earlier in this paper. These side effects may be detected by monitoring the Birth and Abortion Tapes of the NYC Department of Health. However, determination of the extent to which the program may have been responsible for such side effects would require special studies.

A side effect that must be carefully watched for is that funds for services to individuals with Down syndrome might be curtailed. This would be unfortunate since the majority of individuals with Down syndrome are born from women under 35 and since some women over 35 bearing Down syndrome fetuses would choose to carry the pregnancy to term. Services for individuals with Down syndrome are markedly underfunded as it is. Therefore, it is important to monitor state and local budgets as well as reports of planning bodies and legislative committees and to prevent such decrease in funding.

The progress, cost, quality, and outcomes of NYC's PCSP should be compared with those of other prenatal cytogenetic diagnostic programs elsewhere in the nation. In analyzing these comparative findings, it will be important to take into account not only the size of the laboratory, but also the public or private governance of the program, the system of integration and quality control of the program's components, and the geography and resources of the area served.

ACKNOWLEDGMENTS

A large number of people participated in the making of NYC's PCSP. I wish to thank all of them. Among them are: my co-chairs in the SCPI task force, Drs. Kurt Hirschhorn, Zena Stein, and Mervyn Susser; administrators who helped in the transition from plan to reality, Drs. Roger C. Herdman, Ian H. Porter and Ernest B. Hook, Donna O'Hare, Shirley Mayer, Jean Pakter, the late Dr. Frederick Eagle, Mrs. Lucille Rosenbluth, and Mr. Joseph Weingold; the program's laboratory director, Dr. Lillian Hsu; the members of the specialized working groups of the SCPI task force and of the advisory committees to the program, cytogeneticists Arthur Bloom, Rody Cox, Jessica David, Ed. Gendel, Mel. Gertner, Ed. Jenkins, Hyon Kim, Ernest Lieber, O.J. Miller, Harold Nitowsky, Lawrence Shapiro, Edward Schutta, Ram Verma, and Dorothy Warburton, obstetricians, Fritz Fuchs, Thomas Kerenyi, Desider Rothe, Joseph Rovinsky, Zoltan Saary, Morton Schiffer, George Solish, and Bruce Young; ultrasound specialists, Melvin Becker, Ellen Campos, Barbara Walker, and the late Lajos von Micsky; genetic counselors, Jane Engleberg, Gary Frohlich, Lynn Godmilow, Audrey Heimler, Phyllis Klass, Barbara Krauskopf, Elsa Reich, Sylvia Rubin, Lorraine Suslak, Eva Taben, Felice Yahr, and the Director of the Human Genetics Program at Sarah Lawrence College, Joan Marks; immunologist, Eugene Ainbinder; psychiatrist, Naomi Leiter; public health specialists, Gary Barringer, Holger Hansen, Susan Margolis, Frieda Nelson, Andrea Scheidt, Melvin Schwartz, Judith

Shapiro, Mary Lou Skovron, and Barbara Strobino; computer specialist, Henry Policare; medical sociologists, Howard Kelman and Leopold Lippman; medical economists, Irving Levinson, Charlotte Muller, and Ed. Salzberg; consumers, Gilda Abramowitz, Mary Batten, William Boss, Zita Fearon, and Carole McCauley; laboratory administrators, Bernard Davidow, Paul May, and Vito Scardino; and many others who participated more briefly, or in a more limited way, in the planning or implementation of the project. I also wish to thank Ms. Frieda Nelson, Ms. Deborah Katz, Ms. Penny Liberatos, Dr. Leon Landowitz, Dr. Leopold Lippman, and Dr. Melvin Schwartz for their help and encouragement in the analysis of the NYC Birth and Abortion records data. Finally, I wish to thank the staff and secretaries who have helped at various stages in the development of the project, Ms. Diane Bethke, Bernice Lefrak, Judy Mejias, Linda Snyder, and Carmen Vasquez.

With respect to agency support, I wish to acknowledge the support given in the early stages of the project by a grant of the Greater New York Chapter of the National Foundation-March of Dimes to SCPI (Dr. Jahiel) in 1975-76, and by the Maternal and Child Health Services, Health Resources Administration, U.S. Department of Health, Education and Welfare to the NYU Medical Center (Dr. Selma Snyderman), in 1976-77, and the support given in the implementation of the project by the New York State Department of Health, the New York City Department of Health, and the New York City Health Systems Agency.

REFERENCES

1. R.I. Jahiel, Z. Stein and K. Hirschhorn, Availability of Prenatal Cytogenetic Screening: A Public Health Responsibility. Paper presented at the 103rd Annual Meeting of the American Public Health Association, November 20, 1975.
2. Prenatal Cytogenetic Screening Services for the Detection of Chromosomal Defects. Report of the Task Force on the Prevention of Down's Syndrome and Neural Tube Defects, N.Y. Scientists' Committee for Public Information, New York, March 23, 1976.
3. G.P. Oakley, Prenatal Chromosomal Diagnosis Ratios in Four United States Communities. Poster No. 43, Fifth International Conference on Birth Defects, National Foundation-March of Dimes, Montreal, August, 1977.
4. E.B. Hook and A. Lindsjo, *Am.J. Hum. Genet. 30*, 19, 1978.
5. E.B. Hook and J.L. Hamerton, *in* Population Cytogenetics: Studies in Humans, E.B. Hook and I.H. Porter (Eds.), Academic Press, New York, p. 63, 1977.
6. A. Milunsky, The Prenatal Diagnosis of Hereditary Disorders, C.C. Thomas, Springfield, Ill., p. 37, 1973.
7. E.B. Hook, *in* Proceedings of the 1977 Birth Defects Conference, Memphis, Birth Defects Original Article Series, Vol. 14, 6C, D. Bergsma and R.L. Summitt (Eds.), Alan R. Liss, Inc., New York, pp. 249-267, 1978.

8. Cytogenetics Advisory Committee, New York City Prenatal Screening Program and Centralized Laboratory. Guidelines for Cytogenetics, tenth draft, 1978. Available from Dr. Lawrence Shapiro, Director of Cytogenetics, Letchworth Village, Thiells, N.Y., 10984.
9. The NICDH National Registry for Amniocentesis Study Group, *J.A.M.A.* *236*, 1471, 1976.
10. N.E. Simpson *et al., Canad. Med. Assoc. J. 115*, 739, 1976.
11. R. Breg, Monitoring Quality Control in Prenatal Cytogenetic Diagnosis Under Pressure of Large Volume of Service. Paper presented at the Workshop on Quality Assurance in Cytogenetics at the Birth Defects Institute, New York State Department of Health, Albany, N.Y., November 14, 1977.
12. Genetic Counseling Advisory Committee, New York City Prenatal Cytogenetic Screening Program and Centralized Laboratory. Guidelines for Amniocentesis Counseling, 1978. Available from Ms. Phyllis Klass, Genetic Counseling Program, New York Hospital-Cornell Medical Center, 525 East 68th Street, New York, N.Y., 10021.
13. Obstetrics Advisory Committee, New York City Prenatal Cytogenetic Screening Program and Centralized Laboratory. Guidelines for Amniocentesis, 1978. Available from Dr. Bruce Young, Department of Obstetrics, NYU Medical Center, 550 First Avenue, New York, N.Y., 10016.

MATERNAL SERUM ALPHA-FETOPROTEIN SCREENING FOR NEURAL TUBE DEFECTS: STRUCTURE AND ORGANIZATION

James N. Macri
Robert R. Weiss
Boris Libster

Anencephaly and spina bifida (NTD) collectively occur within the United States at a frequency of two per thousand births.[1] For some time, amniotic fluid biochemical parameters have been sought as a means of prenatally diagnosing these severe and common congenital malformations. Most important among them were the amniotic fluid evaluation of bilirubin,[2] 5′hydroxy-indole acetic acid,[3] amino acids,[4] β marker protein of cerebrospinal fluid,[5] fibrinogen degradation products,[6] β lipoprotein, and α_2 macroglobulin.[7] None, however, possess the degree of accuracy and specificity required for utilization in prospective prenatal diagnosis. Certain biophysical evaluations such as diagnostic ultrasonography,[8] amniography,[9] and direct fetoscopy[10] have also been applied to NTD diagnosis with varying degrees of success.

High-Risk Management

Since 1972 a high degree of correlation has been recognized between elevations in amniotic fluid alpha-fetroprotein (α-fp) and the presence of open NTD.[11] This correlation has been used in developing highly successful high-risk management plans directed at preventing the recurrence of NTD.[12] Such a management plan illustrated in Figure 1, however, can only be applied to families demonstrating significantly elevated risk factors because of a strong history. Within these high-risk families the use of diagnostic ultrasonography, amniocentesis, and possibly further confirmatory visualization techniques are justified.

Currently, we have prospectively evaluated amniotic fluid in 300 families at high risk for recurring NTD utilizing 2 standard deviations above the mean as our upper limit of normal. We have prospectively diagnosed recurring NTD within this group at a rate of 1 in 30. This recurrence rate deviates from previous risk

---

Neural Tube Defect Laboratory supported by: The Bureau of Maternal and Child Health and Crippled Children's Services, The National Foundation-March of Dimes, and the National Easter Seal Society for Crippled Children and Adults.

ISBN 0-12-562650-9

factors associated with high-risk families reported to be within the range of 1 in 20.[1]

There is little question that programs designed to evaluate high-risk families for recurring NTD will be extremely successful. Within our high-risk series to date, no false positive amniotic fluid results have been observed. A single false negative amniotic fluid level was seen in association with a sacral skin-covered meningocele with no neurological involvement. Open lesions, therefore, representing over 90% of all NTD should be accurately detectable. It has been estimated, however, that potentially greater than 90% of future NTD fetuses will stem from the non-risk pregnant population.[13] Clearly, amniocentesis on such an unselected population is not feasible. Screening procedures directed at this great majority of potentially defective fetuses have been proposed[14] and evaluated[15] within the United Kingdom. These procedures involve evaluation of maternal serum α-fp as the initial phase of testing.

Screening for Neural Tube Defects

In July of 1976, a model screening program for NTD was iniated within the United States. Prior to actual prospective testing, a normal distribution curve for maternal serum α-fp was established on over 500 singleton pregnancies.[16] In doing so, the serum upper limit of normal was arbitratily designated at the 98th percentile. It was reasoned that within a screening population of 10,000, 200 pregnancies would demonstrate elevated maternal serum α-fp levels. If a high degree of correlation exists between maternal serum α-fp elevations and NTD, it could be inferred that all mothers carrying a fetus with NTD would fall within this group of 200 elevations.

Within the same screening population of 10,000 pregnancies, local surveys indicate the incidence of NTD to be 1-2/1,000. We should, therefore, expect to find 10 to 20 NTD fetuses within our screening population. Furthermore, these 10 to 20 NTD fetuses would be expected to fall within the projected group of 200 mothers demonstrating elevations in maternal serum α-fp. Therefore, if these projections were correct, any mother demonstrating elevated maternal serum α-fp levels could theoretically assume risk factors for NTD of between 1 in 10 and 1 in 20. The task which then remains is to effectively identify those mothers carrying an affected fetus. Within this context, any program undertaking screening must be constantly aware of all possible factors which can potentially elevate maternal serum α-fp falsely.

Factors Influencing Maternal Serum Alpha-Fetoprotein

The single most important factor in generating a false interpretation of maternal serum α-fp levels is the incorrect estimation of gestational age. Almost invariably, errors in gestational age dating based on the last menstrual period will give rise after sonographic correction to a more advanced gestational age assessment. Within the context of screening, if this advance in gestational age esti-

NEURAL TUBE DEFECT - FAMILY HISTORY
HIGH RISK PREGNANCY
diagnostic ultrasonography
abnormal
anencephaly
amniocentesis
AMNIOTIC FLUID
BIOCHEMICAL EVALUATION
ALPHA-FETOPROTEIN
KL. B. - C.I.E.P. - T.P.
visualization of defect
by amniography
ELECTIVE PREGNANCY
INTERRUPTION
normal
amniocentesis
AMNIOTIC FLUID
BIOCHEMICAL EVALUATION
ALPHA-FETOPROTEIN
KL. B. - C.I.E.P. - T.P.
abnormal
spinal lesion
suspected
normal
ROUTINE OBSTETRICAL
CARE

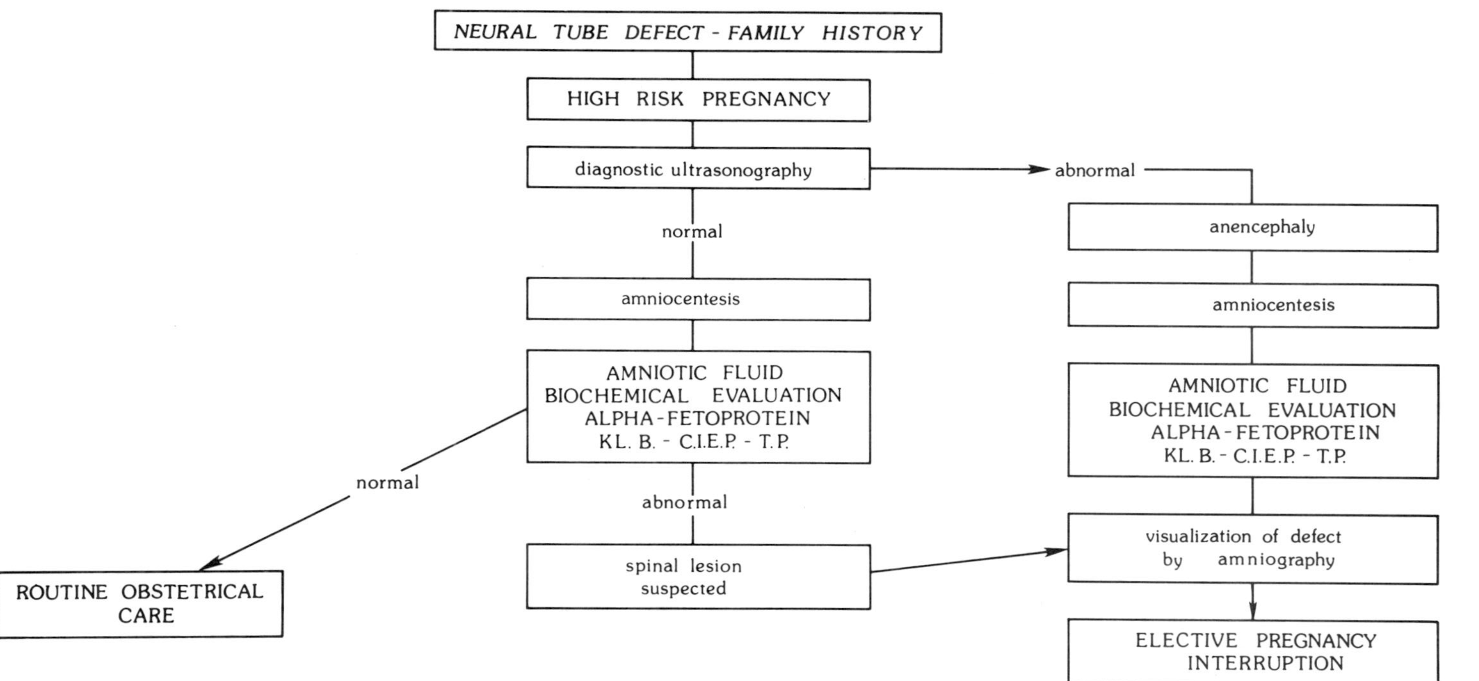

Figure 1.

mation is greater than two weeks and, additionally, renders the maternal serum α-fp level normal, no further evaluation should be necessary.

Two additional clinical entities which can significantly alter maternal serum α-fp levels are multiple pregnancy and impending or actual fetal demise.[17] Once again the utilization of diagnostic ultrasonography in identifying these fetuses is of vital importance to the overall screening process. It is important to note that the accurate detection of multiple pregnancy through screening might serve as a very important adjunct to a process initially intended for birth defects detection. This concept can be fully appreciated when one considers the greatly increased risks associated with multiple pregnancy identified late in gestation.

Other congenital malformations not associated with the formation of the neural tube may also influence the level of maternal serum α-fp. Superficially placed gross lesions of the fetal body which allow for fetal serum leakage or transudation can mimic the NTD diagnostic picture. Such non-neural tube congenital malformations which have been reported in association with raised amniotic fluid α-fp levels include gastroschisis,[18] omphalocele,[19] and sacrococcygeal teratoma.[20] Additionally, disruption of the normal fetal glomerular integrity, such as is seen in congenital nephrosis, can create fetal proteinuria resulting in exceedingly elevated amniotic fluid α-fp levels.[21] Finally, certain upper gastrointestinal atresias interfering with amniotic fluid swallowing and the normal metabolic route for amniotic fluid α-fp can result in elevations.[22] Whether all or some of these defects will influence maternal serum levels of α-fp remains questionable. Normal fetal serum contains milligrams per milliliter levels of α-fp. Any clinical situation, therefore, creating a feto-maternal transfusion can significantly alter the maternal serum levels of α-fp. This type of transfusion can occur actively during amniocentesis or in other unknown ways. For maternal serum levels to be accurately evaluated, therefore, blood samples must be drawn prior to amniocentesis.

With the consideration of all known factors that can influence maternal serum α-fp we can now concentrate our diagnostic efforts on those mothers demonstrating true elevations in maternal serum levels. In doing so, an expansion of the high-risk management plan (Fig. 1), as illustrated in Figure 2, can be applied to all pregnancies. It should be noted that once a pregnancy has been designated as high-risk through the screening procedure, the diagnostic flow in confirming the presence of a neural tube defect is identical to the family with a positive history with the exception of the initial screening process.

Implementation of the Screening Process

In implementing such an expanded management scheme, careful consideration must be given to local health care systems as well as the local practice of obstetrics. Within the United States, the majority of prenatal care involves private office visits. The screening process, therefore, must be initiated currently by the private obstetrician on a voluntary or optional basis. In doing so, the private

NON-RISK PREGNANT POPULATION
MATERNAL BLOOD SERUM
BIOCHEMICAL EVALUATION
ALPHA-FETOPROTEIN
rormal
abnormal
2nd MATERNAL BLOOD
SERUM EVALUATION
rormal
abnormal
HIGH RISK
FOR NEURAL TUBE DEFECT
diagnostic ultrasonography
corrected gestational age
> 2 weeks
multiple pregnancy
abnormal
anencephaly
amniocentesis
AMNIOTIC FLUID
BIOCHEMICAL EVALUATION
ALPHA-FETOPROTEIN
KL. B. - C.I.E.P. - T.P.
visualization of defect
by amniography
ELECTIVE PREGNANCY
INTERRUPTION
normal
amniocentesis
AMNIOTIC FLUID
BIOCHEMICAL EVALUATION
ALPHA-FETOPROTEIN
KL. B. - C.I.E.P. - T.P.
normal
ROUTINE OBSTETRICAL
CARE
abnormal
spinal lesion
suspected

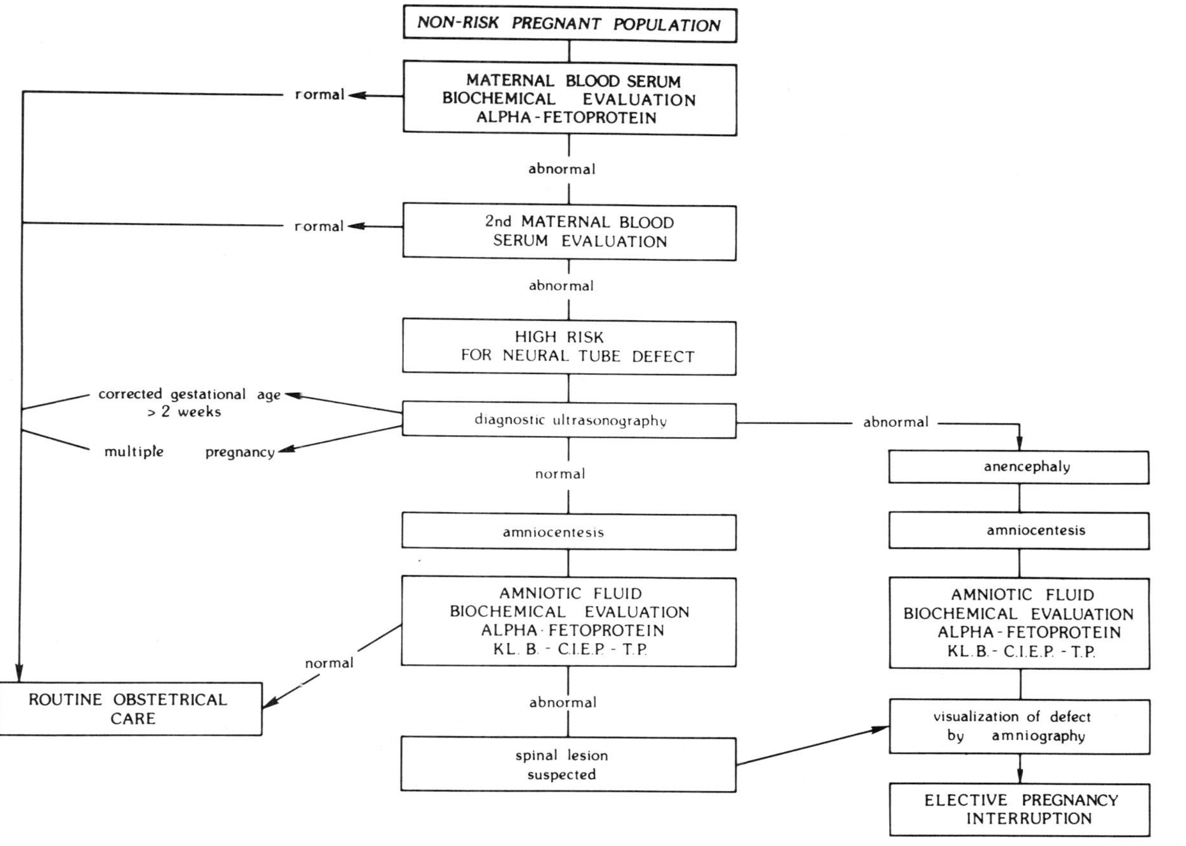

Figure 2

physician must be capable of providing his patients with all pertinent information concerning screening prior to the obtaining of an initial blood sample. Additionally, at present voluntary patient participation within scrrening must involve the obtaining of informed consent.

With physician and patient participation coordinated, a major problem intrinsic to the screening process is the smooth and orderly establishment of a sample collection system. In the Nassau County experience, as illustrated in Figure 3, we have utilized the existing Department of Health laboratory as an established link between the private physician and clinical laboratory testing. We have, therefore, been able to take advantage of the Department of Health blood mailing system. Because most obstetrical offices are not equipped with clinical blood centrifuges, it is fortuitous that whole maternal blood can be forwarded by routine postal service without altering the levels of maternal serum α-fp. Within our geographic area, this mailing system is adequate during most months of the year with caution being necessary only during extremes of temperature. All maternal whole blood samples received by the Department of Health laboratory are coded for NTD screening and undergo logging and serum partitioning. On a daily basis, all maternal sera are forwarded by courier to the NTD laboratory. This direct mailing system is only utilized within the Nassau County screening program for initial maternal blood evaluation.

Mothers demonstrating elevated maternal serum α-fp levels in the first blood sampling initiate direct communication from the screening program to the private participating obstetrician. At this time the obstetrician is urged to schedule that particular mother for a second blood drawing at least one week after the initial sampling. This second maternal serum is not mailed but rather picked up directly by special courier of the NTD screening program. The second blood is delivered directly to the NTD laboratory and receives priority analysis. In the event that the second maternal serum α-fp maintains an elevation, the full diagnostic services of the high-risk NTD testing center are made available to that mother. Any mother electing to take advantage of the high-risk testing service is immediately scheduled for diagnostic ultrasonography.

Should a re-evaluation of gestational age, based on fetal biparietal diameter, advance the gestation greater than two weeks and render the maternal serum α-fp level normal, no further diagnostic procedures are warranted. Additionally, the presence of multiple gestation based on ultrasound examination would require no further testing. Mothers carrying a single fetus whose last menstrual period gestational age is consistent with that derived by ultrasound, are offered amniocentesis and amniotic fluid α-fp evaluation.

In those mothers undergoing amniocentesis the screening process is abandoned in lieu of the highly accurate diagnostic evaluation of amniotic fluid. In spite of the elevated risk factor in mothers demonstrating elevated maternal serum α-fp levels, a normal amniotic fluid α-fp level would strongly suggest the absence of a NTD and preclude further evaluation. Recently, however, evidence has been presented which would indicate that such mothers may be at a higher risk of

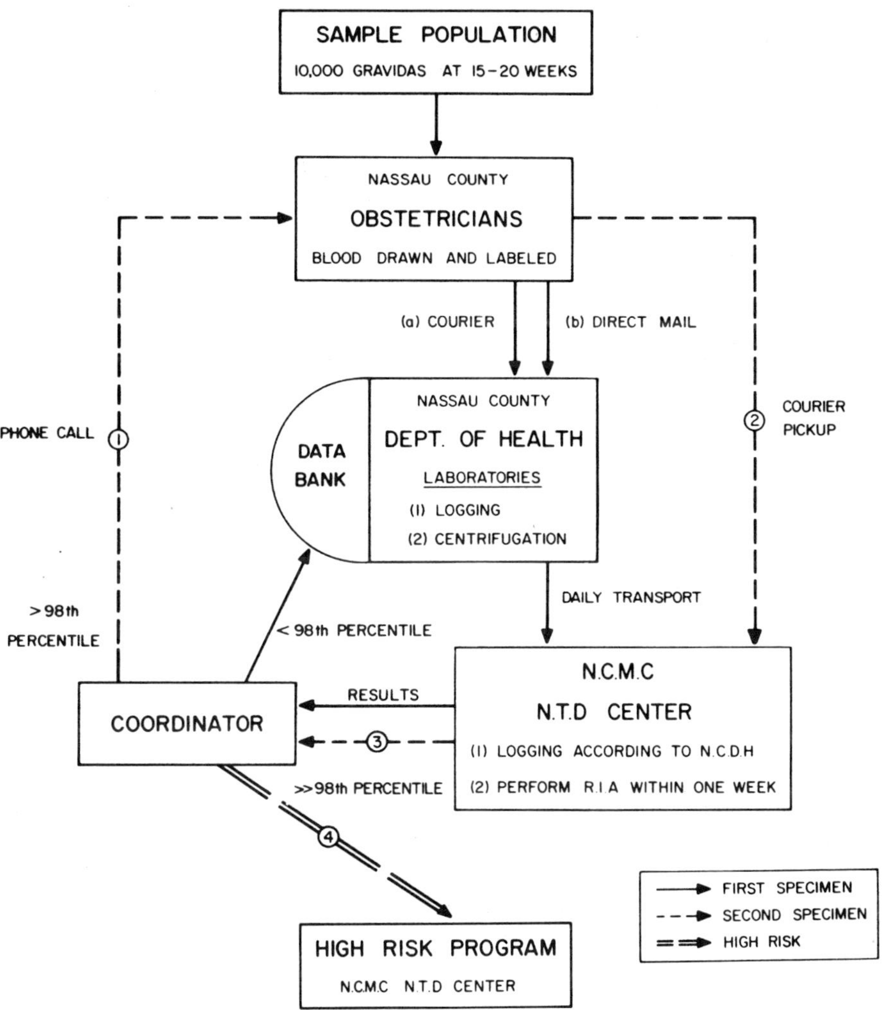

Figure 3.

Reprinted courtesy of *Birth Defects: Original Article Series, Vol. VIII, No. 3D*, 193, 1977.

delivering low birthweight children.[23,24] If this concept is accurate, this parameter may prove to be an additional important adjunct to the screening process.

In those mothers demonstrating elevations in amniotic fluid α-fp, it has been the policy of the Nassau County NTD program to further evaluate the pregnancy by attempting to visualize radiographically potential lesions prior to the irreversible termination of pregnancy. In our opinion this policy can be extremely helpful in the confirmation of NTD as well as aiding in the reduction of possible false positive results.

Figure 4 represents amniography performed in three separate pregnancies all of which demonstrated elevations in amniotic fluid α-fp. The normal amniographic view in Figure 4A, associated with borderline elevations in amniotic fluid α-fp, allowed the family to make a judgement in favor of continuing the pregnancy, resulting in the delivery of a normal male at term. The clear view of anencephaly (Fig. 4B) and spina bifida (4C) were associated with significant elevations in amniotic fluid α-fp. Both of these defects were confirmed at abortion. These results would suggest that NTD is not associated with minimal amniotic fluid α-fp elevations.

Establishing the Upper Limit of Normal

Recently, based on similar data, some investigators have called for an elevation of the amniotic fluid upper limit of normal to the 5th standard deviation above the mean.[25] We have not supported this concept on the grounds that no NTD program, to date, has sufficient experience with the detection of all forms of open lesions. Our data on over 2,000 amniotic fluid α-fetoprotein evaluations might have supported this alteration in cutoff levels until a recent prospective diagnosis of spina bifida demonstrated amniotic fluid α-fp levels between the second and third standard deviation above the mean. In our opinion, much greater emphasis must be placed on the accurate establishment of normal cutoff limits rather than arbitrarily placing such limits in a range which would conveniently eliminate false positive results. Additionally, NTD detection programs should place more emphasis on visualization techniques to minimize such false positive results.

Within the context of screening, the establishment of maternal serum cutoff limits face similar problems. The spina bifida fetus visualized in Figure 4C, while demonstrating significantly elevated amniotic fluid α-fp, was associated initially during screening with maternal serum elevations between the second and third standard deviation above the mean. Had the maternal serum cutoff level been higher than 2 standard deviations above the mean, this non-risk mother would not have been considered at elevated risk. In turn, amniocentesis and amniotic fluid α-fp evaluation would not have been performed. Once again, extreme care must be taken in the establishment of maternal serum cutoff levels in an effort to maximize the efficiency of the maternal serum evaluation.

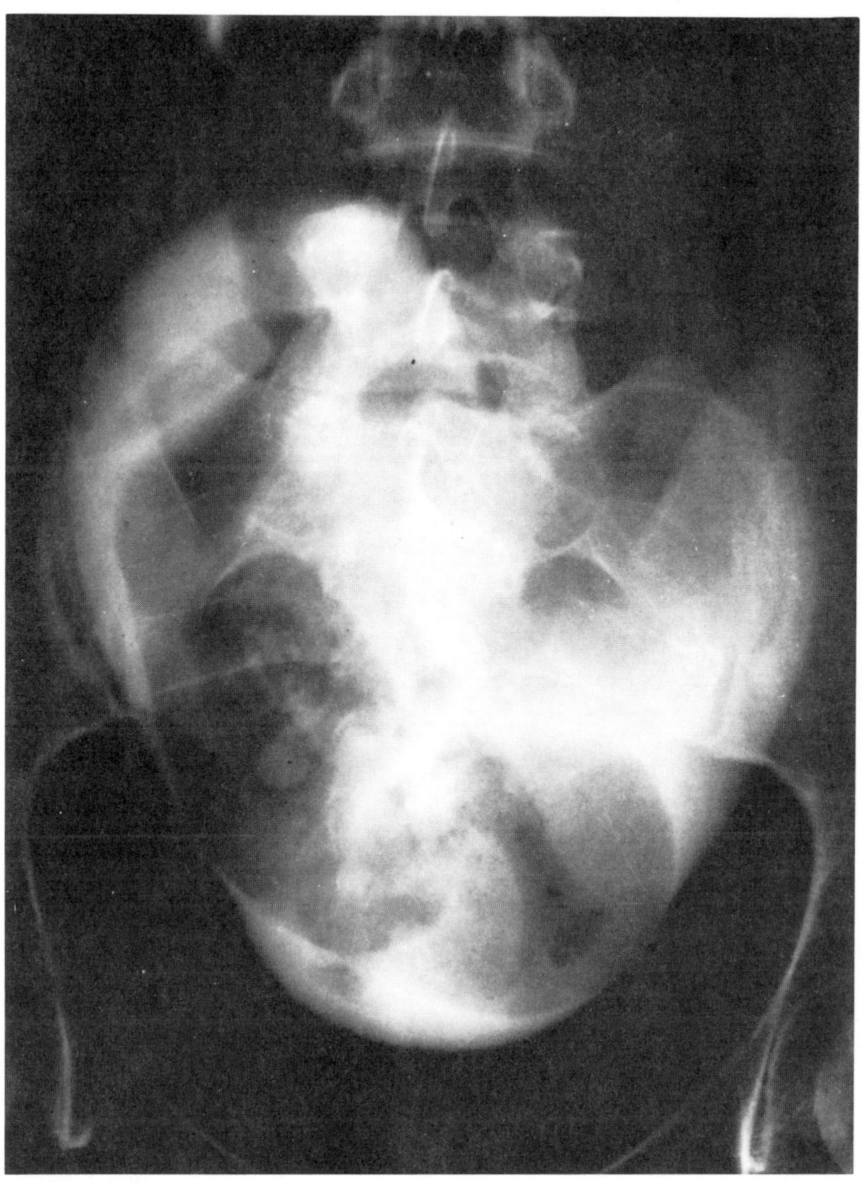

Figure 4A.

(Reprinted courtesy of *J.A.M.A. 236*, 1251, 1976.)

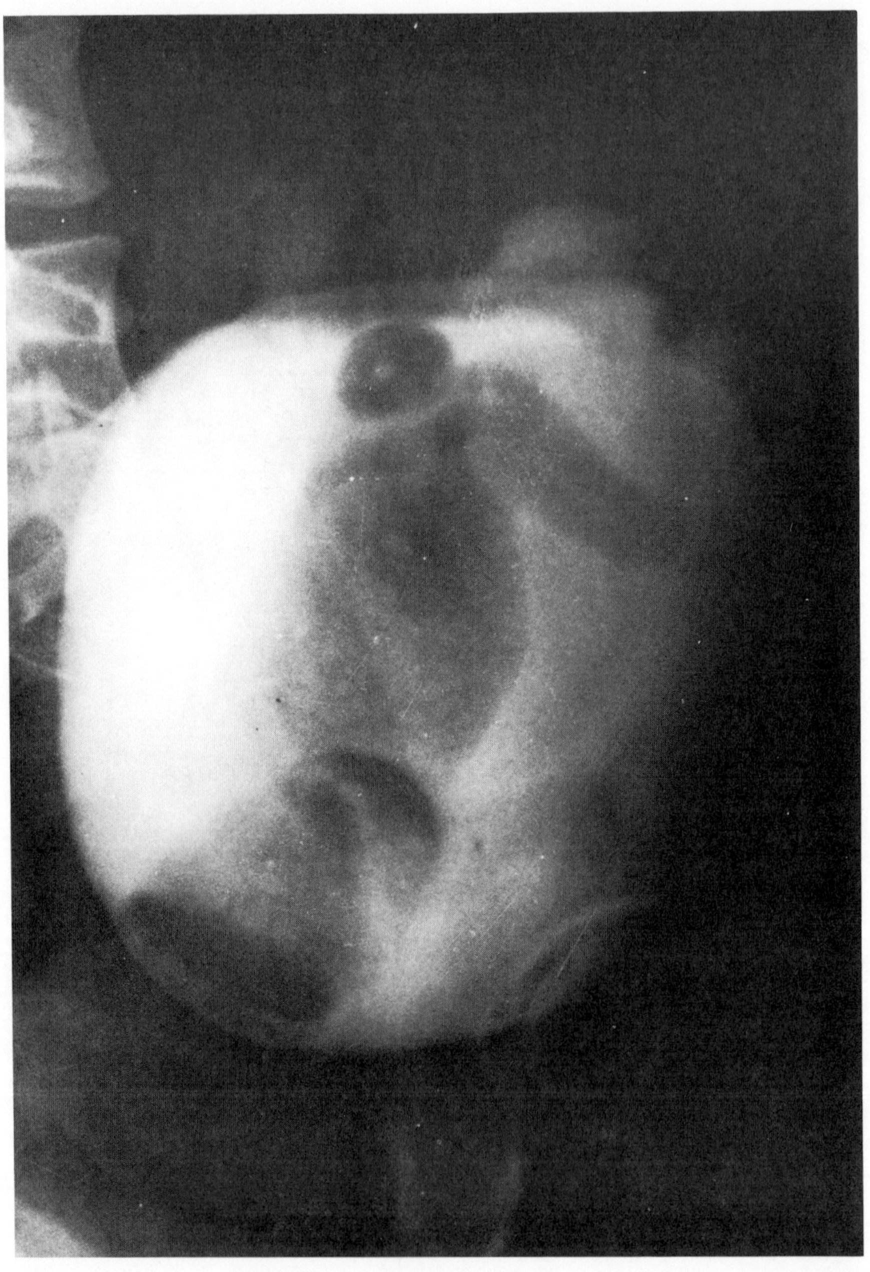

Figure 4B.
(Reprinted courtesy of *J.A.M.A. 236*, 1251, 1976.)

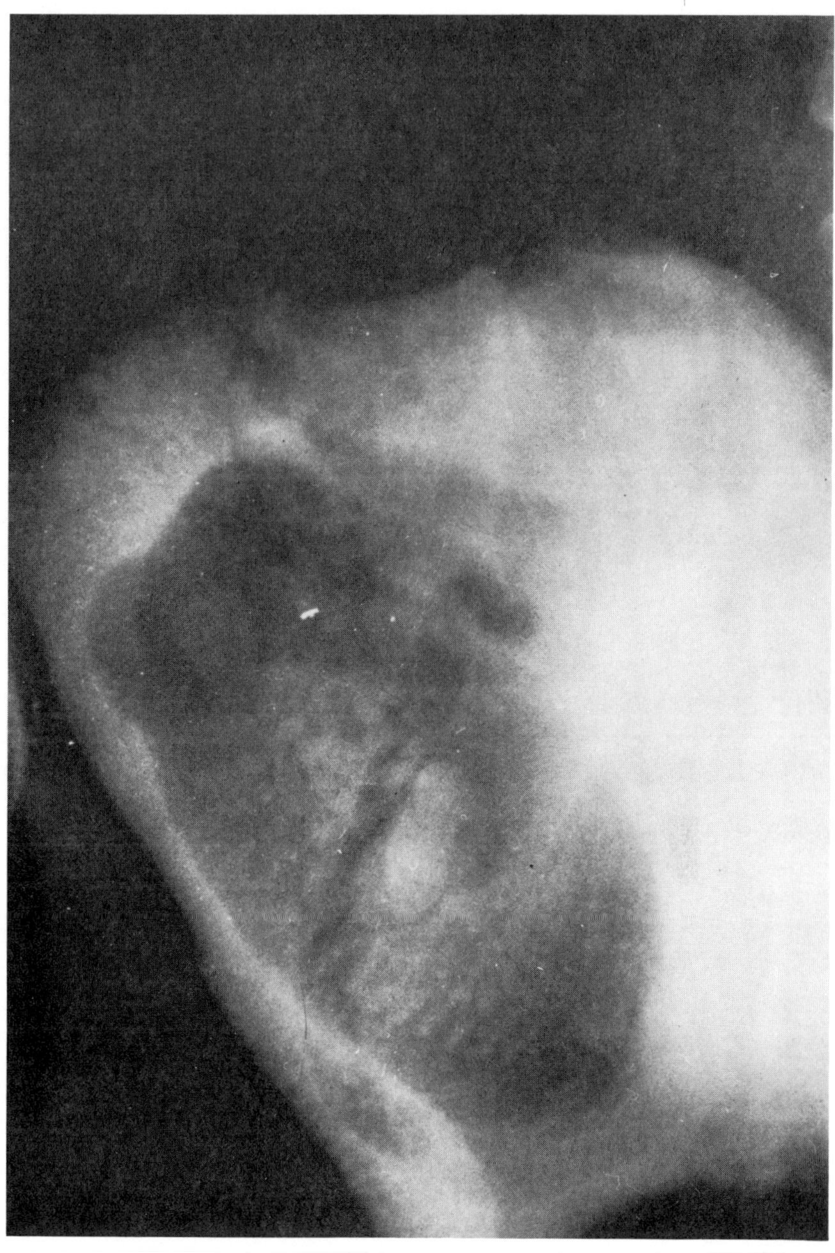

Figure 4C.
Reprinted courtesy of *Obstet. Gynecol. 51*, 301, 1978.

Screening Yield

To date, the Nassau county NTD model program has prospectively screened 5,000 non-risk pregnancies (Table 1). Within this group, 7.6% (382) mothers demonstrated elevated maternal serum α-fp in their initial blood sampling. Of those mothers re-tested, 145 demonstrated serum levels now within normal limits. Serial elevations in maternal serum α-fp sampled at least one week apart were, therefore, observed in 4.3% (216) of the initial screened population. Within this group, 5 spontaneous abortions were recorded before these mothers could be scheduled for diagnostic ultrasonography. Of 204 ultrasound examinations performed, 54 pregnancies demonstrated errors in gestational age assessment sufficient to warrant no further evaluation. Thirty-five twin and two triplet pregnancies were identified by ultrasound representing .74% of the original screened population. An additional five intrauterine fetal deaths were also identified. These additional evaluations and corrections left 105 (2.1%) singleton pregnancies with accurate gestational age to be further evaluated by amniocentesis and amniotic fluid α-fp determination.

Amniotic fluid α-fp levels were measured in all 105 pregnancies considered at risk through screening. Ninety-three of these samples demonstrated levels considered to be normal. Twelve individual samples were found to have significantly elevated α-fp levels, three of which were associated with intrauterine fetal demise not initially detected by ultrasound. Of the nine remaining abnormal amniotic fluid levels, seven pregnancies elected to undergo amniography. Five abnormal amniographies resulted in the elective termination of those individual pregnancies and confirmed open NTD. Two normal amniographies allowed the family the option to continue the pregnancy, one of which has now delivered without NTD. Two additional patients refused amniography and electively terminated their pregnancies again confirming open NTD at abortion.

Discussion

Within the initial screening population, seven open NTD fetuses were accurately prospectively diagnosed. It is of interest to note that by utilizing the 98th percentile cutoff, maternal serum levels gave rise to 105 mothers (2.1%) actually undergoing amniocentesis. In our estimation it is of even greater interest that every mother undergoing amniocentesis because of maternal serum screening was at a 7/105 or 1 in 15 risk of carrying a child with a NTD. These actual findings are consistent with the theoretical projection of risk factors within a screened population previously alluded to. The significant power of the maternal serum α-fp evaluation can be fully appreciated when one considers that mothers demonstrating true elevations in maternal serum levels are at greater risk (1/15) of carrying a child with a NTD than mothers having had a previously affected child (1/30).

Three additional NTD's were observed witin the initial screening population of 5,000 during the process of fetal outcome determination. In one case, maternal

TABLE 1

Neural Tube Defect Screening Program

Total Number of Pregnancies Screened	5,000	
Specimens with elevated AFP first time	382	(7.6%)
Repeat specimens not obtained	21	
Specimens normal AFP second time*	145	
Specimens high AFP second time	216	(4.3%)
Patients refusing sonography	7	
Spontaneous abortions prior to sonography	5	
Number of Sonograms	204	
Corrected dates*,**	54	
Multiple gestation*,**	37	(0.74%)
Intrauterine demise**	5	
Patients refusing amniocentesis	3	
Number of Amniocenteses	105	(2.1%)
Normal AFP levels*	93	
Abnormal AFP levels	12	
Intrauterine demise	3	
Patients refusing amniography***	2	
Number of Amniographies	7	
Normal amniogram	2	
Abnormal amniogram ***	5	

* No further evaluation
** Confirmed by sonography
*** Elective termination of pregnancy

SCREENING YIELD = 7 NEURAL TUBE DEFECTS

5 ANENCEPHALY/ 2 SPINA BIFIDA

serum associated with anencephaly was evaluated at 13 weeks of gestation which now has been documented to be outside of the optimal time frame for maternal serum evaluation. Maternal serum from a second anencephalic pregnancy at 17 weeks of gestation was determined to lie at the 96th percentile. When one considers the very favorable ratio of unnecessary to necessary amniocenteses performed as illustrated in Table 1, it is conceivable that a downward displacement of the maternal serum cutoff may yield greater efficiency and include the detection of such cases. Maternal serum from a third anencephalic pregnancy again at 17 weeks of gestation demonstrated α-fp levels at the 49th percentile. This case is totally unexplainable and will in all likelihood exemplify that percentage of open defects which will, in the future, remain undetectable. These added malformations define an overall NTD frequency within those outcomes currently known of 10 in 5,000 or 2/1,000.

Comment

It has become increasingly clear that maternal serum screening of the unselected pregnant population can be as effective in preventing the occurrence of NTD as amniotic fluid α-fp testing is in preventing the recurrence of NTD. Within the general scope of such a screening design the successful detection of additional obstetrical complications can only serve to enhance its implementation. The high degree of accuracy in the identification of multiple pregnancies supports this concept. The potential for additionally identifying pregnancies at significant risk of delivering low birthweight babies may represent still another important adjunct. Only when one considers the total potential yield of this process can the full power of maternal serum α-fp screening be fully realized.

10. J.C. Hob

REFERENCES

1. K. Shulman, *in* Birth Defects, Atlas and Compendium, D. Bergsma (Ed.), Williams and Wilkins Co., Baltimore, p. 161, 1974.
2. A.E.H. Emery, D.J.H. Brock, D. Burt and D. Eccleston, *J. Obstet. Gynaecol. Br. Commonw. 81*, 512, 1974.
3. A.E.H. Emery, D. Eccleston, J.B. Scrimgeour and M. Johnstone, *J. Obstet. Gynaecol. Br. Commonw. 79,* 154, 1972.
4. A.E.H. Emery, D. Burt and J.B. Scrimgeour, *Lancet 1*, 970, 1973.
5. J.N. Macri, R.R. Weiss and M.S. Joshi, *Lancet 1*, 1108, 1974.
6. D.W. Burdi, P.W. Howie, W. Edgar, C.D. Forbes and C.R.M. Prentice, *Lancet 1*, 1013, 1975.
7. D.J.H. Brock, *Hum. Hered. 26*, 401, 1976.
8. S. Campbell, J. Pryse-Davies, T.M. Coltart, M.J. Seller and J.D. Singer, *Lancet 1*, 1065, 1975.
9. F.D. Frigoletto and N.T. Griscom, *Obstet. Gynecol. 44*, 286, 1974.
10. J.C. Hobbins, M.J. Mahoney and L.A. Goldstein, *Am. J. Obstet. Gynecol.*

118, 1069, 1974.

11. D.J.H. Brock and R.G. Sutcliffe, *Lancet 2*, 197, 1972.
12. J.N. Macri, R.R. Weiss, R. Tillitt, D. Balsam and K.W. Elligers, *J.A.M.A. 236*, 1251, 1976.
13. Leading Article, *Lancet 1*, 907, 1974.
14. D.J.H. Brock and R.G. Sutcliffe, *Lancet 2*, 197, 1972.
15. Report of U.K. Collaborative Study Alpha-fetoprotein in Relation to Neural Tube Defects, *Lancet 1*, 1323, 1977.
16. J.N. Macri, R.R. Weiss, N.A. Starkovsky, K.W. Elligers and D.B. Berger, *Lancet 2*, 719, 1975.
17. J.N. Macri and R.R. Weiss, *in* Embryology and Pathogenesis and Prenatal Diagnosis, R.B. Lowry and D. Bergsma (Ed.), Alan R. Liss Publishers, New York, p. 191-199, 1977.
18. D.L. Douglas, *Lancet 1*, 42, 1977.
19. H.W.A. DeBruign and H.J. Huisges, *Lancet 1*, 525, 1975.
20. W. Schid and F.P. Muhlethaler, *Humangenetik 26*, 353, 1975.
21. B. Kjessler, S.G. Johnsson, M. Sherman, K.H. Gustauson and G. Hultquist, *Lancet 1,* 432, 1975.
22. M. Seppala, E. Laes and M. Narvo-Noponen, *J. Obstet. Gynaecol. Br. Commonw. 81*, 827, 1974.
23. D.J.H. Brock, L. Barron, P. Jelen, M. Watt and J.B. Scrimgeour, *Lancet 2,* 267, 1977.
24. N. Wald, H. Cuckle, G.M. Stirrat, M.J. Bennett and A.C. Turnbull, *Lancet 2,* 268, 1977.
25. M.E. Kimball, A. Milunsky and E. Alpert, *Obstet. Gynecol. 40*, 532, 1977.

CYSTIC FIBROSIS: PROSPECTS FOR PROSPECTIVE GENETIC SCREENING

S.L. Sklower
R.J. Desnick

INTRODUCTION

The practice of medicine is ideally directed to the prevention of disease. The success of immunization and public health strategies for the control of infectious diseases has demonstrated the effectiveness of preventive medicine. Recent concern for early intervention in the management of disorders such as hypertension, diabetes, and heart disease has focused physician efforts toward the detection of individuals with insidious or subclinical manifestations. Within this perspective, strategies designed to prevent tragic genetic disorders have generated increased medical and public attention. Since genetic diseases cannot be cured, and since specific therapy for most remains elusive, emphasis has been directed toward screening for detection and prevention.

Genetic screening can be either retrospective or prospective. Retrospective screening involves the detection of individuals affected with an inherited disease; retrospective screening is particularly important when early therapeutic intervention will improve the patient's prognosis. Indeed, the extensive experience with retrospective screening for phenylketonuria (PKU) has documented the effectiveness of this approach as well as its critical limitations.[1] In contrast, the goal of prospective screening is the identification of individuals or couples who are at high risk for having offspring with a serious inherited disease. In this case, previously unsuspecting couples can be counseled concerning the nature of the disease, their risk of having an affected child, and the various reproductive options available. The prototype for prospective genetic screening has been Tay-Sachs disease (TSD), a fatal, inherited neurologic disorder of children. The crucial finding that made prospective screening for TSD feasible was the elucidation of the disorder's basic defect, the defective activity of the lysosomal enzyme, β-hexosaminidase A.[2] Assay of this enzymatic activity provided for the identifi-

*This review was supported by grants (1-273 and C-155) from the National Foundation-March of Dimes. Dr. Desnick is the recipient of an NIH Research Career Development Award (K04-AM 00042) and Dr. Sklower is the recipient of an NIH Postdoctoral Fellowship in Medical Genetics (IT32 HD 07105).

ISBN 0-12-562650-9

cation of the normal individuals who were heterozygous carriers of the disease causing gene, the ability to prenatally diagnose fetuses affected with this tragic disease as well as biochemical diagnostic confirmation of affected infants.

The successful experience with prospective screening for TSD[3,4] has direct implications for the screening of other relatively common genetic diseases. Among these, cystic fibrosis (CF) stands out as a prime candidate. CF is one of the main causes of chronic disease and death in children and adolescents, occurring in about one in every 2,500 Caucasian babies. The manifestations of the disease are related to a generalized dysfunction of exocrine glands. Affected individuals suffer from the triad of chronic pulmonary disease, pancreatic deficiency with steatorrhea and azotorrhea, and abnormally high sweat electrolytes. Additional manifestations include hepatic cirrhosis, intestinal obstruction, nasal polyps, rectal prolapse, and other complications secondary to pulmonary or gastrointestinal obstruction. To date, therapy for these patients remains supportive. Approximately one in every 25 Caucasian individuals is a carrier of the disease-causing gene. Efforts to identify the specific defect have not been successful, although research endeavors in several areas appear promising.[5–14] When this breakthrough occurs, prospective screening for CF should become feasible.

Since comprehensive reviews of genetic screening, both retrospective and prospective, are available,[1,15,16] the following discussion will review some of the major lessons learned from past experiences and emphasize the essential requisites of future screening endeavors. In addition, considerations for the rapid implementation of prospective screening for CF are presented, assuming that the specific biochemical/enzymatic defect will be delineated in the future.

PAST EXPERIENCE: LESSONS AND REQUISITES FOR PROSPECTIVE GENETIC SCREENING

Retrospective Screening

Phenylketonuria: Mass retrospective screening for genetic diseases began in the early 1960's with PKU. This autosomal recessive disorder, caused by the defective activity of phenylalanine hydroxylase, is characterized primarily by mental retardation. The suggestion that a phenylalanine-restricted diet might prove therapeutic stimulated efforts to detect hyperphenylalaninemia in newborn infants. Development of a rapid, reliable and inexpensive diagnostic test provided the rationale for mass genetic screening.[17,18] Subsequently, legislation was rapidly enacted for the compulsory screening of newborns for PKU; currently 43 out of 50 states have PKU screening laws.[1] The impact of PKU screening has been impressive; early intervention has resulted in significant therapeutic benefit. However, the experience has provided important lessons for future genetic screening programs (Table 1). These concern the sensitivity of the diagnostic assay, the implications of genetic heterogeneity and the need for adequate follow-up.

TABLE 1

Genetic Screening: Lessons From Past Experiences

Phenylketonuria:	
1. Rapid Substrate Assay:	Hyperphenylalaninemia Variants
2. Genetic Heterogeneity:	Phenylalanine Hydroxylase Dihydropteridine Reductase
3. Lack of Follow-up:	Maternal PKU
Sickle Cell Anemia:	
1. Screening Legislation:	Mandatory vs. Voluntary
2. Public Education and Counseling:	Uninformed – Confused (disease vs. trait) Stigmatization
Tay-Sachs Disease – Model for Prospective Genetic Screening:	
1. Defined At-Risk Population	
2. Reliable Heterozygote Discrimination by Enzyme Assay (genetic variants detectable)	
3. Prenatal Detection Available	
4. Effective Education: Medical and Public Communities	
5. Voluntary Mass Screening Program	
6. Genetic Counseling and Follow-Up	

The diagnostic assay detected newborns with elevated levels of blood phenylalanine; however, not all neonates with hyperphenylalaninemia proved to have classical PKU. Variant forms of hyperphenylalaninemia have been recognized which do not cause mental deficiency and the use of dietary restriction for these children is contraindicated.[19,20] In 1975, Kaufman and associates reported a child in whom dietary restriction failed to prevent neurologic manifestations.[21] This child had hyperphenylalaninemia; however, his level of phenylalanine hydroxylase was normal. Further evaluation demonstrated a deficiency of dihydropteridine reductase, the enzyme required to generate tetrahydrobiopterin, an essential cofactor for hydroxylase activity. This finding underscored the fact that screening and/or early therapeutic intervention programs must be cognizant of genetic heterogeneity; although a disease may have the same clinical or chemical characteristics, the basic genetic defects may differ. Thus, efforts must be tailored to identify and specifically treat, if possible, the variant forms of the disease (see Addendum).

Another problem related to PKU screening has become of more concern in recent years. In 1957, the first cases of mentally retarded offspring of untreated mothers affected with PKU were described.[22] Subsequently, maternal PKU was documented in almost all of the heterozygous offspring of PKU mothers. With the advent of screening and treatment, more mentally normal women will reach childbearing age and and number of infants affected by maternal PKU will increase. It is possible that reinstitution of phenylalanine restriction during pregnancy will minimize the fetal insult.[23,24] However, it is more unfortunate – and an important lession – that many PKU women, treated during childhood, have been lost to follow-up. These women, therefore, remain unaware of the risk to their offspring as well as potential treatment. Clearly, close follow-up and counseling of these women during adolescence and early adulthood is necessary. The requisite of adequate follow-up is obviously important for all screening programs.

Sickle Cell Disease: Considerable controversy has resulted from efforts to screen for sickle cell disease.[25,26] This disease, which is inherited as an autosomal recessive trait, has a carrier frequency of about 1 in 11 Black Americans. Most affected children develop clinical manifestations by 6 months of age and, at present, there is no specific therapy.

Although heterozygous carriers of the sickle cell gene are clinically normal, they can be identified by a rapid and inexpensive blood test. Individuals detected by this screening test must have a hemoglobin electrophoresis performed in order to discriminate sickle cell heterozygotes from homozygotes and individuals with other hemoglobin variants. Though screening in infancy might identify affected individuals who should be medically evaluated and closely followed, early therapeutic intervention is not available to alter the progressive course of the disease. Therefore, many screening advocates consider adolescence, prior to marital plans, to be the best time for carrier detection. At the inception of mass screening efforts in the late 1960's, antenatal diagnosis of affected fetuses was unavailable. Recently, the use of fetoscopy to obtain placental blood for globin chain synthesis studies has demonstrated the feasibility of prenatal detection; however, at present these methods are limited to a few expert centers[27,28,29] (see Addendum).

A major lesson learned from sickle cell screening resulted from the rush to compulsory screening legislation. Several states required premarital sickle cell testing, but few provided funding or adequate genetic counseling. Of more concern, public and physician education regarding sickle cell disease was, and to a lesser degree remains, grossly inadequate. This lack of understanding resulted in the psychological and/or social stigmatization of the normal individuals identified as being carriers. Breech in confidentiality by testing agencies caused job loss and discrimination, elevated insurance premiums, and heightened anxiety levels among carriers.[15,25,26] These psycho-social issues evolved in spite of the fact that carriers of the recessive sickle cell gene almost never have disease manifestations.

Prospective Screening

Tay-Sachs Disease: TSD has provided the prototype for the control and prevention of tragic genetic diseases.[30] This disorder, inherited as an autosomal recessive trait, is caused by the defective activity of the lysosomal enzyme β-hexosaminidase A,[2] resulting in the progressive neural accumulation of its substrate G_{M2} ganglioside. Onset of the disease occurs at about four to eight months of life and is characterized by the loss of developmental milestones. The psychomotor retardation is progressive and affected children usually expire by five years of age. Since there is no treatment available for infants affected with TSD,[31] efforts have been directed toward the prevention of this disease by prospective identification of the heterozygous carriers of the TSD gene.

The rationale for prospective screening was based on three major facts: (1) the gene for TSD has a high frequency (0.016) in a defined and accessible population (Jewish individuals of Central and Eastern European descent);[32,33] (2) carriers of the gene can be detected by determining the β-hexosaminidase A activity in easily obtained sources including plasma, tears and/or isolated peripheral leukocytes; and (3) prenatal diagnosis can accurately identify affected fetuses by the 15-18th week of gestation. Thus, previously unsuspecting carrier couples, at risk for offspring with TSD, can be prospectively identified and counseled as to their various reproductive options.

Mass prospective screening of at-risk families was initiated in 1971 in the Washington-Baltimore Jewish Community by Dr. Michael Kaback and colleagues. This voluntary program was designed to screen Jewish individuals in the reproductive age range (18-45 years of age). Screening followed intensive educational and publicity programs directed at the at-risk population as well as the medical community. This successful program served as the model for over 50 Tay-Sachs

TABLE 2

Tay-Sachs Disease – Prototype for Prevention of Genetic Disease[3]

Heterozygote Screening – 1971-1976

- Over 150,000 adults screened
- Over 6,000 heterozygotes identified
- Heterozygote frequency = 0.037 (1 in 27.3)
- 125 at-risk carrier couples identified

Prenatal Diagnosis – 1969-1976

At-Risk Carrier Couples	Pregnancies Monitored	Normal	Affected
With a previously affected child	371	278	93
Identified by screening programs	90	68	22
	461	346	115

TABLE 3

Pathway for Screening, Prevention and Treatment of Cystic Fibrosis

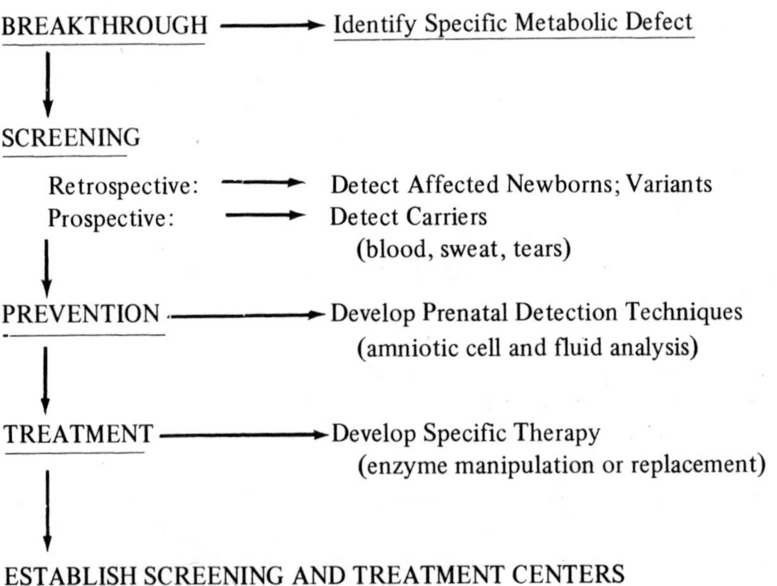

screening programs undertaken in Jewish communities throughout the United States, Canada and several other countries. Each of these programs was voluntary, had "saturation-type" educational and publicity programs, and provided genetic counseling and appropriate follow-up for detected carriers and particularly for carrier couples.

The international experience with Tay-Sachs screening programs has been reviewed recently by Kaback[3,30] and the pertinent data have been summarized in Table 2. During the five-year period from 1971 to 1976, over 150,000 Jewish adults voluntarily participated in Tay-Sachs screening programs. Over 6,000 heterozygous carriers of the Tay-Sachs gene were detected, a carrier frequency of about 1 in 27 screened. Most importantly, 125 previously unsuspecting carrier couples were identified and counseled as to their risk of having a child affected with this disease.

Prenatal diagnosis of fetuses at risk for TSD became available in 1969, shortly after the specific enzymatic defect was identified.[2] From 1969 to 1976, 461 pregnancies at risk for TSD were monitored; of these, 371 were in families that previously had an affected child, and 90 were in previously unsuspecting families who were identified by carrier screening programs. Of these 461 at-risk pregnancies, prenatal studies diagnosed normal fetuses in 346 (which were confirmed postnatally) and affected fetuses in 115.[3] With two exceptions, the families with the pregnancies carrying affected fetuses elected to terminate. It is notable that many of the parents who had a Tay-Sachs child indicated that they had not contemplated another pregnancy until the availability of prenatal diagnosis for TSD. The TSD experience to date documents the effectiveness of prospective screening and counseling for the prevention of this disease. Thus the availability of prenatal diagnosis for TSD allowed parents of affected children and unsuspecting carrier couples identified by screening the choice to have only unaffected children.

PROSPECTS FOR PROSPECTIVE SCREENING FOR CYSTIC FIBROSIS

Prospective screening for CF is dependent on a major breakthrough in the search for the basic defect, presumably a defective enzyme. There are no methods currently available to reliably detect heterozygous carriers of the CF gene or to prenatally detect affected fetuses. As outlined in Table 3, a breakthrough in the elucidation of the specific metabolic defect would most likely lead to: (1) retrospective screening for accurate diagnosis of affected newborns; (2) prospective detection of heterozygous carrier couples using conveniently obtained enzyme sources for assay; (3) prevention by prenatal diagnosis of affected fetuses and selective termination; and (4) the development of rational treatment focused at the molecular defect – enzyme manipulation and/or replacement. The initiation and evaluation of screening, prevention and therapeutic endeavors for CF will require the establishment or utilization of regional screening and treatment centers in major medical institutions.

The magnitude of mass screening for CF carriers is underscored when the gene frequency for CF is compared to those for PKU, TSD, and sickle cell disease (Table 4).[34] Although the estimated gene frequencies for CF and TSD are similar (0.02 versus 0.016, respectively), the fact that the population at risk for CF includes all Caucasians of Northern European ancestry primarily accounts for the vast difference in the estimated yearly number of affected fetuses conceived in the United States (1,000 versus 40). Thus, if the entire Caucasian population (185,000,000)[35] in the United States was screened, over 7,400,000 heterozygotes for the CF gene would be detected. More significantly, if we estimate the Caucasian reproductive population to be 42,000,000 then over 67,000 at-risk carrier couples would be identified. Clearly, in terms of prospective screening, the number of individuals to be tested and the number of heterozygotes and carrier couples that will be detected are staggering. In view of the immense number of individuals to be screened, an effective strategy must be devised if prospective screening for CF is to succeed.

A MODEL FOR THE PROSPECTIVE SCREENING OF CYSTIC FIBROSIS

Program Requisites

Table 5 outlines the proposed requisites for effective screening for CF. These requisites are based in part on the lessons learned from previous screening experiences and can be considered generally applicable to screening endeavors for other genetic diseases. First, a rapid and inexpensive test, preferably a sensitive enzyme assay, must be developed and automated using conveniently obtained enzyme sources such as serum and/or tears. Initially affected individuals from hundreds of CF families must be tested to determine if CF is a genetically heterogenous disorder and if so, the extent and nature of this heterogeneity must be defined. Ideally, the test must be adaptable to the routine screening of all newborns, concomitant with other screening tests for PKU, galactosemia, etc. Next, obligate heterozygotes for CF must be studied to evaluate and optimize the test for carrier detection. The test should then be made available to members of CF families; these individuals may have a chance as great as 2/3 (sibs of affected individuals) of being CF carriers. Having established the reliability of the test for heterozygote detection, prospective screening can be undertaken, perhaps using the strategy proposed below. In addition to the screening test, a more sensitive confirmatory or backup assay should be developed. Presumably, this test will use another enzyme source and/or the natural substrate, etc., and will permit discrimination of borderline or ambiguous results obtained from the screening test.

Second, a massive educational program must be launched, using a multiple media approach, to inform the public as well as the medical community about the disease, the availability of voluntary retrospective and prospective screening, and what it means to be a carrier for a genetic disease such as CF.

TABLE 4

Frequency and Incidence Estimates for Selected Autosomal Recessive Disorders in Defined Ethnic Groups in the United States*

Disease	Ethnic Group	Gene Frequency	Carrier Frequency	At-Risk Couple Frequency**	Disease Frequency	Incidence of Affected Newborns in USA***
Phenylketonuria	Europeans	0.008	0.016	1 in 4,000	1 in 16,000	160
Sickle Cell Anemia	Blacks	0.040	0.080	1 in 150	1 in 600	500
Tay-Sachs Disease	Ashkenazi Jews	0.016	0.032	1 in 900	1 in 3,600	30
Cystic Fibrosis	Northern Europeans	0.020	0.040	1 in 625	1 in 2,500	1,040

*Modified from Kaback.[34]

**Likelihood that both members of a couple are heterozygous for the same recessive gene (assuming nonconsanguinity and that both are of the same ethnic group).

***Based on 2,500,000 Caucasian newborns/year, 300,000 Black newborns/year, and 110,000 Jewish newborns/year.

Third, centers must be established for the implementation of screening, treatment, appropriate counseling and follow-up. Ideally, a program would be cordinated nationally with geographically distributed regional centers. Each center would have a laboratory which performed all the tests for that region. A single national reference and quality control laboratory would periodically monitor the performance of the regional laboratories, standardize laboratory values for inter-laboratory data comparisons, and serve as the consultant to resolve technical problems. Each center would provide genetic and family counseling; these services would be made available to all identified carriers, and particularly to carrier couples.

To insure the success of the program, each center would record the name, test results, and other pertinent data on each affected individual and carrier detected. This information would be compiled in the central national laboratory; strict confidentiality would be maintained. The national registry would be updated yearly, and access to this information would be restricted. Should a new treatment or other beneficial information become available, the registry would provide ready access to affected individuals. Furthermore, if a physician wanted to determine if the patient had been tested previously, the information would be retrievable with written consent.

The final requisite for effective screening involves a continued commitment to research. For both retrospective and prospective screening, pilot trials of various screening strategies must be carried out and evaluated. These pilot screening trials will establish the feasibility of mass screening programs and identify the limitations and concerns which must be incorporated into the large-scale collaborative programs. New and improved screening methods must be developed and evaluated. Finally, with the elucidation of the basic defect, efforts to develop specific therapy for individuals suffering from CF would become a major research focus.

IMPLEMENTATION OF PROSPECTIVE MASS SCREENING FOR CYSTIC FIBROSIS

Demographic Considerations

The following prospective screening strategy for CF is designed to fulfill the above requisites. Because of the magnitude of the undertaking, realistic efforts to detect carriers would be directed to couples who have initiated a pregnancy. Table 6 summarizes the following demographic considerations. Based on vital statistics data,[35] about 5% of Caucasian women between the ages 15-44 years are pregnant each year. Initial screening efforts would be directed to this group of 2.5 million women. With an estimated heterozygote frequency of 0.04 for CF, 100,000 pregnant carriers would be detected annually. Subsequent testing of

TABLE 5

Requisites for Effective Genetic Screening for Cystic Fibrosis

1. Accurate Screening Test:	
a. Retrospective:	Affected Newborns; Variants
b. Retro/Prospective:	CF Families for Heterozygotes
c. Prospective	At-Risk Population (Caucasians; 18-45 years)
d. Accurate:	Confirmatory Diagnostic Test for Homozygotes and Heterozygotes
2. Educational Program:	
a. Public	
b. Medical Community	
3. Screening, Treatment and Counseling Centers:	
a. Regional Centers	
b. Centralized Laboratory Facilities	
c. Reference/Quality Control Center	
d. Genetic and Family Counseling	
e. Appropriate Follow-Up	
4. Research:	
a. Pilot Screening Trials	
b. Improved Screening Methodology	
c. Therapeutic Endeavors	

their spouses would be accomplished to identify carrier couples; approximately 4,000 pregnant carrier couples would be identified yearly. Since each of these couples has a 25% risk of an affected child, prenatal diagnostic studies could identify about 1,000 affected fetuses annually. Genetic counseling and the discussion of various reproductive options would be offered to each couple.

TABLE 6

Demographic Considerations for Prospective Screening for Cystic Fibrosis*

Total U.S. Population	213,000,000
Caucasian Population	185,000,000
Reproductive Population (women 15-44 yrs.)	42,000,000
Pregnant Women (5%/year)	2,500,000/year
Heterozygotes Identified (carrier frequency = 0.04)	100,000/year
Screen for Carrier Spouses	100,000/year
Carrier Couples Identified	4,000/year
Affected Newborns Prevented	1,000/year

*Based on Vital Statistics Data for 1976.[35]

Economic Considerations

The cost of such a program is difficult to estimate. Table 7 compares the annual costs of the above screening program with the medical costs involved in the lifetime care of the CF patients born each year. The yearly cost for screening 2.6 million people, assuming a $5 automated test, would be 13 million dollars. This estimate does not include the initial purchase of equipment or expenditures for educational and counseling programs. An average cost to monitor each pregnancy, including ultrasound, amniocentesis, and amniotic fluid and cell analyses would be about $300, or a total of 1.4 million dollars.

With good supportive medical care, a baby born with CF today can be expected to survive about 20 years.[36] A conservative estimate of the yearly medical costs per patient is $2,500. Thus, the lifetime medical care for the 1,000 CF patients who would be born each year would be approximately 50 million dollars. In no way can these estimates account for the psycho-social costs of this debilitating and progressive disease for affected children and their families. Thus, the cost of screening, prenatal diagnosis, and termination of affected fetuses

TABLE 7

Cost-Effectiveness of Prospective Screening for Cystic Fibrosis

Screening Tests:	
Total Screened/year (2,600,000) @ $5/test =	$13,000,000/year
Prenatal Diagnostic Studies:	
4,000 At-Risk Pregnancies @ $350/test =	$ 1,400,000/year
Patient Costs:	
CF Births/year x yrs of survival x cost/yr 1,000 x 20 x $2,500 =	$50,000,000/year

TABLE 8

False Negatives ⟶ Affected Newborns

Population Screened: (pregnant women)	2,600,000/year
Assume 5% False Negatives: Heterozygotes Missed	5,000/year
Carrier Couples Missed:	200/year
Affected Newborns:	50/year

would be approximately 1.5 million dollars per year, or 38.5 million dollars less than the costs that would be incurred from the lifetime medical care of the CF babies born that year.

Finally, a critical consideration in any mass screening and prevention program is the occurrence of false negatives. At a maximal false negative rate of 5%, 5,000 heterozygotes would defy identification, as shown in Table 8. This would result in the failure to identify 200 carrier couples and to prenatally detect 50 affected newborns. The additional medical costs for these CF patients would be about 2.5 million dollars.

PROSPECTUS

Although the basic defect in CF remains elusive, the search continues on several fronts and prospects for a breakthrough are encouraging. Once the defect in CF is discovered, the application of this knowledge to genetic screening will be an obvious objective. It was the purpose of this paper to consider this prospect, to emphasize the magnitude of the task, and to propose a strategy for the rapid implementation of prospective screening. If unsuspecting carrier couples can be identified early in pregnancy and if prenatal diagnostic techniques can determine the genotype of the fetus, then these couples can choose to prevent the tragedy of CF by termination of these pregnancies. Furthermore, the elucidation of the basic defect should result in efforts to develop rational therapy for those already suffering from CF or for newborns who are detected retrospectively, whether born to couples who were not screened prospectively or others who had false negative screening results. Clearly, the control of CF will require two strategies: prevention by prospective screening and prenatal diagnosis, and continued efforts to develop effective therapy for those individuals who suffer from the disease.

REFERENCES

1. National Academy of Science, National Research Council, Assembly of Life Sciences, Division of Medical Sciences, Committee for the Study of Inborn Errors of Metabolism: Genetic Screening: Programs, Principles, and Research, Washington, D.C., 1975, National Academy of Sciences.
2. S. Okada and J.S. O'Brien, *Science 165*, 698, 1969.
3. M.M. Kaback, *Pediat. Res. 11*, 458, 1977.
4. M.M. Kaback, R.S. Zeiger, L.W. Reynolds, and M. Sonneborn, *in* Progress in Medical Genetics, A. Steinberg and A. Bearn (Eds.), p. 103, 1974.
5. National Academy of Sciences, National Research Council, Assembly of Life Sciences, Division of Medical Sciences, Committee for a Study for Evaluation of Testing for Cystic Fibrosis, *J. Pediat. 88*, 711, 1976.
6. J.A. Mangos and R.C. Talamo (Eds.), Cystic Fibrosis: Projections into the Future, Symposia Specialists, Miami, 1976.
7. G.J.S. Rao and H.L. Nadler, *Pediat. Res. 9*, 739, 1975.

8. L. Chou and H.L. Nadler, *Pediat. Res. 10*, 176, 1976.
9. E. Shapira, Y. Ben-Yoseph and H.L. Nadler, *Biochim, Biophys. Res. Comm. 864,* 1310, 1976.
10. E.J. Conod, J.H. Conover and K. Hirschhorn, *Pediat. Res. 9*, 724, 1975.
11. G.B. Wilson and H.H. Fudenberg, *Pediat. Res. 10*, 87, 1976.
12. K.Y.H. Chan, D.A. Applegarth and A.G.F. Davidson, *Clin. Chim. Acta 74*, 71, 1977.
13. B.H. Bowman, B.J. Lankford, G.M. Fuller, S.D. Carson, A. Kurosky and D.R. Barnett, *Biochim, Biophys. Res. Comm. 64*, 1310, 1975.
14. S.D. Carson, B.L. Harper, D.R. Barnett, A. Kurosky, B.J. Lankford and B.H. Bowman, *Tex. Rep. Biol. Med. 34*, 210, 1976.
15. D. Bergsma (Ed.), Ethical, Social and Legal Dimensions of Screening for Human Genetics Disease, Birth Defects Original Article Series, Vol. X(6), Symposia Specialists, Miami, 1974.
16. H.L. Levy, *in* Advances in Human Genetics, H. Harris and K. Hirschhorn (Eds.), Vol. 4(1), Plenum Press, New York, 1973.
17. R. Guthrie, *J.A.M.A. 178*, 863, 1961.
18. R. Guthrie and A. Susi, *Pediatrics 32*, 338, 1963.
19. J.L. Berman and R. Fard, *J. Pediat. 77*, 764, 1970.
20. H.L. Levy, V.E. Shih, V. Karolkewicz, W.A. French, J.R. Carr, V. Cass, J.L. Kennedy, Jr., and R.A. MacCready, *N. Engl. J. Med. 285*, 424, 1971.
21. S. Kaufman, N.A. Holtzman, S. Milstein, I.J. Butler and A. Krumholz, *N. Eng. J. Med. 293*, 785, 1975.
22. C.E. Dent, *in* Etiologic Factors in Mental Retardation, Report of 23rd Ross Pediatric Research Conference, Nov. 8-9, 1956, p. 32, 1957.
23. T.L. Perry, B.A. Hansen, B. Tischler, F.M. Richards and M. Sokol, *N. Eng. J. Med. 289*, 395, 1973.
24. R.M. MacCready and H.L. Levy, *Am. J. Obstet. Gynecol. 113*, 121, 1972.
25. B.J. Culliton, *Science 178*, 283, 1972.
26. C.F. Whitten, *N. Engl. J. Med. 288*, 318, 1973.
27. Y.W. Kan, A.M. Dozy, B.P. Alter, F.D. Frigoletto and D.G. Nathan, *N. Eng. J. Med. 287*, 1, 1972.
28. J.C. Hobbins and M.J. Mahoney, *N. Engl. J. Med. 290,* 1065, 1974.
29. Y.W. Kan, M.S. Golbus and R. Trecartin, *N. Engl. J. Med. 294*, 1039, 1976.
30. M.M. Kaback (Ed.), Tay-Sachs Disease: Carrier Screening and Prevention, Birth Defects Original Article Series, A.R. Liss Publishing Company, New York, 1977.
31. R.J. Desnick and J.D. Goldberg, *in* Tay-Sachs Disease: Carrier Screening and Prevention, Birth Defects Original Article Series, D. Bergsma and M.M. Kaback (Eds.), A.R. Liss Publishing Company, New York, pp. 129-141, 1977.
32. S.M. Aronson and B.W. Volk, *in* Cerebral Spingolipidosis, S.M. Aronson and B.W. Volk (Eds.), Academic Press, New York, pp. 375-394, 1962.
33. N.C. Myrianthopoulos, *in* Cerebral Sphingolipidoses, S.M. Aronson and B.W.

Volk (Eds.), Academic Press, New York, pp. 359-374, 1962.
34. M.M. Kaback, *in* The Prevention of Genetic Disease and Mental Retardation, A. Milunsky (Ed.), W.B. Saunders, Philadelphia, p. 98, 1975.
35. U.S. Bureau of the Census, Statistical Abstract of the United States, (97th edition), Washington, D.C., 1976.
36. M.J. Robinson and A.P. Norman, *Arch. Dis. Child. 50*, 962, 1975.

ADDENDUM

During the publication of this manuscript, the genetic heterogeneity in PKU was further underscored by the description of another variant which was due to a deficiency of biopterin biosynthesis (S. Kaufman, S. Berlow, G.K. Summer, S. Milstein, J.D. Schulman, F. Orloff, S. Spielberg and S. Pueschel, *N. Engl. J. Med. 299*, 673, 1978).

Recently a new method for the prenatal diagnosis of sickle cell anemia which does not require fetal blood aspiration, but uses amniotic fluid cells, has been reported (Y.W. Kan and A.M. Dozy, *Proc. Natl. Acad. Sci. USA 75*, 5631, 1978).

GENETIC SERVICES WITHIN A STATE HEALTH DEPARTMENT

Ian H. Porter

I. Introduction

The aims of a state (or regional) genetic service are:

A. prevention through genetic counseling for reproductive options,

B. treatment and management of children detected in newborn screening programs and of patients seen in genetic diagnostic and counseling centers, and

C. research for the development of public health policies and for the generation of scientific progress.

The difficulty in achieving these aims lies in the independent administrative development and unrelated financial support of the Physically Handicapped Children's program, the Newborn Screening Program, and the genetic diagnostic and counseling centers. I believe the principal, though unstated, purpose of the National Genetic Disease Act is the amalgamation of these programs.

II. Physically Handicapped Children's Program

At the turn of the century the plight of crippled children was a philanthropic matter but, in 1901, New York State built a 25-bed hospital in Tarrytown for the care of crippled children. It was moved to West Haverstraw in 1904, and is known today as the Helen Hayes Hospital. The Health Department also organized clinics in various regions for the rehabilitation of patients with poliomyelitis. Most of the children cared for were the victims of poliomyelitis and TB, infectious diseases being the major concern of the State Health Department at that time. Thus, the establishment of the then Haverstraw Hospital and the organization of the Health Department's clinics provided treatment and rehabilitation for physically handicapped children in a regional setting.

The Physically Handicapped Children's Program was introduced in 1919 and was administered until 1940 by the: courts (eligibility), Health Department (determination of need), and Education Department (fiscal management). Since 1940 the Program has been administered by the Bureau of

ISBN 0-12-562650-9

Medical Rehabilitation in the State Health Department.

The Physically Handicapped Children's Program was originally for the care of patients with poliomyelitis and TB, gradually took on a more orthopedic orientation with the State's involvement in rehabilitation, and as poliomyelitis and TB disappeared, congenital abnormalities became the greater concern. Not until 1976 were diagnosis and treatment of inborn metabolic diseases included in the Program.

State Aid for Physically Handicapped Children was introduced in 1926. The program now receives funds from two sources and is divided into two parts.

A. Diagnosis and evaluation is part of the Crippled Children's Program which was started in 1935 and is financed by a Federal Grant to the State Health Department under Title V of the Federal Social Security Act.

B. The treatment program is financed by:

1. State Aid, 50% of which is appropriated by the State and 50% by the Counties, and
2. Medicaid, 50% of which is appropriated by the Federal Government, 25% by the State, and 25% by the Counties.

This is a decentralized county-run state aid program in which the local county health departments determine both financial and medical eligibility. All medical services must be given in approved centers.

III. Newborn Screening Program

A. Inborn Metabolic Diseases (IMD)

Spurred by the poor community services for retarded children and the deplorable conditions in many state institutions, parents of retarded children banded together to improve the lot of the mentally retarded, and in 1950 this movement coalesced into the National Association for Retarded Children (NARC).

In 1961, Guthrie reported his method for assaying blood phenylalanine and the Children's Bureau approved his proposal to use his method to demonstrate the value of screening for PKU in newborns the following year.

In October 1964, NARC's Public Health Services Committee, after reviewing the results of the PKU collaborative study, recommended mandatory screening for PKU and drew up a model law for such a program which immediately was adopted in New York State, although both the American Academy of Pediatrics and the American Medical Association were against it.

New York State amended the Public Health Law in September 1974 to include six more inherited metabolic diseases: maple syrup urine disease, homocystinuria, histidinemia, galactosemia, adenosine deaminase deficiency, and sickle cell disease, and in July 1977 it was further amended to include hypothyroidism.

The screening laboratories are situated in New York City (Health Department) which screens 113,000 births per year, Buffalo (Erie County Health Department) which screens 40,000 births per year, Syracuse (Onondaga County Health Department) which screens 25,000 births per year, and Albany (Birth Defects Institute) which screens 71,000 births per year.

In addition to testing, there are four additional aspects of the program.

1. The promotion of research tied up with the development of methods, evaluation of the effectiveness of the program, and quality control.
2. Education tied up with a recognized need for the State to inform physicians about the diseases and to enlist their cooperation in the program.
3. The establishment of a registry. A few states require a registry; others, however, merely require the test results to be reported to a state official.
4. Finally, treatment.

The purpose of newborn screening is to prevent mental retardation by early detection and treatment, but the statute mandating newborn screening makes no provision for confirmatory tests, genetic counseling, or treatment and follow-up. And herein lies the weakness of the program. As the purpose is to find, to treat, and to follow affected individuals, and to get answers to many unanswered questions, the screening program must be a comprehensive one and not merely a laboratory service. Guthrie has repeatedly pointed out that the essence of success in an effective screening program lies in the integration of the screening laboratories with the diagnostic and treatment centers – it means close cooperation between health departments and medical centers. To foster this collaboration between the laboratory and the treatment centers, the newborn screening program came under the aegis of the New York State Health Department Birth Defects Institute in 1977.

B. Sickle Cell Disease

In 1972, Congress passed the Sickle Cell Prevention Act, which resulted in the institution of sickle cell anemia centers and a series of screening, education and counseling centers throughout the country, and in September 1974 sickle cell disease was included in the amended New York State Public Health Law.

The purpose of screening for the inborn metabolic diseases included in the newborn screening program, and for hypothyroidism, is early detection and *treatment* before irreversibly harmful effects have become established. But this was not the purpose of screening for sickle cell disease, for which only symptomatic and not definitive treatment is available. So, the purpose is *prevention* through genetic counseling, including prenatal diagnosis.

As it turns out, the detection of children with sickle cell disease before onset of symptoms may reduce early mortality but, of course, only if these children can be followed reliably in centers where they can receive comprehensive pediatric care.

One therefore needs public health nurses to keep track of the affected children, genetic counselors to help their parents, and facilities for prenatal diagnosis, particularly where incidence is high. The overall incidence in New York State is 1:5,000, but in New York City it is 1:2,500, whereas in Syracuse it is 1:25,000.

Finally, the scope of the program should not be limited to sickle cell disease, but expanded to include all hemoglobinopathies that also are detectable in the newborn screening program.

In addition to finding the expected prevalence of sickle hemoglobin and hemoglobin C, other mutant hemoglobin genes are also uncovered. Many of these are not associated with disease but merely reflect normal genetic diversity. Many people have difficulty understanding that though they have an abnormal hemoglobin gene, they themselves are not ill or abnormal. The solution lies in education at all levels so that the normal existence of genetic diversity is recognized.

C. Hypothyroidism

Congenital thyroid hormone deficiency is the most recent example of a condition for which we can now screen because of reliable screening and diagnostic tests, and availability of treatment. In July 1977, legislation for statewide hypothyroid screening was approved. Starting in March 1978, hypothyroid testing was conducted as a pilot program, and on December 1, 1978, the statewide program was implemented.

Although the rationale for screening for congenital hypothyroidism in the newborn infant is early treatment, it is not yet known whether early treatment of congenital hypothyroidism can completely overcome the effect of hormone deficiency up to the time of diagnosis. This is one reason mass T_4 testing should be promoted as part of a comprehensive service consisting of screening laboratories integrated with facilities, and support for long-term follow-up and evaluation. Another reason is to establish the physiologic dose of thyroxine for newborns and infants, which is still not known. Too low a dose will, of course, not produce the optimal clinical response, and recently it has been learned that too high a dose may produce premature synostosis. The final reason is to determine the best method for discriminating between the neonate with primary hypothyroidism and those who have low serum T_4 levels due, for example, to prematurity, respiratory distress syndrome, sepsis, and low thyroxine binding globulin.

In spite of the published reports from the New England Regional Hypothyroidism Screening Program and the Quebec Network for Genetic Medicine, field trial was conducted before initiating statewide screening to determine:

1. cost of study;
2. the best methods for T_4 and TSH determination;
3. the most appropriate instrumentation;
4. the design of protocols for the handling of specimens, reporting of results, and documentation of clinical findings (a great deal of care has been taken with this part of the program, to avoid clerical errors which have resulted in cases being missed in other programs, and to obtain the essential information for ongoing evaluation of all parts of the program);
5. the software necessary to reduce laboratory and clinical data;
6. the requirements for the follow-up centers; and
7. time to train technicians, buy equipment, and write and design educational material.

To improve the operation of the newborn screening program, it has been recommended that an advisory committee under the authority of the State Health Department be set up consisting of:

1. representatives of hospitals who send specimens;
2. specialists in metabolic, endocrine, and genetic diseases;
3. a nurse and/or nutritionist involved in management of patients;
4. representatives of practicing physicians;
5. the directors of the laboratories performing the tests; and
6. consumers;

and having the following responsibilities:

1. determination of conditions to be screened;
2. education and evaluation of informed consent procedures; and
3. regular evaluation of the program.

D. Cost[1]

The total cost of the IMD screening program includes (1) hospital collection of blood specimens and recordkeeping, (2) laboratory analysis of blood specimens, and (3) follow-up of inadequate blood specimens and presumptive positive tests.

Hospital Costs. The hospital costs incurred from collecting blood specimens, mailing of specimens, recording results, and follow-up are the most serious reasons for underestimating the cost of the IMD program. The cost of collecting a single blood specimen in 1977 was estimated at $3.25, and the total expenditure for the 241,000 births in the State was estimated at $783,000.

Laboratory Costs. Cost usually associated with the State mandated IMD screening program are those for laboratory services. The Albany laboratory is operated by the State, and the three local laboratories contract with the state to provide the service. The average cost of an IMD blood specimen analysis was estimated at $2.99 during 1977, and the total expenditure for the 245,855 specimens analyzed would have been $735,000.

Follow-up Costs. The IMD screening program incurs follow-up costs for inadequate specimens and presumptive positive results. In 1977, about $15,000 was required for this portion of the program.

Diagnostic Evaluation and Treatment Costs. Federal funds are available to the IMD centers for diagnosis and evaluation, and State aid is available for treatment on a 50-50 matching formula with localities. In 1977, the cost of diagnosis and evaluation was about $4,000, and the cost of treatment was about $73,000. The latter did not, however, include the full cost of medical consultations or hospitalizations when these were required.

Total Program Costs. The estimated total expenditure in 1977 for New York State's IMD screening program, therefore, was:

Category	Amount
Hospital blood collection	$ 783,000
Laboratory testing	735.000
Follow-up	15,000
Diagnostic evaluation	4,000
Treatment	73,000
Total	$1,610,000

So, collection of blood specimens accounted for 49 cents, laboratory tests for 46 cents, and follow-up, diagnosis and evaluation, and treatment for 5 cents of every dollar in the screening program. The cost of identifying the 20 infants with inherited metabolic disorders born in 1977 was $80,500 per confirmed case.

Left untreated, these diseases usually result in severe retardation. If institutionalized, the lifetime costs are calculated at approximately $800,000 (in 1977 dollars) per severely retarded individual. Given the estimated $80,000 cost to identify and treat a patient, the potential savings to the State would be approximately $720,000 per case.

E. Problems in a Newborn Screening Program:

1. Determining the number of babies missed by the program.
2. Inability to find patients who need repeat testing after discharge from hospital.[2]
3. Screening babies:
   a. who are discharged from hospital before the third day (*i.e.*, too early),
   b. who require long-term hospitalization and are screened too late, if at all, and
   c. who are born outside hospitals.

4. Insuring uniform standards of care in treatment centers, particularly with regard to social services, genetic counseling, and education.
5. Evaluation of program effectiveness.
6. Built-in support for appropriate research and development.

F. Regionalization of Prenatal Diagnosis

1. Cytogenetics

The Secretary of HEW suggested the establishment of regional networks for prenatal diagnosis to improve efficiency, standards, and availability. The New York State Health Department anticipated the Secretary's recommendation, spurred on by the Task Force on Prevention of Down Syndrome of the New York Scientists' Committee for Public Information (SCPI), under the leadership of Jahiel, and with the support from geneticists in New York City. The recommendation was to establish a regional cytogenetic laboratory screening service for the prenatal detection of Down and related syndromes in high risk pregnant women in New York City.

The basis of the recommendation was that:

a. less than 20% of the 7,000 women at high risk, in New York City, availed themselves of prenatal diagnosis;
b. the existing prenatal diagnostic laboratories in New York City were working at full capacity and could not handle additional cases, particularly as several laboratories are using research funds to support this activity;
c. there was a need for an expansion of laboratory capabilities that could process 4,000 specimens a year, and provide service for about 60% of high risk pregnant women;
d. a cost analysis of the procedure by cytogeneticists on the Task Force on Prevention of Down Syndrome of SCPI showed that if there is a sufficient number of specimens, considerable economy of scale could be achieved;
e. a massive increase in laboratory facilities would best be achieved by creating one centralized laboratory. To achieve individualized treatment of the pregnant woman, however, ongoing care, ultrasound studies, amniocentesis, and genetic counseling will be done by obstetricians and counselors in approved medical centers under contract with the laboratory.

In 1977, the State Health Department allocated funds for the project. The State and City Health Departments and related agencies, with the aid of committees of experts and consumers in cytogenetics, obstetrics, counseling, records and statistics, and policy and research, advise on and oversee the program, with particular emphasis on maintaining a high level of safety, accuracy, efficiency and privacy.

As recommended for the Newborn Screening Program there is, in addition, an advisory committee with the same kinds of responsibilities and composed of representatives from state and local agencies, representatives from the scientific committees, and consumer representatives. Ongoing monitoring and evaluation of all components of the program will be performed at two levels:

a. internal evaluation by the Director and her staff and by consultants retained by the five committees, and
b. external evaluation by a panel of out-of-state experts, and proficiency testing by the State Health Department.

The following statistics provide an absolute and a relative quantification for this population at risk in Upstate New York:

TABLE 1

Women Age 35 and Over at Delivery With Live Births During 1973-1975 By Health Systems Agency

Health Systems Agency	Number of Women	Percent of Total
No. 1 Western N.Y.	3,308	4.9
No. 2 Finger Lakes	2,061	4.3
No. 3 Central N.Y.	3,030	5.2
No. 4 N.Y.-Penn. (N.Y. counties only)	624	5.2
No. 5 Northeastern N.Y.	2,734	5.2
No. 6 Hudson Valley	4,601	6.9

In the Rochester regional program for prenatal detection of birth defects, for example, only 13% of pregnant women 35 and older, and 18% of pregnant women 40 and older, have received second trimester prenatal diagnostic counseling and amniocentesis for detection of fetal abnormality. These figures are probably representative for the whole state and indicate that amniocentesis has not yet gained widespread use even for a clearly identified population at risk, and yet all prenatal cytogenetic laboratories are experiencing a logarithmic increase in demands for service; but we do not know when the demands will level off; *i.e.*, we do not yet know what percent of the population at risk will eventually avail themselves of this service. An area serving 2 million people may need laboratory capacity to do the cytogenetics for about 1,000 amniocenteses per year.

Recommendations for prenatal diagnosis have to be reviewed regularly as new epidemiological information becomes available. Thus, for example, it now appears that:

a. the average age of mothers of children with Down syndrome is decreasing,[3] so that whereas 13% of pregnancies occurred in women 35 and older and resulted in 50% of children with Down syndrome, now only 7% of pregnancies occur in women 35 years and older, and they give birth to only 35% of children with Down syndrome;[4] but
b. the age-specific risk for a woman of having a child with Down syndrome is increasing, and the age-specific risk of mothers under 15 years of age may be as high as those for 30-35 year old women.[5]
c. In 20-25% of couples with a child with Down syndrome,[6] the non-disjunctional event takes place in the father, and in fathers over the age of 55 years, there appears to be an age-dependent risk.[7]
d. The second trimester spontaneous abortion rate in mothers carrying fetuses with Down syndrome is 24%.[8]

2. Neural Tube Defects

Neural tube defects (NTD) are among the most common major congenital abnormalities in New York State, having an incidence of 1-2 per 1,000 births. So, between 200 and 400 affected infants are born in New York State each year. Of the half that survive the first 24 hours, 75% will have severe handicaps, and 20% will be moderately or severely mentally retarded.

Antenatal diagnosis of NTD's by alpha-fetoprotein (AFP) assay of *amniotic fluid* was introduced in 1972 as a method of detecting 90% of NTD's. This approach to prevention is, of course, suitable only for high risk couples, *i.e.,* those who already have an affected child, and accounts for only 10% of children born with NTD's. As 90% of children with NTD's stem from couples not known to be at high risk, the results of the United Kingdom Collaborative Study of *maternal serum* AFP screening is particularly important.[9] The experience from this study and the Nassau County Neural Tube Defects Program, however, raises the following points of caution:[10]

a. The serum AFP radioimmunoassay is difficult; the precision required for this assay is greater than radioimmunoassays currently applied to other clinical tests. Also, each laboratory screening for NTD's must establish a normal distribution curve for maternal serum AFP for each week of gestation within the diagnostic range as the AFP levels vary with gestational age. This test should, therefore, not be conducted on a hospital-by-hospital basis that lacks adequate volume, or in commercial laboratories that lack appropriate services for communication and information.
b. The public must be made to understand the difference between screening and diagnostic tests.
c. A screening center must not only provide a reliable assay for

amniotic fluid and serum AFP but also ultrasound, cell culture facilities for chromosome studies, and genetic counseling.

d. A state plan offering such service must emphasize equal access and voluntarism.
e. Accurate cost-benefit ratios must be calculated. We do not know, for example, what proportion of pregnant women would elect to be screened. If some potentially detectable NTD's were missed because an as yet unknown percentage of women decided not to be screened, the costs might outweigh economic benefits (the decision on a state screening program aimed at lowering the incidence of NTD cannot, of course, be taken solely on the basis of economic arguments).

Many questions remain to be answered about whether a state program should be introduced and if so, how it should be operated. Regional centers such as the Nassau County Neural Tube Defects Program should, therefore, be supported to provide a service under limited and controlled circumstances from which all may learn, as maternal serum AFP screening, after FDA licensing of reagents, may eventually become part of routine obstetric practice.

IV. Genetic Diagnostic and Counseling Centers

Introduction

Physiology, biochemistry, molecular biology, and other biological sciences were developed in medical schools, and students and physicians were exposed to the newest ideas as they unfolded. Genetics, however, was developed by zoologists and botanists, some of whom – unlike their clinical colleagues – saw its relevance to man. So genetic counseling was begun by nonmedical geneticists, or by physicians trained in genetics but working in departments or clinics not directly engaged in patient care. Thus, counseling developed apart from clinical medicine with serious clinical, educational, and financial consequences.

A traditional principle of genetic counseling is the neutrality of the counselor in decisions about reproduction. This is unusual in medical practice, and is a difficult attitude for many physicians to adopt, and may even be confusing to some patients who expect to be guided by their physician. This attitude of neutrality originated in counselors not engaged in patient care and who felt some reluctance to enter into the lives of their counselees in the way practicing physicians do.

Few American medical schools provided formal instruction in genetics until the 1960's. The prevailing view was that hereditary conditions were so rare that most physicians saw perhaps only a single case during their entire career. But physicians gradually became more receptive to developments in genetics. This was, in part, because infectious diseases, which until then had been the most important cause of death, now produced a less significant proportion of deaths. Children were better nourished and protected by one means or another against infection. The death rate was lower, and the expectation of life at birth was increasing. But genetic conditions did not share in this amelioration and became, therefore, relatively more important. At the turn of the century, tuberculosis, pneumonia, and gastrointestinal infection accounted for 75% of all deaths. Now they account for only 10%. In contrast, approximately 4% of infant deaths were then attributed to congenital malformations, now about 20% are. To put it another way, in 1900 one infant death in approximately 25 was due to congenital malformations; now it is about one in five. It is, in other words, not the absolute but the relative rate of congenital malformations which is increasing. Medical school curriculum committees could, therefore, no longer argue that instruction in genetics would overload the curriculum with irrelevant material.

And then the philosophical basis of medicine broadened to include the concept of prevention. The application of genetic principles to medical problems harmonized well with this philosophical shift. With a knowledge of heredity, the physician could counsel prospective parents with genetic conditions and thereby prevent the unwitting passage of a disease to subsequent generations.

Most of the existing genetic centers in New York State were established in the 1960's, following the rapid expansion of clinically relevant medical genetics in that era. In 1968, the Regional Genetics Program of Western New York, supported by the RMP, was a prototype of its kind. Other centers followed suit but, partly because of lack of reimbursement from Medicaid and third party carriers, services often were supported by non-service related funds and, therefore, difficult to develop adequately. Only recently have fee schedules been approved by Medicaid, and in several regions, notably in the Northeastern and Central New York regions, Blue Cross/Blue Shield and other third party carriers are now reimbursing for genetic diagnostic and counseling services.

A. Birth Defects Institute

The Birth Defects Institute (BDI) was enacted into law in 1968 and funds were appropriated through the State Health Department. This was no doubt spurred on by the growth of genetics in the 1960's, the need for genetic services in the Physically Handicapped Children's and screening programs, and because of the public's greater understanding of the relationship between genetics, birth defects, and congenital abnormalities. The intent of the law was to create a research institute and laboratory services, but from its inception an attempt was made to establish a regionalized program for genetic diagnostic and counseling centers. At present, there are eight such centers with contracts from the BDI.

As of 1978, all chromosomal analysis must be reported to the New York State Birth Defects Institute Chromosome Registry. All concerned meet regularly to discuss matters related to the registry, to develop programs for quality assurance, and to formulate requirements for genetic diagnostic and counseling centers to be approved for Medicaid reimbursement.

B. Voluntary Agencies

There are a large number of voluntary agencies in New York that have been helpful, directly or indirectly, with providing genetic services. The National Foundation-March of Dimes is foremost among these in providing leadership and money. At present, they support nine centers in New York State.

C. Problems

There are four main problems that have to be dealt with to fulfill the needs of an integrated network of genetic services:

1. How to provide genetic services in a large, mixed urban-rural community.

New York State occupies 49,576 square miles and, as of July 1976, there were 18,084,000 people, of which 41.6% lived in New York City. There were 235,176 live births to New York State residents, of which 182,349 were White live births and 52,379 were non-White live births. The median age of mothers was 25.9 years.

Clearly, regionalized programs centered in medical centers, with an ability to deliver the appropriate services at the local level, are the most efficient.

A well-tested delivery system is the center-satellite model: a centralized medical genetics unit with comprehensive specialty and laboratory services, clinics in local communities to make the services accessible to the residents, and a public and professional education program. This model has been tested in three areas: The University of California in northern and central California, Wyoming Regional Genetic Counseling Program, and eastern Pennsylvania.

A center-satellite program serving two million people, the size of several of New York State's regional programs, ideally should be staffed by:

3 medical geneticists
2 cytogeneticists
1 biochemist
1 obstetrician whose principal interest is prenatal diagnosis
2 clinical fellows
3 genetic counselors
10-12 cytogenetic technicians
2-4 biochemical technicians
3 secretaries

This model has several advantages. Genetic counseling is frequently and routinely available over large areas. The motivation of patients or families to travel long distances, or of their physicians to refer them, is often insufficient to initiate a visit to a distant center since the problems

TABLE 2

Birth Defect	Annual Incidence	Prevalence	Cause	Detection	Treatment	Prevention
Down syndrome (mongolism)	5,100	44,000	chromosomal abnormality	amniocentesis, chromosome analysis	corrective surgery special physical training and schooling	genetic services
Muscular dystrophy	unknown (late appearing)	200,000	hereditary; often recessive inheritance	apparent at onset	physical therapy	genetic services
Spina bifida and/or hydrocephalus	6,200	53,000	hereditary and environmental	amniocentesis, prenatal x-ray, ultrasound, maternal blood test, examination at birth	corrective surgery, prostheses, physical training special schooling for any mental impairment	genetic services
Cleft lip and/or cleft palate	4,300	71,000	hereditary and/or environment:	visual inspection at birth	corrective surgery	genetic services
Cystic fibrosis	2,000	10,000	hereditary: recessive inheritance	sweat and blood tests	treat respiratory and digestive complications	genetic services
Sickle cell anemia	1,200	16,000	hereditary: incomplete recessive – most frequent among Blacks	blood test	transfusions	genetic services
Hemophilia (classic)	1,200	12,400	hereditary: sex-linked recessive inheritance	blood test	clotting factor	genetic services
Phenylketonuria (PKU)	310	3,100	hereditary: recessive inheritance	blood test at birth	special diet	carrier identification genetic services
Tay-Sachs disease	30	100	hereditary: recessive inheritance – most frequent among Ashkenazi Jews	blood and tear tests, amniocentesis	none	carrier identification genetic services
Thalassemia	70	1,000	hereditary: incomplete recessive inheritance	blood test	transfusions	carrier identification genetic services
Galactosemia	70	500	hereditary: recessive inheritance	blood and urine tests, amniocentesis	special diet	carrier identification genetic services
Turner syndrome	575	2,100	chromosomal abnormality	amniocentesis, chromosomal analysis	corrective surgery medication	genetic services

Source: The National Foundation-March of Dimes, "Birth Defects: Tragedy and Hope", 1977. Incidence and prevalence figures for the United States

for which counseling is appropriate are not acute. Finally, the center-satellite system is a financially effective way of delivering a service which must have significant but limited resources in specialized personnel and facilities by avoiding duplication of resources.[11]

While every attempt is made to make access to the central clinic available to all, irrespective of income, the patient population is middle class, with a small admixture of less affluent families drawn principally from the clinic populations of the medical centers and their affiliated hospitals. In the satellite clinics, on the other hand, the mix tends to be broader, particularly in those which are located in agricultural areas.

2. How to determine the number of individuals at risk for presenting at birth or developing a genetic problem later in life, and how to determine the number of individuals who receive appropriate treatment and counseling; *i.e.*, a needs assessment study.

Disease with a genetic component is now quite prevalent (Table 2). Approximately 9.4 individuals out of every 100 liveborn suffer at some time in their lives from a serious disease or handicap that is genetic in etiology, and another 2.7 persons out of every 100 born alive suffer from disorders of unknown etiology.

But frequency varies with geographic region and ethnic group. For example, sickle cell disease is 10 times as common in New York City as it is in Syracuse, and of the 2½ million Jews in the State, 2 million live in the Metropolitan area. Multifactorial congenital malformations also show variation in regional and ethnic frequency, and age may confer increased risk for chromosomal nondisjunction in older women, and new dominant mutations in older men.

The prevalence of the sickle cell and hemoglobin C gene in Blacks is 77% and 2% respectively, and the beta-thalassemia gene in Mediterranean-American populations is 2.5-5.0%, the Tay-Sachs gene in Ashkenazi Jews is about 1.3-1.6%, the cystic fibrosis gene in the White population is 5-6%, and the PKU gene is about 2%.

Chromosomal mutations occur in about 5 of every 10 spontaneously aborted fetuses, in about 5% of stillbirths and of infants dying within 7 days of birth, and in about 5 per 1,000 surviving live births.

About 10% of liveborn infants have some form of genetic variation that could be responsible for a handicap during the person's lifetime; approximately 12% of pediatric hospital admissions are for single gene, chromosomal, or multifactorial disease with a significant genetic component. Among those with severe mental retardation, 15% of diagnoses are Mendelian and 45% reflect a genetic component. Down syndrome accounts for 20-25% of retarded people.

It is difficult to obtain specific estimates on the number of individuals with genetic problems or birth defects in New York State, although there are some data available from selected areas of the State which enable approximate needs for genetic services to be determined.

For example, data from the Finger Lakes Area Region provide approximate figures for a variety of hereditary conditions that have been developed using available incidence figures for the United States and other populations of Western European origin. Data also are available about the incidence of birth defects and perinatal mortality and morbidity for the Hudson Valley Region, and similar data also were found by case finding and examination of birth certificates in Suffolk County. A review of the case histories of 2,000 children followed by the Suffolk County Physically Handicapped Children's program shows that more than 50% of the families concerned would benefit from genetic counseling.

3. How to inform the public and educate the profession[12,13]

Screening and subsequent counseling is a new form of medical practice, novel both to the public and to the medical profession. In many cases, the family doctor would be the most appropriate person to do the counseling since he knows the family, its attitudes, and the socio-economic background, but physicians (especially graduates of more than ten years) do not know much about genetics and do not perceive its relevance to their work.

Although diseases with a genetic component form a large portion of the medical care burden, individual patients with a specific genetic diagnosis are not common in office practice. Of the medical problems seen by the typical family practitioner, half fall under 22 diagnostic headings, and among those, the genetic problems likely to be encountered are complex and multifactorial. The other half is made up of 550 other diagnostic headings, which means that Mendelian and chromosomal conditions are rare.

The ideas of prevention of disease and promotion of good health are implicit in the predictive function of genetics. So, if genetics is to play a part in health maintenance, its pertinence must be recognized by the profession and public alike. The most certain way is to improve the genetic content of health services is to educate the consumer. So, it is disconcerting to realize that biology is not required in high school, that less than 10% of the average biology text is devoted to genetics, and that only half of the examples used to illustrate genetic principles has a human orientation. The result is that students are ignorant about human genetics, although they do believe genetic screening is important, understand the value of prenatal diagnosis, and perceive that heterozygosity may be of etiologic significance in disease.[14]

4. Cost-benefit analyses

Economic benefit components are difficult to evaluate. There are almost no data on how effective genetic counseling is and how much money is saved. Nevertheless, the case of chronically ill children is expensive, and the savings achieved by genetic counseling must be appreciable. The most frequently quoted and generally considered the best analysis estimated a cost of $100,000 per affected individual. Thus, for example, in Westchester County, an average of 4 cases of Down syndrome per year are reported on birth certificates but, according to a study done by Hook,[15] only 35% of cases with Down syndrome are reported on birth certificates in New York State. There are, therefore, an estimated 11 cases for Westchester County alone, or an estimated 22 in the Hudson Valley region per year. This amounts to a yearly cost to society of $1,220,000. Prevention through the counseling, educational, and case identification aspects of the genetic diagnostic and counseling centers could save large amounts of money.

V. Conclusion

An advisory committee to the Commissioner of Health on genetic programs should advise the Commissioner on impending legislation (such as the recently proposed, ill-conceived bill on screening for Cooley's anemia, HSS 10634), make recommendations about which conditions should be included and which should be excluded from the program, and about where and for which conditions diagnostic laboratories and reference laboratories should exist. It should, in other words, plan a three-tiered progam consisting of statewide screening laboratories, regional diagnostic laboratories, and single reference laboratories for rare disorders. The committee should: (1) ensure that laboratory, clinical, and genetic services are well integrated, that high quality is maintained, and that adequate funding is provided for all phases of the program, including comprehensive health care for children detected in the screening program; (2) plan information for the public, particularly expectant mothers, to improve on follow-up of results following the delivery of their child, and improved education of physicians and paraprofessionals in hospitals and health departments to ensure better cooperation in the recall of samples for retesting; and (3) acquire reliable and accurate statistical data from the screening program, diagnostic laboratories, and genetic diagnostic and counseling centers upon which to base public policies as they relate to genetic services.

REFERENCES

1. The Legislature – State of New York, Legislative Commission on Expenditure Review, Newborn Metabolic Screening Program, 1978.
2. G. Ranjeet *et al.*, *Pediatrics 61*, 740, 1978.

3. J.A. Evans, A.G.W. Hunter and J.L. Hamerton, *J. Med. Genet. 15*, 43, 1978.
4. L.B. Homes, *N. Engl. J. Med. 25*, 1419, 1978.
5. D.J. Erickson, *Ann. Hum. Genet. 41*, 289, 1978.
6. A. Hansson and M. Mikkelsen, *Cytogenet. Cell Genet. 20*, 194, 1978.
7. E. Matsunaga, A. Tonomura, H. Oishi and Y, Kikuchi, *Hum. Genet. 40*, 259, 1978.
8. E.B. Hook, *N. Engl. J. Med. 299*, 1036, 1978.
9. U.K. Collaborative Study on Alpha-fetoprotein in Relation to Neural Tube Defects, *Lancet 1,* 1323, 1977.
10. A. Milunsky, *N. Engl. J. Med. 298*, 738, 1978.
11. C.J. Epstein, R.P. Erickson, B.H. Hall and M.S. Golbus, *Amer. J. Hum. Genet. 41,* 289, 1978.
12. Biological Sciences Curriculum Study, B.S.C.S./National Foundation-March of Dimes, Boulder, Colorado, 1977.
13. Trends and Teaching in Clinical Genetics, Birth Defects: Original Article Series, XIII, No. 6, Alan R. Liss, New York, 1977.
14. C.R. Scriver, D.E. Scriver, C.L. Clow and M. Skok, *Amer. Biol. Teacher* (in press).
15. E.B. Hook and G.M. Chambers, *in* Birth Defects Original Article Series, Vol. 13, No. 3A, D. Bergsma, R.B. Lowrey, B.K. Trimble and M. Feingold (Eds.), Alan R. Liss, Inc., New York, pp. 123-141, 1977.

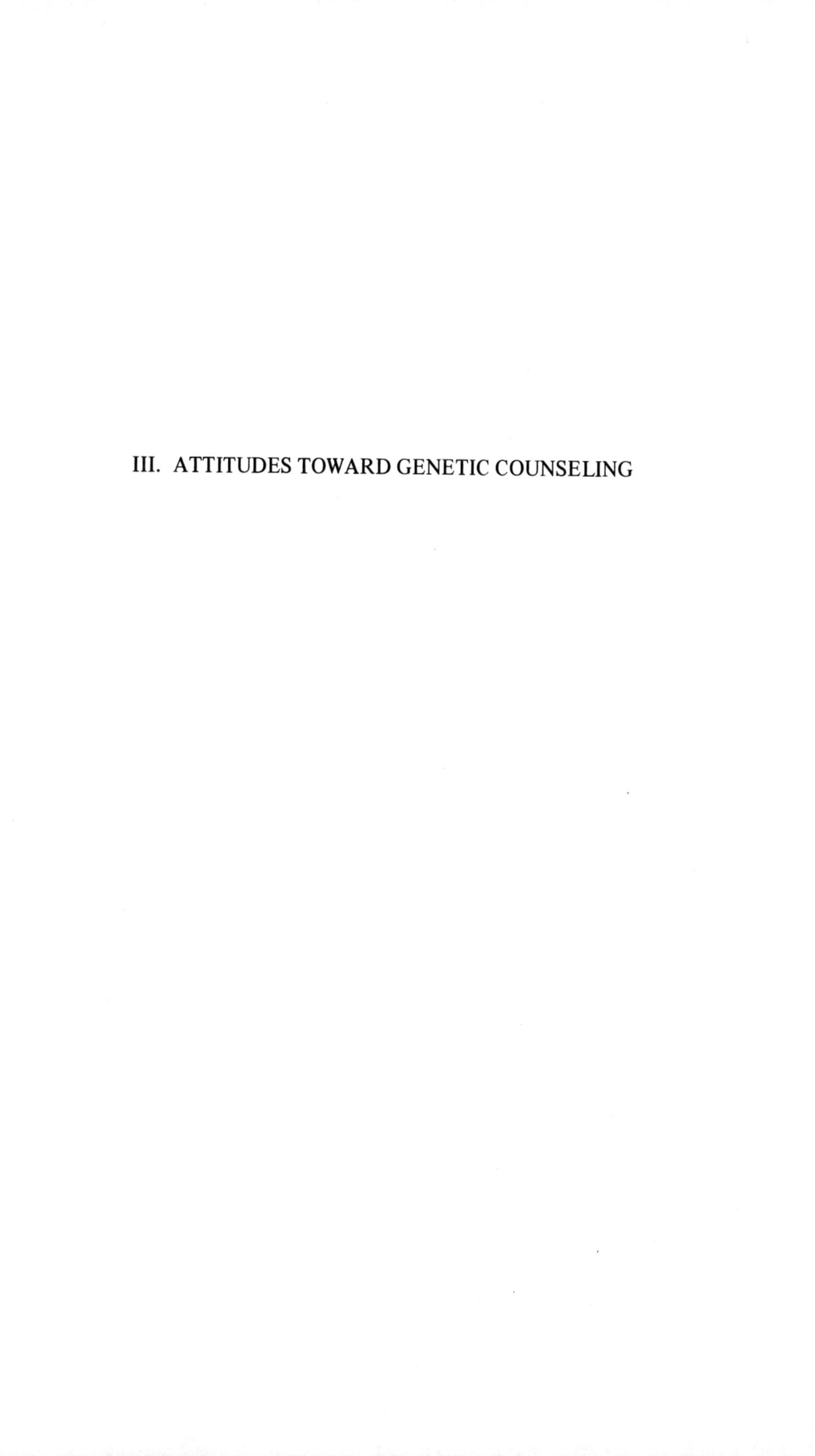

III. ATTITUDES TOWARD GENETIC COUNSELING

FAMILY PHYSICIAN, PUBLIC HEALTH ADVOCATE, OR NEW EUGENICIST: SOME ATTITUDES AND VALUES OF AMERICAN GENETIC COUNSELORS

James R. Sorenson

Introduction

The title of this symposium is "Service and Education in Medical Genetics". The title of my presentation is "Family Physician, Public Health Advocate, or New Eugenicist: Some Attitudes and Values of American Genetic Counselors". The themes of the symposium and my presentation come together in a series of questions that are at once both philosophical and practical. These are questions that relate both to what experts in applied human genetics are trying to achieve, what laymen, in their varied pursuits of genetic information, need and expect.

At a general level these questions take the following form: What is the purpose of medical genetics generally, and genetic counseling specifically? For whom are services to be provided, and to what end? What are tomorrow's practitioners of medical genetics to be taught? What might the public expect of medical genetics? At the philosophical level such questions might be approached rhetorically. From the perspective of the practicing genetic counselor or the genetic patient, however, these can be pressing questions. For some, such questions appear solvable in the increasing statistical precision and technical sophistication of contemporary applied human genetics. For others, however, questions remain; questions, in fact, made more complex by the increasing capacity of medical genetics to predict or diagnose variation in the human animal before and after birth.

I do not attempt, obviously, to provide answers to such questions in the discussion to follow. Rather, what I hope to provide is some perspective on how contemporary experts in clinical genetics approach such issues, and how their various approaches may condition or relate to the manner in which they provide medical genetic services.

Let me begin with some observations, some comments about genetic counseling as a type of professional helping behavior. My first observation is that genetic counseling is, as professional activities go, a type of hybrid strain. It is the product of the intermarriage among a number of diverse groups. Upon close inspection we see that some of these have been marriages of the heart while for

ISBN 0-12-562650-9

others only marriages of convenience, at best. If one tries to construct a family pedigree of this professional activity, several different families appear. Perhaps the main branches of the family tree are composed of the following: passionate eugenicists, scholarly academicians, practical clinicians, and devoted researchers.[1] The influence that each of these branches of the family tree has had on contemporary clinical genetics is complex. Nevertheless, genetic counseling remains today a hybrid activity, reflecting its varied origins.

My second observation is that even though genetic counseling has a rich ancestry in terms of diversity, it is at least today a kind of orphan, professionally. Perhaps some of the alliances referred to above were not really marriages but simply arrangements, and there is some question as to the legitimacy of genetic counseling. Be that as it may, genetic counseling is not yet a recognized medical specialty, at least not formally. Medicine has not fully adopted clinical genetics, although I do think that we can see the early signs of interest in adoption.[2] In short, genetic counseling has had to reside in a number of foster homes to date, and has not yet become fully established. Yet, as with most hybrid strains, genetic counseling has exhibited amazing hybrid vigor, particularly recently. Certainly the number of conferences, professional as well as public, is a sign of considerable survival fitness. Recent passage of the National Genetic Diseases Act by Congress signals continuing interest, not only among professionals but among politicians at a national level as well.[3]

My third observation is that if one tries to define or describe the activity called genetic counseling it becomes immediately apparent that counseling has wide variability. This is an important observation, I believe, because it highlights some problems for medical genetic professionals. For example, which programs should be used as models, and which revised? Shortly I will document some of the diversity that exists. For the present, however, one might view this diversity as a good thing, at least initially, for it permits a process of natural selection to occur among the variety of approaches to counseling. Theoretically the better or more effective programs will naturally come to dominate and the poorly designed or executed programs will falter. Unfortunately, the process of natural selection that we observe in the biological kingdom apparently does not have a natural analogue in the world of social affairs, be they medical or otherwise. For selection to occur there must be some assessment, some comparative weighing and balancing of the costs and benefits of various approaches. Small inroads are being made in this area, but we are as yet far from appreciating the optimal mix of professionals and procedures, technological and otherwise, for meeting the only partially documented and understood genetic health needs of the public.[4]

Taken together, these observations suggest a number of concerns and issues, only two of which I want to emphasize at this time. The first is the marked diversity in the goals and purposes of genetic counseling as it is practiced in this country, which raises some problems for attempts to develop more elaborate training and genetic service programs. The second consideration is that the develment of clinical genetics has taken place largely without systematic assessment of the needs of the users of such services, and of the ways in which genetic counseling, as variously practiced, helps or fails to help patients. A natural progression at this time would be to carefully interrelate variation in service provision with patient outcome assessments. Such studies would be particularly relevant for any attempt to increase or strengthen both professional training programs and clinical services.

Applied Human Genetics: A Study in Diversity

In order to more fully appreciate the diversity of approaches to clinical genetics I would like to review briefly four topics: (1) the early context of applied genetics to this country; (2) contemporary definitions of genetic counseling; (3) some assessments of the effectiveness of genetic counseling; and (4) some results of an attitudinal study of about 450 professionals in genetic counseling.

Some Early History

Historically, genetic counseling in this country dates back formally to at least 1910, when it was offered as one of the services at the Eugenics Record Office at Cold Spring Harbor, New York.[5] The early context of applied human genetics was typified by at least three main concerns: the eugenic implications of unrestricted procreation, especially among those deemed unfit; the social and economic impact of diseased and defective individuals; and disease avoidance *per se.*[6] In terms of their importance as rationales underlying the eugenic movement, the first two concerns were by far the most important. In fact, while individual physicians achieved some fame and stature in the eugenics movement, medicine as an organized group was not conspicuously present. As has been documented elsewhere, the goals of the eugenics movement were more genetically and socially/economically oriented than medical.[7] A spirit of social reform typified the movement, and the leaders of the movement constituted a group of diverse professionals and laymen, having in common their self-appointed status as experts in social reform and eugenic purification.

It is interesting that geneticists, while they are enthralled with the past in terms of what it can tell them about the present and what it can predict about the future, as a group do not seem to engage in ancestor worship. In fact, when it comes to that period of history when genetics as a scientific discipline was linked with applied genetics, geneticists have mixed feelings about their history.[8] This is important for understanding the context of applied human genetics today.

An important symbolic event for contemporary applied human genetics took place in 1947.[9] At that time, Dr. Sheldon Reed, an early genetic counselor, noted that genetic counseling was conducted under a variety of names, including genetic consultation, genetic advice, and genetic hygiene. Reed rejected these names for a variety of reasons, but two were particularly important.[10] The first reason was that the existing labels reflected a concern or emphasis on social and eugenic topics that were not typical of the more traditional concern of the physician in his patients and their individual problems. Second, he thought that such words as hygiene connoted an interest in health issues that were not reflective of the concerns of the doctor and patient in genetic counseling. Reed suggested the name genetic counseling, hoping it would remove the possible eugenic and hygienic implications of existing labels.

The name genetic counseling was widely adopted. Two things about the new labels are worth noting, however. First, the label remains, even today, more the one selected because it is in opposition to earlier prevailing labels than because it accurately reflects what actually happens when doctor and patient meet. Second, the label is quite vague, and has multiple meanings for both professionals and laymen. As we will see shortly, genetic counseling means a variety of things to the professionals who provide it, some giving more emphasis to the word genetic than to the word counseling, while others give equal or more emphasis to the word counseling. For patients, the word counseling may connote that they will receive direct advice or counsel about what to do, while other patients may be at considerable loss to understand what type of medical service they are to receive.

Since the 1930's, when applied genetics began to move out ot the eugenics context, it has come to be applied increasingly in the world of medicine. Ludmerer notes, in a recent study of genetics in this country, that a number of developments helped to spur the movement of applied genetics into medicine.[11] These included: (1) discoveries of the genetics of blood groups; (2) a rapid and continuing expansion in understanding the role of genetics in a wide spectrum of diseases; and (3) with the advent of atomic energy in the 1940s, medical interest in the mutational and genetic impact of atomic radiation. In looking over these developments, Ludmerer comments on their significance for applied human genetics. He writes:

> "These discoveries were important for more than purely intellectual reasons. They gave human genetics a start in medicine, which is an ideologically neutral field. Insofar as human genetics became part of medicine, it too became ideologically neutral, and this justified the faith of geneticists that human genetics could stand as an independent discipline apart from eugenics."[12]

Ludmerer's statement is an assertion that, in moving into medicine, applied human genetics has become ideologically neutral. This assertion probably means that the traditional interests of the doctor in his patient are relatively more important in shaping the goals and activities of the medical genetic counselor than are larger social, economic, or genetic concerns. In terms of the rationales identified above that underly the eugenics movement, we would expect to find today a reverse ordering of importance in which concern with disease prevention takes on paramount importance, and concern with the social, economic, and genetic issues take on much less, if any importance. We will examine this argument by looking first at some definitions of counseling provided by contemporary genetic counselors.

Genetic Counseling: Some Definitions

Several dozen articles on genetic counseling have been published to date, and a significant number of these contain explicit or implicit definitions.[13] It would be impossible to discuss all the various definitions of genetic counseling that exist. However, a summary of the major orientations suggests three definitional groupings.

The first set of definitions involves a commitment to genetic counseling as a form of preventive medicine. The emphasis or goal of counseling, such definitions suggest, is the prevention of the birth of children with predictable birth defects.[14]

There are limits, of course, to the extent to which this goal ought to be pursued. If a child may be born with a genetic disease that is treatable, then there is a less compelling reason to prevent the birth unless, of course, there is some interest in the genetic implications of such births. In general, however, this orientation to counseling argues that the best method of assessing the effectiveness of genetic counseling would be to note changes in the incidence of predictable birth defects in a population subsequent to the introduction of genetic counseling services.

How this goal relates to the actual practice of genetic counseling in general, and to the directiveness of the individual counselor *vis a vis* the individual patient are important issues. It is possible, of course, for the individual counselor to identify with this goal at the population level, yet in terms of how he relates to his individual patients, to be non-directive. Such a counselor would hope that by whatever criteria he may hold up as constituting a high risk or burdensome disease, the majority of couples that find themselves in such situations would refrain from reproduction.

It is probable, however, that endorsement of a disease prevention goal would be related to a counselor being willing to directly advise his individual patients about what he/she feels is appropriate reproductive behavior. We will examine this with some data below. For the present, however, regardless of the level at which the individual genetic counselor wants to assess his counseling, population of discrete pregnancy outcome, a counselor with a disease prevention orientation is primarily interested in reducing the number of pregnancies which result in the birth of a child with a predictable defect.

A second major definitional grouping focuses less on the prevention of the birth of children with predictable defects and more on facilitating the reproductive decision-making process of individuals and/or couples seeking genetic counseling. The goal of such counseling is providing information that patients will find useful, regardless of the actual decisions they make. In particular, such an orientation to genetic counseling places much emphasis on patient education, and then helping patients place this often newly acquired information into an individual decision-making framework that they will find useful.

The definition of genetic counseling provided by Fraser *et al.* in *The American Journal of Human Genetics* is a definition in which this counseling orientation seems to have high saliency. Counseling is defined here as:

> "A communication process which deals with the human problems associated with the occurrence, or risk of occurrence of a genetic disorder in a family. This process involves an attempt by one or more appropriately trained persons to help the individual or the family to (1) comprehend the medical facts, including the diagnosis, the probable course of the disorder and the available management; (2) appreciate the way heredity contributes to the disorder and the risk of recurrence in specified relatives; (3) understand the options for dealing with the risk of recurrence; (4) choose the course of action which seems appropriate to them in view of their risk and their family goals and act in accordance with that decision; and (5) make the best possible adjustment to the disorder in an affected family member and/or to the risk of recurrence of that disorder."[15]

Adoption of this counseling goal suggests that the criteria one might hold up to assess counseling effectiveness would consist not of changes in the incidence of predictable birth defects after introduction of a counseling program, but rather in the extent to which counseling patients found the counseling experience of use to them in making decisions, reproductive and otherwise. There are a variety of ways in which one could make assessments of how effective counseling had been in achieving this. For example, couples could be asked about whether or not the counseling provided needed information, and if counseling put this information into a personal perspective patients found useful.

However one wants to formulate such criteria, the emphasis this counseling orientation takes is on informing and assisting the decision-making of patients, not necessarily on altering the incidence of children born with predictable birth defects.

A third major orientation that comes out of the literature views the goal of counseling as not just the transmission of information and assistance in helping patients make decisions. In addition, particular emphasis is given to the psychological implications of genetic counseling. This orientation argues that there are significant psychological needs that exist in patients who obtain genetic counseling, and these psychological needs cannot be met simply by educating the patient and providing him/her with health care assistance. Rather, it is important that the genetic counselor be sensitive to the special psychological needs of the counseling patient, and that he/she structure into counseling the provision of psychological counseling.

There is a rather large impressionistic literature on psychological and psychiatric issues in genetic counseling.[17] Of recent interest is the argument that some patients in counseling who have a defective child will naturally go through a five-stage process of psychological coping and adaptation.[18] In light of this hypothesized coping sequence, it is argued that counseling should be delivered in accordance with the stage that the patient is in. In addition, some patients may be so psychologically distraught as to require significant psychiatric treatment.

From this psychologically oriented perspective, an evaluation of the effectiveness of genetic counseling would have to focus on a number of things. There is concern, of course, that counseling result in the acquisition and retention of accurate information. There is also concern that counseling enable patients to make decisions and to cope with their problems. In addition, however, this orientation would require some assessment of the psychological health or psychological functioning of patients subsequent to counseling. As with the previously described counseling orientation, the psychological orientation does not seem to concern itself with impacting on the incidence of predictable birth defects in a population subsequent to counseling.

The three orientations identified above constitute very brief descriptions of major orientations toward genetic counseling. In the actual practice of counseling it is highly likely that any individual counselor would exhibit elements of each of these orientations. What would probably vary significantly and what would shape the impact of his/her counseling, however, would be the *relative* importance that the counselor attaches to achieving each of the different goals identified.

Some Evaluations of Counseling Effectiveness

Perhaps a more direct indicator of the goals of genetic counseling than definitions are the criteria that genetic counselors use to assess the effectiveness of their undertaking. To date about thirty studies of the impact of genetic counseling have been published, almost all of which were studies conducted by individuals who themselves are involved in the provision of genetic counseling. It seems instructive to look at the criteria against which these individuals assess the effectiveness of their counseling.

In examining these studies, a brief methodological note is required. The majority of studies published to date permit, at best, only limited inference about the actual effectiveness of genetic counseling, variously defined. To a large extent these studies suffer from one or another significant design, statistical, or inference problem that makes it difficult to draw firm conclusions about counseling effectiveness. This does not mean, however, that we can not look to these studies and the criteria they employ as indicators of what genetic counselors are trying to achieve.

As one looks across the several published studies it appears that they can be grouped into one of three groupings, groupings not totally inconsistent with the three major orientations identified in our discussion of prevailing definitions.[19]

One set of these studies seems to emphasize the educational aspects of genetic counseling and imply, in so doing, that effective genetic counseling is equivalent to effective medicogenetic education.[20] According to this position the counseling has been effective – to the extent that genetic counseling has been successful in providing and educating patients about the genetics of their situation and some of the medical aspects of the disease. To a large extent these studies focus on the acquisition of two general sets of information: (1) the genetic mode of inheritance for a disease in a family and, in particular, the occurrence or recurrence risk; and (2) some understanding of the disease, often reported simply as patient conception of the burden the disease imposes on the affected. In the several studies that look at these criteria, it is not possible to infer how well counseling inculcates such knowledge since, as suggested, these studies assess such knowledge only after, not before, genetic counseling. In such situations we can say that after counseling patients know certain things, but it is not possible to infer that counseling educated patients since we do not know the level of knowledge with which patients entered the counseling situation.

A second series of studies begins by looking at the level of genetic and disease knowledge patients have after counseling, but proceeds one step further and looks at either or both the reproductive intentions and/or behavior of couples subsequent to counseling.[21] In so doing, these studies imply that the goals of counseling are more complex than simple education. In fact, these studies suggest that counseling should ultimately be related to the reproductive intentions and behavior of individuals. In some studies criteria are proposed as to what constitutes a high risk and what is a burdensome disease, and patient reproductive intentions, contraceptive behavior, and actual reproduction are examined in terms of these criteria. Two things are worth noting. First, the criteria specified as to what constitutes a high risk or what is a burdensome disease are mostly set by the professionals, not the patients. Patient behavior is examined in light of these criteria and, for example, positive reproductive intentions or behavior when a risk of recurrence is one in 10 or greater is considered less than successful counseling.[22] Second, while some of these studies attempt to impute or infer causation between recurrence risk, disease burden, and reproductive intentions and behavior, it is extremely difficult to do so, given the study designs. Had these various studies ascertained patient perceptions of risk and burden, not professional perceptions, then a stronger case could be made for inferring causation.

As a group, however, these studies suggest that effective counseling results in lowered reproductive intentions and behavior under conditions of high risk and great burden, defined professionally. In so doing, they imply that the appropriate decision matrix that individuals and couples should employ in making reproductive decisions is a limited matrix, defined in terms of risk and burden. Apparently such a consideration as parental desire for a child is not a legitimate concern to enter into the decision-making equation.

Finally, a third set of studies are those which attempt to focus on the sociopsychological aspects of genetic counseling. These studies are concerned also with knowledge acquisition and retention, but in addition, they make various attempts to assess the psychological impact of counseling on the people receiving counseling. In such studies phenomena such as parental self concepts and anxiety are examined, in terms of how counseling alters such psychological states, as well as how such psychological variables related to the process of education in counseling.[23]

While these studies to date do not relate directly to those definitional orientations identified above which focus on such issues as psychological coping in counseling and returning counseling patients to a state of psychological homeostasis, in the long run this would appear to be one of the goals of such evaluation strategies. To date, the major impact of studies in this area is to alert counselors to the manifest and latent psychological functions of genetic counseling. In so doing, these studies imply that effective genetic counseling is that in which the genetic counselor is sensitive to such issues in his/her counseling, and the good counselor is one who attempts to utilize such psychological issues when they can augment the educative aspects of counseling and ameliorate them when they threaten this function. In terms of counseling and outcomes, this orientation would consider effective counseling as that which educates the patients, both in terms of medicogenetic knowledge, and more broadly in terms of the social and psychological aspects of the health problems faced. Effective counseling would entail working with patients to lessen their anxiety and sustain or improve their self concepts, particularly in reference to their reproductive competency.

Several additional studies have taken slightly different tracks in attempting to assess the effectiveness of genetic counseling but, by and large, the three orientations identified above predominate in the evaluation literature. It is interesting that a health services orientation is absent in this literature which focuses on such things as the fit between the problems patients bring to counseling and the nature and extent of services provided or, more globally, the degree of patient satisfaction with genetic counseling. Perhaps as the assessment of counseling expands, and those involved in such efforts are not counselors themselves, we might expect to see a stronger emphasis on consumer view in this literature.

Some Counselor Attitudes

Finally, a national questionnaire survey and selective interview study of practicing genetic counselors was undertaken by the author between 1973 and 1975, to look at various facets of contemporary counseling.[24] While the full results of this study are not published at this time, some limited data have appeared that are directly relevant to this discussion of variation in counseling orientations.

Just as was the case when we examined various definitions of genetic counseling, and when we looked at several studies of counseling effectiveness, results of the national survey suggest considerable diversity of opinion among contemporary genetic counselors, both as to what they want their counseling to achieve and about their role *vis a vis* patients in counseling.

In an article based on the national survey that appeared in the recent book *Genetic Counseling*,[25] Sorenson and Culbert identified three varying orientations of counselors toward their patients. These orientations are first a guiding strategy in which the counselor feels it appropriate to guide patients in their decision making, particularly in assuring that counseling results in disease prevention. The second strategy, termed supportive, is one in which disease prevention does not predominate. Rather, the major concern of such counselors appears to be to help patients realize their goals and values and to see that patient decision-making, reproductive or otherwise, is cast in a decision matrix that contains personal patient concerns and desires, not just medical-genetic criteria such as magnitude of recurrence risk and burden of the disease risked. Finally, the third counseling orientation, labeled an advising strategy, is one in which the counselor appears to be interested not only in disease prevention but, in addition, has an interest in both the genetic and the social implications, economic and otherwise, or reproduction among those at risk for having a genetically diseased child. As was commented by Sorenson and Culbert, while the first two orientations are ones which constitute variation on the traditional model of the doctor/patient relationship in our society, the third orientation is one which departs from this model in some important respects.[26] Perhaps one of the most important deviations is that the third orientation endorses a kind of public health perspective on the part of the counselor, not normally one of the views of the doctor when he meets with a patient. Discussions of this position have appeared in the medical literature on genetic counseling and constitute one of the points of conflict over the appropriate goals of counseling and the role of the counselor in achieving those goals.[27,28]

As is suggested in the discussion by Sorenson and Culbert, each orientation appears to be related to a different view of the genetic counselor *vis a vis* his directiveness in counseling. The more a counselor endorses the public health stance, the more willing he is to advise patients. Those with strong endorsements of counseling as a form of preventive medicine are only somewhat less willing to directly advise patients. The counselors who adopt the supportive position are much less willing to view their role as an advisor. Their orientation is apparently one of helping patients realize their personal goals and expectations. These sometimes may entail disease prevention, and at other times a mix of disease avoidance and strong desires to be a parent.

In short, the data from this national survey of some 450 professionals in genetic counseling finds some evidence to support the variations in orientations that suggested themselves when we examined definitions of counseling and different attempts by several counselors to assess their effectiveness. The national survey does suggest, in addition, that of the approximately 450 counselors surveyed, the majority, or about 60%, adopt a disease prevention orientation, about 24% view their role as essentially educative-supportive, while the smallest group, about 15%, are much concerned with preventing both somatic as well as genetic abnormality.[29]

Conclusion

After briefly noting the historical origins of genetic counseling in this country, this article has focused on three sets of data regarding the goals and orientations that counselors may have toward their professional activity. While there is not perfect agreement among the orientations so identified, the discussion suggests variation on three central themes. Sometimes counseling is viewed as essentially preventive medicine, and to the extent that it results in a reduction in the birth of children with predictable birth defects, it has been effective. Second, counseling is sometimes viewed as preventive medicine in a broader, public health and genetic perspective. From this view, counseling should lead to a reduction in the birth of predictable defects, whether at the level of phenotype or genotype. Finally, counseling is sometimes viewed as a form of patient education and counseling in which the goal is not so much to reduce the incidence of children born with predictable defects, but rather to permit parents in risky situations to make decisions that are both technically informed and reflective of the values and goals of the parents.

Consideration of these orientations and others is important as we move toward strengthening and enlarging professional training programs as well as clinic services. Such expansion needs to be premised on a clear notion of what applied human genetics is trying to achieve, and what are the most effective ways of so doing. It is no longer permissible to continue support of various approaches to counseling unless we are at the same time making some attempt to see how effective the various approaches are. To continue so is to fail to recognize that genetic counseling, in its present status, is experimental medicine. It is experimental in that a variety of approaches exist and we are presently operating without a sophisticated sense of how well each approach is working. Genetic counseling constitutes an intervention into the lives of thousands of patients, and expanded educational and service programs should be premised on a far more complete and sophisticated understanding of the effects of these interventions.

Finally, as referenced at the outset, it is critical at this stage of development that we obtain a better understanding of both the problems patients bring to counseling, as well as the problems they encounter thereafter. In reviewing the literature on genetic counseling, it was not possible to locate studies of patient needs or problems. The improvement of professional training and patient services is dependent on such studies. To use a medical analogy, to continue to train professionals and provide services in the absence of information on patient needs and problems is to run the risk of developing a "diagnosis" and instituting a "therapy regimen" (counseling services) in the absence of a good diagnosis of what the patients' problems are. Our sophistication in the service delivery and human issues in genetic counseling must be at a comparable level with the purely technical advances and refinements in applied human genetics.

REFERENCES

1. K.M. Ludmerer, Genetics and American Society: A Historical Appraisal, The Johns Hopkins University Press, Baltimore, 1972.
2. D. Bergsma (Ed.), Advances in Human Genetics and Their Impact on Society, *Birth Defects: Orig. Art. Ser., Vol. VIII, No. 4*, July, 1972.
3. Public Law 94-278: Title IV: National Sickle Cell Anemia, Cooley's Anemia, Tay-Sachs, and Genetic Diseases Act.
4. H. Lubs and F. De la Cruz (Eds.), Genetic Counseling, Raven Press, New York, 1977.
5. M.H. Haller, Eugenics: Hereditarian Attitudes in American Thought, Rutgers University Press, New Brunswick, 1963.
6. *Ibid.*
7. J. Sorenson, *in* Law and Genetics, A. Milunsky and G. Annas (Eds.), Plenum Press, New York, pp. 467-485, 1975.
8. K.M. Ludmerer, *op. cit.*
9. S.C. Reed, *Soc. Biol. 24,* 332, 1974.
10. M. Griffin, C. Kavanaugh and J. Sorenson, *Social Work in Health Care 2 (2)*, 171, 1976-77.
11. K.M. Ludmerer, *op. cit.*
12. *Ibid.*
13. J. Sorenson, Social and Psychological Aspects of Applied Human Genetics: A Bibliography, DHEW Publication No. (NIH) 73-412, 1973.
14 V. Riccardi, The Genetic Approach to Human Disease, Oxford University Press, New York, 1977.
15. F.C. Fraser, *Am. J. Hum. Genet. 26*, 636, 1974.
16. M. Antley, R. Antley and H. Hartlage. *J. Psychol. 83.*, 335-1973.
17. J. Sorenson, cit. No. 13.
18. A. Faleck and S. Britton, *Soc. Biol. 21*, 1, 1974.
19. J. Sorenson and A. Culbert, *in* Genetic Counseling, H. Lubs and F. de la Cruz (Eds.), Raven Press, New York, pp. 131-156, 1977.
20. Y.E. Hsia, *in* Genetic Responsibility, M. Lipkin and R.T. Rowley (Eds.), Plenum Press, New York, pp. 43-60, 1973.
21. C. Carter, K. Evans, J.A. Fraser-Roberts and A. Buck, *Lancet 1*, 281, 1971.
22. *Ibid.*
23. Antley, *op. cit.*.
24. See Sorenson and Culbert, ref. cit. No. 19.
25. *Ibid.*
26. *Ibid.*
27. R.E. Stevenson and R.R. Howell, *Annals of American Academy of Polital Social Sciences,* 30, December, 1972.
28. B. Childs, *Yale J. Biol. and Med. 46*, 297, 1973.
29. J.R. Sorenson, unpublished results of national questionnaire study of professionals in genetic counseling, Boston University School of Medicine, 1977.

GENETIC COUNSELING IN THE CONTEXT OF GENETIC SCREENING*

Peter T. Rowley
Mack Lipkin, Jr.
Lawrence Fisher

Introduction

A committee of the U.S. National Academy of Sciences has reported:

> "When a disease is discovered through the usual medical channels, the mechanisms for moving the patient on to management and treatment are usually well worked out and, as one aspect of management, counseling has its times, places, and methods. But the role of genetic counseling in genetic screening programs is only now being clarified; and while it is clear that the service is essential, the exact procedures governing where and how it is best done, and how often and by whom, are not yet worked out."[1]

Some studies of counseling following genetic screening suggest that subjects learn little. Most studies do not illuminate the response to genetic information of the population at large because of subject selection bias. Individuals who seek genetic counseling, whether because of a symptomatic family member, or in response to a public education effort, are self-selected for interest in genetic information. Studies using them under-represent those individuals for whom identification of genetic risk is threatening. For health planning purposes, data is needed on the response of unselected persons to defined genetic information.

To accomplish this goal we have studied response to genetic screening for a single entity in a health maintenance organization. Its members accept an orientation toward prevention and expect to be screened for conditions not individually specified. The heterozygotes detected are thus not selected for interest in receiving genetic information. The individual identified is asked for informed consent for participation in the study just prior to the offer of counseling and before the name of the condition is mentioned.

The condition studied here, beta-thalassemia trait, is suitable for a study of the

*This study was supported by N.I.H. Grant No. 3 R01 HL 17465 and by New York State Health Research Council Grant No. 664.

ISBN 0-12-562650-9

DIAGRAM OF STUDY
SCREEN
NON-BETA-THALASSEMIA
BETA-THALASSEMIA TRAIT
NOTIFY BY
Letter
Telephone
Unresponsive
INVITE STUDY PARTICIPATION
CONSENT
No further involvement with study
Counsel if patient desires
Declines
RANDOMIZE (on basis of age, sex, & marital status)
Not counseled
PRETEST
Health Check List
Medical Attitude and Experience Questionnaire
Thalassemia and Genetics Knowledge Questionnaire
Probability Questionnaire
Marital Adjustment Scale
Self-Concept Scale
Mood Adjective Check List
I.Q. and Personality Scales
COUNSEL
Conventional
Programmed
IMMEDIATE ASSESSMENT
Mood Adjective Check List
Test of Comprehension
Assay of Plans
2 MONTH ASSESSMENT
Open-Ended Interview
Thalassemia Knowledge Questionnaire
Health Check List
Medical Attitude and Experience Questionnaire
Marital Adjustment Inventory
Self-Concept Scale

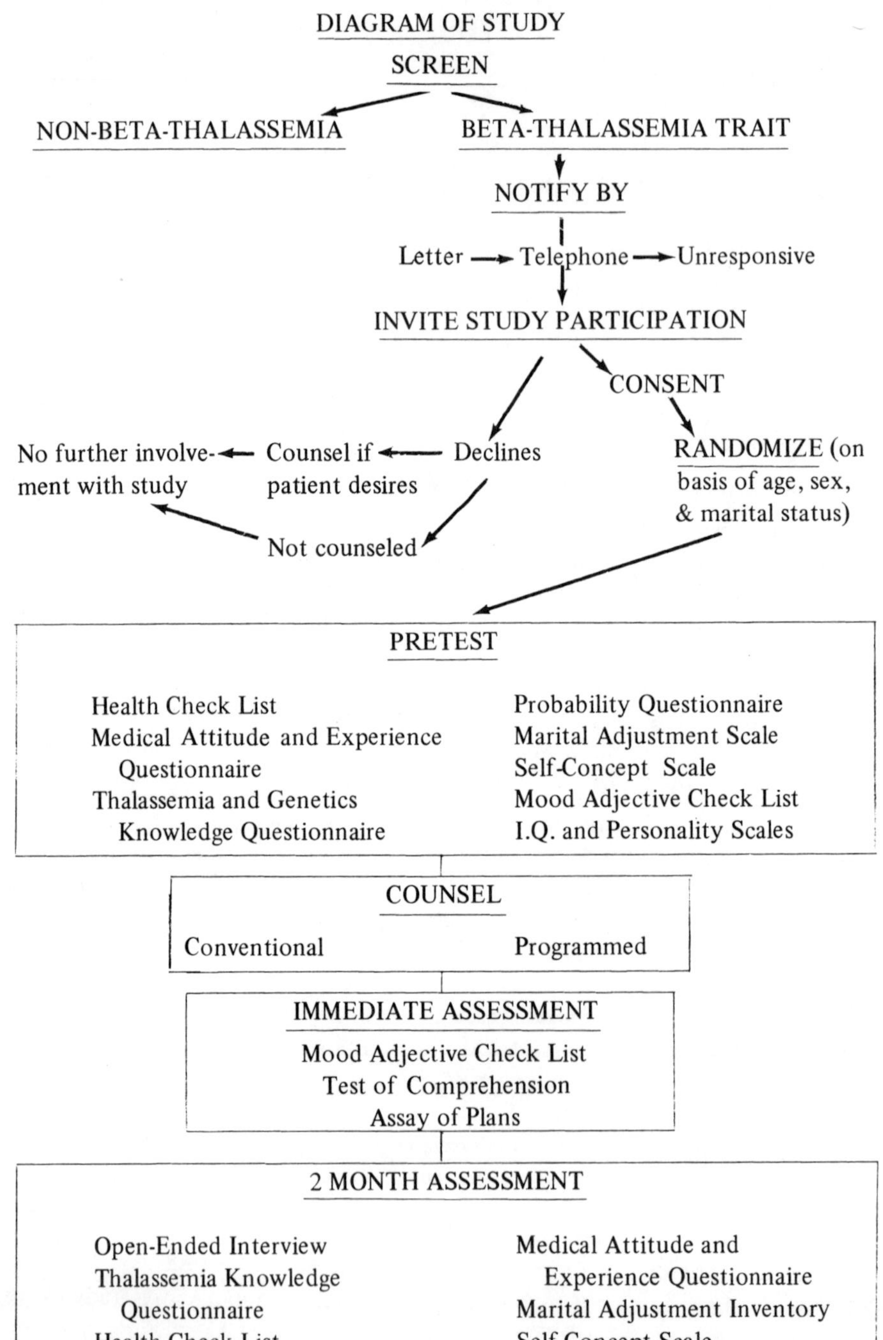

Figure 1.

impact of genetic counseling in the setting of genetic screening for several reasons. First, it is common enough for the collection of an adequate number of subjects. Second, the homozygous state is serious and without satisfactory treatment. Finally, new diagnostic methods suitable for large-scale application now permit recognition of the majority of individuals at risk for affected offspring.

This project attempts to answer the question, "Is it a genuine service to identify beta-thalassemia trait individuals among a population not specifically requesting identification?" It attempts to answer this question by assessing effects on knowledge, mood, attitudes, and behavior. This report addresses only the first of these – effects on knowledge. It asks, "Does the subject learn?"

With the emphasis today on containment of health care costs, the best counseling method is the method of achieving an acceptable result most economically. We have compared two methods, identical in information presented, called here *programmed counseling* and *conventional counseling.* The former involves viewing a specially produced videotaped self-instructional program. This method was introduced because it minimizes the expenditure of counselor time, an important consideration in any large-scale program.

Design of the Study

A flow diagram of the study is shown in Fig. 1. The population being screened is that of the Genesee Valley Group Health Association (GVGHA) in Rochester, New York – New York's first federally certified health maintenance organization. Its subscribers, currently numbering 32,000, represent a cross section of the population of the region.

Red cell indices were determined for all patients aged 18 to 65 years having a phlebotomy for initial health assessment or for any reason. Each individual with a mean corpuscular volume (MCV) < 78, had a hemoglobin A_2 determination by DEAE cellulose microcolumn chromatography[2] or, earlier, by isoelectric focusing.

Each patient with an elevated hemoglobin A_2 was sent a letter by his own GVGHA physician stating that a "laboratory abnormality" had been found and inviting him to come in for an explanation. Prior to counseling each patient was asked to participate in a study of how doctors can best explain health information to patients. Of 54 patients with beta-thalassemia trait identified, 50 agreed to participate. This high percentage of participation enhances the degree to which results of the study may be generalized.

Following consent, all subjects were tested to collect baseline information on health, medical attitudes and experience, knowledge of thalassemia, of genetics, and of probability, marital adjustment, self-concept, mood, I.Q., and psychological characteristics.

Immediately following testing, patients received counseling. To enhance the comparison of counseling methods, we controlled precisely and made identical the information (16 items) that each method was to communicate, *i.e.,* the synonyms for beta-thalassemia, the characteristics of beta-thalassemia trait, the characteristics of thalassemia major, and two mating types with the probabilities

TABLE 1

Content of Counseling

Names for the condition:	
	Thalassemia
	Mediterranean anemia
	Cooley's anemia
Characteristics of trait form:	
	Detected by a blood test
	Mild anemia common
	Usually without symptoms
Characteristics of major form:	
	Transfusions required
	Growth slow
	Life shortened
	Both parents have trait
Risk to offspring of trait individuals:	
	Trait x normal → 50% trait + 50% normal
	Trait x trait → 25% normal + 50% trait + 25% MAJOR

for their offspring, as detailed in Table 1.

We did not present the ethnic distribution of beta-thalassemia (except for mentioning the name Mediterranean anemia) primarily because we did not want the counselee to assume that any child the counselee may have by a non-Mediterranean person must be healthy. When asked, we discussed the world-wide distribution.

Discussion of prenatal diagnosis for thalassemia was not initiated because of its experimental status. Questions about it were fully answered.

The *programmed* counseling method employed a specially produced color videotape depicting an actual counseling session by a physician in which the counselee readily understands the information presented and indicates intent to use it, interspersed by narrator comments. Active learning was promoted by questions directed at the viewer with an interval to record answers. Following viewing, the patient had an opportunity to question a physician-counselor.

In the *conventional* counseling method the physicians were especially trained to present the same information in the same order as the videotape. The 16 items and other information were reviewed and readings were assigned. The trainee counseled surrogate patients until he could do so without errors, as evidenced on review of an audio recording of the counseling session.

Both methods were nondirective; the choices facing the patient were listed, but the patient's inclinations were not elicited. The screening of family members was neither encouraged nor discouraged. This has been called the neutral educator approach.[3]

Each method took about the same time, 40 minutes.

Immediately after counseling, mood, comprehension, and self-concept were assessed.

Two months after counseling, the patient was asked to return for reassessment as shown and asked what impact the new knowledge had had on his life.

Effect of Counseling on Knowledge

Mean scores for all subjects for knowledge in three areas – thalassemia, probability, and genetics – at three times – before, immediately after, and two months after counseling – are shown in Fig. 2. To assess the changes, individual scores were submitted to a time x group analysis of variance with repeated measures on time.

Knowledge in each area increased significantly. In the case of both thalassemia and genetics, increases evident immediately after counseling have largely been retained at two months.

Comparison of Counseling Methods

In order to contrast the two counseling methods, pre/post difference scores in knowledge were assessed by t tests for different scores. As shown in Fig. 3, in regard to knowledge of thalassemia, there was no significant difference between

EFFECTS OF COUNSELING ON KNOWLEDGE
All Subjects
Before Counseling
After Counseling
Immediately
2 Months
TOPIC
THALASSEMIA
F = 59.35
p<.001
54.7
84.0
81.6
PROBABILITY
F = 9.34
p<.01
72.8
82.9
GENETICS
F = 18.12
p<.001
62.3
82.5
79.1

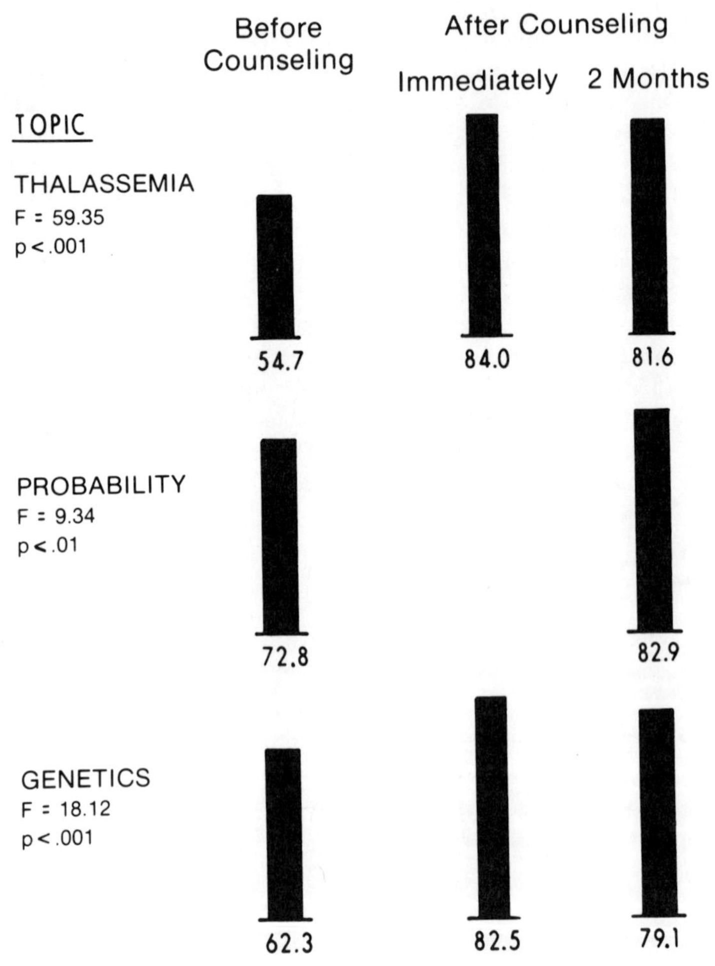

Figure 2.

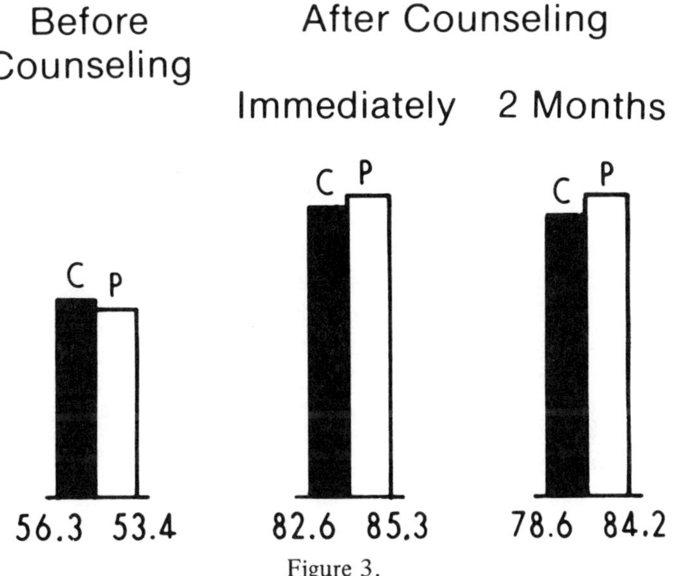

Figure 3.

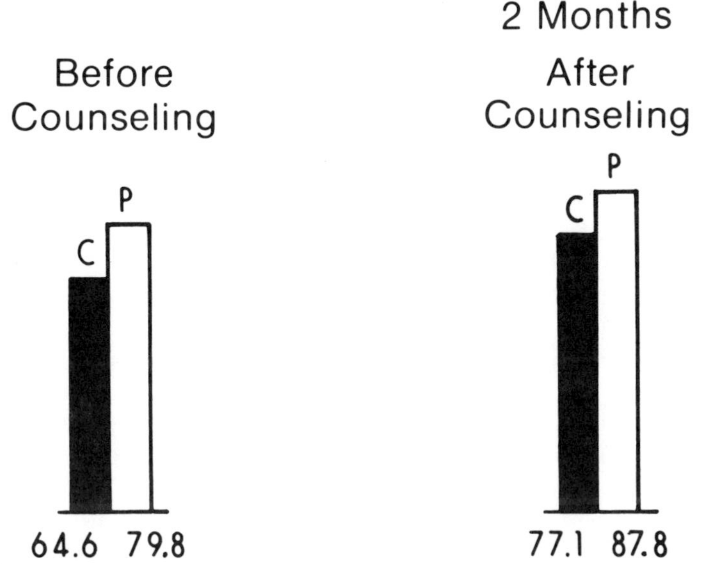

Figure 4.

the two counseling groups, conventional and programmed.

Similarly, in knowledge of probability, the increment in knowledge following counseling, though greater in the programmed counseling group, was not significantly different in the two counseling groups, as shown in Fig. 4.

In knowledge of genetics, however, subjects receiving programmed counseling displayed significantly greater learning than did subjects receiving conventional counseling ($t = 2.41$; $p < .01$), as shown in Fig. 5.

It is uncertain why knowledge of genetics increases more for subjects receiving programmed counseling, whereas no such differential increases occur in knowledge of thalassemia or of probability. Several explanations may be offered. First, it may be that the information about genetics is more complicated and is communicated better by the videotape than than by the live counselor. A second possibility is that the live counselor may be distracted from the orderly presentation of genetic principles necessary for learning when the patient breaks in with questions about their application to his own situation. A third possibility is that the counselee depicted in the videotape permits the subject to think about thalassemia trait in a more objective way than if the information were initially directed at him, or provides a role model for understanding and applying the information provided. A fourth possibility is that the videotape more efficiently fosters learning through its more systematic posing of questions to the subject.

Benefit-Burden Ratio

Is the burden of knowing one's trait status outweighed by the benefit of avoiding the bearing of a homozygous child unless one has consciously accepted the risk? The critical factor is the benefit-burden ratio. We feel that this question deserves an attempt at answering through a comprehensive assessment of benefits and burdens in a relatively unselected population. To the present report of retention of knowledge over a short period, we will later add reports of retention of knowledge over a longer period and of effects on mood, attitudes, and behavioral outcomes.

Conclusions

Information is needed about the response to genetic counseling in the setting of genetic screening in a relatively unselected population.

In a health maintenance organization, all members phlebotomized were tested for beta-thalassemia trait. Nearly all identified wished information and consented to be studied. With regard to learning about thalassemia and probability, each of two counseling methods studied was effective in communicating information with no significant difference between groups. With regard to the teaching of genetics, programmed counseling was superior to trained physicians.

These data, from a study also evaluating the psychological effects of genetic counseling and their relation to behavioral change, suggest that carefully designed instructional devices may both conserve professional effort and improve learning.

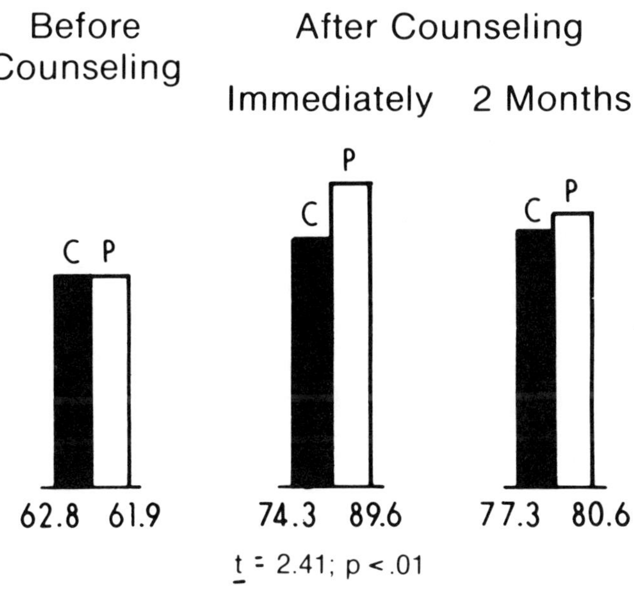

Figure 5.

ACKNOWLEDGMENTS

We thank Dr. James S. Roberts and the staff of the Joseph C. Wilson Health Center, Genesee Valley Group Health Association, for permission to study their patients, and Starlene Dick, Joyce Kofsky, Sandra LaBella, Judy Lee, and Carol Sutera for expert technical assistance.

REFERENCES

1. B. Childs (Ed.), Genetic Screening: Programs, Principles and Research. National Research Council, National Academy of Sciences, Washington, D.C., p. 178, 1975.
2. T.H.J. Huisman, W.A. Schroeder, A.N. Brodie, S.M. Mayson and J. Jakway, *J. Lab. Clin. Med.* *86*, 700, 1975.
3. J. Hall, *in* Ethical Issues in Human Genetics, B.D. Hilton, D. Callahan, M. Harris, P. Condliffe and B. Berkeley (Eds.), Plenum Press, New York, p. 23, 1973.

PSYCHIATRIC CONSIDERATIONS IN GENETIC COUNSELING

John D. Rainer

It gives me great pleasure to take part in this Symposium on Service and Education in Medical Genetics, since what I have to discuss concerns medical genetics as a service to people and involves the education of both the server and the one who is served. About 13 years ago I participated in a similar program here in Albany on Genetics for Physicians. At that time I discussed Genetics in Psychiatry,[1] outlining the role of genetics in psychiatric research, an area which has made considerable advances since that date. At the recent meeting last May of the American Psychiatric Association in Toronto, a panel was held on the Use and Abuse of Psychiatric Genetic Counseling. In that panel, certain questions were raised which are pertinent to the wider issues with which we are concerned today. Among the objectives of the panel were to acquaint the clinician with the psychological factors that influence and permeate the genetic counseling process. The counselor's assessment of the client's ability to cope psychologically with whatever decision he or she entertains was stressed. As I said in the 1964 meeting here, "In the broader sense, the provision of genetic counseling represents the direct link between medical knowledge in this field and the patient and his family. There are no decisions in a patient's life more important and more surrounded by emotion than the one to marry and the one to assume parenthood, and none more consequential with respect to family welfare. If any doubts exist regarding questions of heredity, any person or couple needs to have access to a trained professional person who is able not only to elicit the pertinent facts and evaluate them scientifically, but also to communicate them with understanding and the proper amount of guidance so that the persons will achieve happiness in their ultimate choices."

That genetic counseling is more than the provision of information is something which has been gradually accepted over the past 25 years. There have been two or three streams of input into this expanded concept – one from the behavioral sciences – first psychiatry, then psychology and, lately, social work; one from those concerned with medical ethics; and, to some extent, one from the consumers and families themselves.

In 1952, when there were 7 genetic counseling centers in the United States and Canada, one of the founders and the 5th president of the American Society

ISBN 0-12-562650-9

of Human Genetics, Franz Kallmann, himself a distinguished psychiatrist, said in his presidential address:[2] "...much attention should be given to the careful selection and systematic training of future workers in human genetics. As is true for any other group of specialized guidance workers in the field of public health, a genetic counselor should be selected from the standpoint of both professional qualifications and personal integrity. While in training, he should have ample opportunity to gain practical experience in dealing with people in distress, and he thereby should be taught to broaden his frame of reference from genetic to human problems." Three years later in 1955,[3] before the same Society, Kallmann dealt with the problem of how fearful people face reality as follows: "The tacit assumption – often evidently wishful – is that intelligent people, who are morally entitled to truthful information regarding the prospects of their own health and that of their children, are capable of dealing with their family problems realistically and without special guidance.

"From a psychological standpoint, realism may be defined as the tendency to view things as they are, rather than as what we want them to be. As a principle of adult behavior, this tendency is indicative of a mature mind and a wholesome pattern of adjustment to human imperfection and stress. However, a realistic attitude in the face of severe threats to health and survival can never be divorced from the existing circumstances. Nor can these circumstances be dealt with impersonally.

"In no situation calling for genetic counseling can it ever be taken for granted that the person is realistic or will be able to attain a realistic attitude without the counselor's help. The attainment of this goal is highly desirable, but often requires considerable effort. Even well-educated persons may fail to achieve it without encouragement and guidance. In many instances, unguided reality enforcement is apt to create fear, anxiety, and inner tension, and not realism.

"Frightened people either withdraw from reality by regressing to immature patterns of behavior, or they attempt to neutralize reality by means of pathological defense reactions such as repression and displacement, rationalization and projection. The final outcome will not be on the positive side, and an emotionally disturbed mind is a high price to pay for meek reality testing."

In 1964, writing together, Kallmann and I said: "Of the two main objectives of genetic guidance work – determination of the empirical risk that a pathologic condition may appear in a given individual and comprehension of the impact that this knowledge would have on the person concerned – the second is by no means less important than the first. Actually, since the two objectives are practically inseparable, the aforementioned definition of genetic counseling work seems to require the qualification that when one provides potentially stressful morbidity risk information for married couples and future parents, one should give full consideration to the emotional state of the persons seeking guidance."[4]

In all of these earlier statements, you will notice reference to offering guidance. Perhaps, today, with the increased information available, the counselor's attitude may be somewhat less paternalistic, but in my experience clients can no more today than twenty years ago be provided with risk data alone without full consideration of the psychological and social factors which determine the ability to use these data and the conclusions based upon them. At all times the counselor must avoid creating undue anxiety, and he must be well aware of his own emotional biases and reactions so as to avoid interjecting them into the counseling sessions. People who find reason to suspect even remotely the genetic transmission of undesirable characteristics in their families may be more than ever besieged by guilt, shame, obsessional doubts, and indecision. The psychiatrist has the responsibility for the discussion of these matters in the training of non-psychiatric personnel as well as his fellow psychiatrists in the psychological aspects of genetic counseling. Athough the genetic counseling sessions need not be categorized as a formal program of psychotherapy, they will greatly gain in effectiveness if based on psychological understanding and conducted along established lines of psychiatric interviewing. In essence, sessions of this kind amount to forms of short-term psychotherapy aimed at bolstering the decision-making apparatus and reducing marital anxiety and tension, shame and guilt, depression, hostility, and sexual inhibition.

From the point of view of public thought and feeling, the growing knowledge of genetic factors in disease and the increasing availability of genetic counseling – there are now close to 300 centers compared to the 7 of 1952 – have brought about revolutionary conceptual changes in people's view of themselves. Just as psychoanalysis led people to be concerned about their personality and to suspect their unconscious conflicts, so genetics is causing people to wonder about their constitution and to question their recessive genes. Now more and more parents are asking genetic counselors "Will my baby be normal?"

Although it is not necessary to emphasize the nefarious programs that have been instituted on the basis of pseudoscientific theories, couples today often do measure their own worth against arbitrary, poorly defined standards of genetic perfection. The concept of normalcy – what constitutes "genetic health"? – has been extensively discussed recently from the ethical or humanistic standpoint. Is the carrier of a gene with no clinical manifestations healthy? Is a heterozygote who can transmit a trait only if mated with a similar heterozygote healthy? Genetic disease to some people has become something one *is* rather than something one *has*, although to the medical scientist it may be more correctly seen as a measure of the probability of developing or transmitting illness under various conditions and circumstances.

Summing up this brief historical development of genetic counseling as a health service activity, it is now pretty well agreed that it is a process of communication, that it deals with the human as well as the scientific aspects of genetic risk, and that its aim is to help the individual or family, to help them to understand, to decide, and to cope or adjust. Today, therefore, more serious effort must be given to working out the best techniques and to explore the role of psychiatric theory and practice in this highly charged professional undertaking.

In the language of the psychiatric diagnostic manual,[5] the disturbance associated with unwelcome news about heredity, or with the birth of a defective child, might be characterized as a transient situational disturbance or adjustment disorder. This category is used for more or less transient disorders of any severity (including those of psychotic proportions) that occur in individuals without any apparent underlying mental disorder and that represent an acute reaction to overwhelming environmental stress. The symptoms may be of depression, anxiety, withdrawal, or consist of physical symptoms or conduct disturbances. If the patient has good adaptive capacity, according to the manual description, his symptoms usually recede as the stress diminishes.

The neurochemical and physiological (hormonal) substrate of this syndrome is still to be explored. Meanwhile, moving from a phenomenological to a psychodynamic framework, human feeling and behavior can be interpreted from a number of overlapping points of view. Among these are the structural – Freud's ego, id, superego; the developmental – from dependence to increasing independence; and that based on object relations, the gradual separation from and appreciation of other persons and delineation of an effective self. When threatened with the existential anxiety associated with damage to self-esteem (narcissistic injury), the individual may at first lose the ability to think and act rationally, regress to an infantile dependent status, and lose all sense of worth and human relatedness. If this person has average or good adaptive capacity, he or she will exhibit a variety of mechanisms to stem or contain these painful and unacceptable trends. Among these are the well known defenses of the ego – repression, denial, reaction formation (which is denial of affect), projection, rationalization; the withdrawal reaction typified by depression; and the aggressive one typified by anger or rage. All of these reactions – the disintegrative ones and the attempts at reintegration – may surely be observed in the case load of any genetic counselor.

We have seen those persons who will deny genetic facts and their implications in their desire for natural children or investment in their own "normality". This denial may be based on a grandiose sense of invulnerability or a resigned attitude of helplessness. Such persons do come to clinics at the urging of spouses, other family members, or doctors. The roots of this denial may go deep and brief counseling can do no more than establish the pattern. Further short-term individual or family psychotherapy may in some cases be recommended and accepted. At the other extreme is the person obsessed with the most remote threat to a guaranteed perfect outcome. Both of these attitudes have been known to be aggravated by unknowing physicians or laymen who minimize or exaggerate genetic risks. With the swing of the pendulum in recent years, there is more and more of the latter, and the genetic counselor's job very often is to reassure. This often requires psychodiagnostic insight, in the case of the obsessional pessimist, as well as with the counselee looking for a genetic basis to avoid marriage or parenthood feared on other grounds.

The problems are complicated, of course, in the case of couples, the members of which may disagree in their approach or attitude, or tend to project blame or responsibility onto the other. Sometimes one or both may divert their anger toward the counselor, seen as the bearer of bad news.

In considering some of the ways that genetic counselors can deal with the range of personality vulnerabilities and resistive patterns encountered, obvously there is no question of recommending psychoanalytic psychotherapy as part of genetic counseling. However, it is necessary to be aware that there are these vulnerabilities, aggravated by specific threats to self-esteem and procreativity, that there are conscious and unconscious defense mechanisms and perhaps secret fantasies, and that the response to counseling involves the developmental history and entire personality structure of the counseled individual. There are benefits to be gained from familiarity with some of the psychiatric aspects of genetic knowledge and genetic counseling, and some observations on the application of this total approach to the counseling procedure and the training of counselors are in order. Indeed, the somewhat overworked Hippocratic maxim *nil nocere* contains two parts – it has been translated "As to diseases, make a habit of two things – to help or at least to do no harm". The maxim is always worth heeding, with the first part given equal weight with the second.

First then, a simple admonition, but one often violated, seldom with good results – namely, genetic counseling must be done face to face, in person, and not by phone or mail. There is no good way to understand, to react, or to interact except through personal contact; the results are unpredictable, may often be damaging, and are largely unassessable. Telephone and mail communication may serve adequately in follow-up and, indeed, providing written summaries in the course of counseling has many benefits, but the personal initial encounters are essential. Mail requests from long distances can best be handled by local referral, now that good centers exist throughout the world.

A *second* observation relates to the inevitable problem of the counselor's own emotional reaction and personal involvement as it affects his objectivity and freedom to understand and deal with the persons before him. This includes so-called counter-transference emotion. The same traits and defenses can be seen in the counselor as in the client. The obsessional counselor, supercautious, intolerant of uncertainty may communicate his doubts so effectively that the client can make no decision and leaves confused and angry. Counseling is generally not the place to discuss doubtful procedures and inconclusive tests, or in a largely negative approach, to dwell excessively on the state of our scientific ignorance. Likewise a counselor unaccustomed to or fearful of affect and feeling may stress "realism" and authoritarianism, with detrimental effect to the whole procedure. Excessive anxiety or conversely excessive denial and the tendency to overidentify with the client are characteristics in the counselor not always easy to change, but necessary at least to recognize. Attitudes toward sexual practices, toward roles of men and women, and toward abortion cannot remain unacknowledged.

In the *third* place, the counselor must be free to understand the transference aspects of the client's relationship – not only is the counselor seen as the helpful and knowledgeable professional, but also variously as policeman, as protector or persecutor, as critic, as teacher, as priest, minister, or rabbi, as father or mother. With all these imaginary people in the room, it is no wonder that the counselor's words may not be heard clearly! From a practical point of view, countertransference blind spots or transference stereotyping may be lessened by the practice of having more than one counselor – of various ages and backgrounds and both sexes – involved in the procedure as it progresses.

A *fourth* observation is that there are actually usually two persons, sometimes many more, coming for counsel, perhaps with different underlying motives, often playing their fears and doubts against one another. The application of group methods – that is a group of clients – if skillfully done may uncover, detoxify, and turn to advantage these otherwise confounding crosscurrents.

A *fifth* point is in reference to the timing of genetic counseling. For example, the emergency emotions following the recent birth of a defective child – anxiety, rage, depression – often preclude useful counseling beyond the stage of ventilation. Yet the counselor who is sensitive to these feelings but not threatened by them can establish a working relationship which will extend into a more workable period. Conversely, counseling an individual who is young, unmarried, and has no immediate stake in the result may have little impact; a certain amount of anxious involvement is probably necessary. The experience with screening programs seems to point to avoiding the arousal of such anxiety prematurely in young adolescents.

A *sixth* task – for possibly a sixth sense – is to assess the underlying motives of those coming for counseling. A young woman and her fiance, the latter a son of deaf parents, requested counseling; when a recessive mode of inheritance was established, he was reassured, but she broke off the engagement anyway because "his family was not socially acceptable." Recently there has been a quandary over determining the sex of a child when the parents, admittedly or not, want this information to terminate a pregnancy of the unwanted sex. The ethical and legal aspects of this are under much debate. Psychologically, however, parents often become more attached to an unborn child once sex is known and it ceases to be an "it". Depression following abortion for diagnosed trisomy can be deeper if the sex is divulged, while, paradoxically, the planned abortion for unwanted sex may not take place.

As corollary to much that has been said, a *seventh* point, one with which geneticists should be sympathetic, is to individualize counseling to deal with the characteristic personality type and defenses of the client. Risk figures will be appreciated and dealt with differently according to intelligence, background experiences, and life outlook. Beliefs and attitudes, religious and cultural, cannot be ignored without peril.

Point *eight* involves the counselors ability to diagnose depression and assess its depth. A common if not universal sequel to genetic trauma, depression may occasionally require referral for more intensive treatment, including antidepressive drugs.

In *ninth* place is the admonition that in taking a history, the counselor must allow the client to talk, to cry, to concretize his motives, to come to the point in his own way under skillful but not overintrusive questioning. Finally, and *tenth* in the list of observations, the counselor must combine neutrality with empathy, a skill familiar to most psychiatrists and mental health workers, but not universal to those used to a more guarded or directive approach.

To implement the approach outlined here, there is certainly a need for further investigation of the psychodynamics of counseling, and for training of genetic counselors in the skills to be acquired and the pitfalls to be avoided. Such teaching is called for in genetic counseling training programs, and is best done by working with actual examples of counselor/client interaction.[6]

At the same time, at least in larger centers, psychiatrists themselves have been attached to genetic counseling clinics. At Columbia, where the Psychiatric Institute's department was for decades a center of psychiatric genetics activity (Dr. F.J. Kallmann, Dr. J.D. Rainer), a new clinic is in operation at Babies' Hospital (Dr. A. Bloom) and a part-time psychiatrist (Dr. E. Goldstein) has been participating in counseling sessions talking at greater length to clients when necessary, taking part in conferences, and training and supervising graduate and medical students.

In the larger ethical areas of genetic counseling, the psychiatric contribution is no less important. As I wrote on a previous occasion,[7] "Traditionally, it is not for the psychiatrist to be uneasy in thinking about new and difficult problems. Some of the solutions strike at the root of many human emotions, procreativity, family and social structure. It may very well have to be the job of some psychiatrists to be the caretakers of the human aspects of genetics, to have a voice in the larger issues, and if they do not do the counseling themselves, at least to be concerned, to supervise, and to be involved with it."

REFERENCES

1. J.D. Rainer, *N.Y. State J. Med.* *65*, 1651, 1965.
2. F.J. Kallmann, *Am. J. Hum. Genet.* *4*, 237, 1952.
3. F.J. Kallmann, *Am. J. Hum. Genet.* *8*, 97, 1956.
4. F.J. Kallmann and J.D. Rainer, *Internat. Psychiat. Clinics* *1*, 799, 1964.
5. American Psych. Assoc., Diagnostic and Statistical Manual of Mental Disorders, Second Edition, 1968.
6. S. Firestein, *Social Casework* *57*, 265, 1976.
7. J.D. Rainer, *Res. Publ. Assoc. Res. Nerv. Ment. Dis.* *47*, 222, 1969.

ATTITUDES TOWARD AMNIOCENTESIS: SURVEYS OF FAMILIES WITH SPINA BIFIDA CHILDREN, 1974, 1977*

Y. Edward Hsia
Felix Leung
Linda L. Carter

INTRODUCTION

In 1972, fetal diagnosis for spina bifida and anencephaly became possible by measurement of amniotic fluid alpha-fetoprotein.[1] This expansion of the indications for amniocentesis has meant that one in 600 families who had had a child with anencephaly or spina bifida could now be offered the option of amniocentesis, for a recurrence risk that is higher than that for the maternal age-related risk of trisomy 21.

Much has been reported on the outcome[2,3] and safety[4] of amniocentesis, but little data has been collected about the attitudes of families who could be candidates for the test. A survey for maternal age-related candidates is not easy to obtain, because most women of these age groups are not intending to get pregnant, and only a small minority of these women do become pregnant.

For spina bifida, however, if the affected child survives, there are urgent factors keeping parents in close touch with medical facilities, and powerful motivations for these parents to form special interest groups.

We have contacted three parents groups associated with spina bifida clinics and have assessed the acceptability of amniocentesis to these parents. Our findings about their plans for future children and their attitudes toward the recurrence risk for a neural tube malformation, toward amniocentesis, and toward therapeutic abortion provide predictive data about the potential demand for amniocentesis by parents of children with spina bifida.

METHODS

We surveyed the parents of children attending spina bifida clinics in 1974 and 1977, in Connecticut and Hawaii. Each survey was preceded by an informal open parents' meeting to explain about recurrence risks for spina bifida or anencephaly (3%), about the safety, accuracy, and limitations of the test. A questionnaire was sent, accompanied by a brief written explanation about genetic risks and

*Supported in part by the National Foundation Medical Service Grant C-41 and Genetic Center Grant GM-20124.

ISBN 0-12-562650-9

TABLE 1

Demographic Characteristics of Respondent Families

	Yale 1974	Newington 1974	Newington 1977	Hawaii 1977	Total
Respondent families	23	49	68	27	167
Age of affected child					
<5 years	16	21	16	11	64
5-9 years	7	16	27	5	55
$\geqslant 10$ years	0	12	25	11	48
Sex of affected child					
male	14	19	26	10	68
female	10	16	36	15	77
Number of children in family					
1	7	13	15	3	38
2	7	16	27	12	62
3	6	10	14	7	37
>3	3	10	12	5	30
Youngest child was the affected child	18	26	42	17	103
"Small young families"	14	26	34	10	84
Families no longer fertile	?	?	46	16	62
Had not heard previously about prenatal testing	—	—	14	11	25
Had already had amniocentesis			4	3	7

about the test (Appendix A). It was sent only to families with a living child affected with spina bifida.

In 1974, both clinics in Connecticut, at Yale-New Haven Hospital and Newington Children's Hospital, were surveyed. In 1977, the larger Clinic at Newington, and the Myelodysplasia Clinic in Honolulu were surveyed. We asked about respondents' family compositions; subjective impressions of their risk for having another affected child; safety of the test for mother and fetus; accuracy of the test; whether they planned more children; and whether they would use the test. In 1977, we also asked their reasons for refraining from having more children; their contraceptive practices; and their attitudes toward abortion whenever families chose, or when a fetus was known to be seriously abnormal.

RESULTS

We obtained responses from 72 families in 1974 and 95 families in 1977, including 16 from Newington who had responded to both surveys (Table 1) from a population of approximately 225 families. Two respondent families had adopted an affected child. All respondents had only a single affected child.

Most respondents had understood the written explanation; felt the test was safe for mother and child, felt it was reasonably accurate, and more felt the risk was "big" or "huge"than that the risk was "small" (Table 3). Twelve families felt there was no risk. Eleven of these families were no longer reproductive, including two who had already had testing, and the twelfth intended to use the test. Seventy-eight percent of respondents felt the test should be offered to all at risk, and 69 percent would use the test for a pregnancy. Twenty-five respondents in 1977 claimed no prior awareness of the test; these had far less positive attitudes than those who did claim prior knowledge (Table 2a). Seven had already had amniocentesis for a recent pregnancy; results and outcome were normal in all seven pregnancies.

As for future children, 26 percent were probably or possibly intending to have another child, and 28 percent would or might be influenced by the availability of the test (Table 4).

The attitudes toward abortion of the 1977 respondents showed approval whenever parents chose by 43 percent, and approval for a seriously abnormal child by 68 percent (Table 5).

The contraceptive motives and practices of the 1977 respondents are presented in Table 6. Seventeen percent of the respondents cited recurrence risk as a reason for having no more children. It was apparent that a large proportion of these families were no longer fertile. We therefore looked at two subpopulations, "young small families" where the affected child was under 10 years of age and there were only one or two children in the family, and families contemplating having more children.

Among the 84 "young small families", 57% were no longer fertile, most of these because of voluntary sterilization (one-fifth by vasectomy). Of the

TABLE 2

Attitudes Toward Fetal Testing for Spina Bifida

	Yale 1974	Newington 1974	Newington 1977	Hawaii 1977	Total
Very positive	10	23	41	10	84
Positive	6	16	16	7	45
Undecided	4	7	9	7	27
Negative	3	3	2	3	11

TABLE 2A

1977

	Had heard about test	Had not heard about test	Total
Very positive	46	5	51
Positive	14	9	23
Undecided	6	10	16
Negative	3	2	5

TABLE 3

Subjective Opinions About Fetal Testing

		Yale 1974	Newington 1974	Newington 1977	Hawaii 1977	Total
Did you understand written explanatior?	most	20	45	57	19	141
	some	3	2	8	8	21
	none	0	2	3	0	5
Is test reasonably safe for the mother?	yes	19	38	55	15	127
	undecided	4	8	12	9	33
	no	0	3	1	3	7
Is test reasonably safe for the fetus?	yes	15	38	47	13	113
	undecided	7	6	15	11	39
	no	1	5	6	3	15
Is test reasonably accurate?	yes	16	35	50	12	113
	undecided	6	11	13	11	41
	no	1	3	5	4	13
How do you regard the recurrence risk?	big	11	21	21	5	58
	undecided	6	15	26	14	61
	small	5	11	15	5	36
	none	1	2	6	3	12

TABLE 4

Acceptability of Fetal Testing for Spina Bifida

		Yale 1974 (N=23)	Newington 1974 (N=49)	Newington 1977 (N=68)	Hawaii 1977 (N=27)	Total (N=167)
Should test be offered to all at risk?	yes	18	38	57	18	131
	undecided	3	8	10	8	29
	no	2	3	1	1	7
Would you use the test for a pregnancy?	yes	19	33	45	17	114
	undecided	2	10	16	8	37
	no	2	6	6	2	16
If you had another pregnancy, would you have the test?	yes	18	31	31	14	94
	undecided	2	10	12	6	30
	no	3	8	25	7	43
Are you likely to have another child?	probable	5	10	4	5	24
	possible	4	3	11	1	19
	unlikely	14	36	53	21	124
Will availability of test influence your decision about another child?	yes	2	11	12	5	29
	undecided	5	6	2	5	18
	no	16	32	54	18	120

TABLE 5

Attitudes Toward Abortion

		Newington 1977	Hawaii 1977	Total
Agree with abortion whenever parents choose	yes	31	10	41
	undecided	14	6	20
	no	23	11	34
Agree with abortion for seriously abnormal child	yes	47	18	65
	undecided	14	6	20
	no	7	3	10

TABLE 6

Contraceptive Motives and Practices

	Newington 1977	Hawaii 1977	Total
Reasons for not wanting more children*			
Satisfied with family size	21	11	31
Concerned about recurrence risk	11	8	19
Financial pressures	7	6	13
Current needs of family	12	11	23
Unable to have more children	34	18	52
Contraceptive practices			
Mother sterilized	18	1	19
Father sterilized	15	0	15
Pill	2	6	8
IUD	7	5	12
Diaphragm/condom/foam	16	2	18
Rhythm	2	1	3

*Many families gave more than one reason.

TABLE 7

Respondents Likely to Have More Children or May Be Influenced by Availability of Test

		Yale 1974	Newington 1974	Newington 1977	Hawaii 1977	Total
Number of families		10	19	17	11	57
Age of affected child						
	< 5	10	14	6	6	36
	5-9	0	4	7	2	13
	$\geqslant 10$	0	1	4	3	8
Sex of affected child	male	4	6	6	5	21
	female	6	13	9	6	34
Youngest child was the affected child		8	10	11	4	33
Test would influence decision	yes	2	10	9	2	33
	undecided	5	5	4	8	22
	no	3	4	4	1	12
Test should be offered to all at risk	yes	6	15	14	6	41
	undecided	3	2	3	4	12
	no	1	2	0	1	4
Would use test	yes	7	12	13	6	38
	undecided	2	4	4	4	14
	no	1	3	0	1	5
If pregnant, would use test	yes	7	13	13	4	37
	undecided	1	4	4	5	14
	no	2	2	0	2	6

remaining 43% who appeared able to have more children, only one-third intended to have no more children and would not be influenced by the test.

There were 57 families contemplating more children, or indicating that the availability of the test could alter their decision to refrain from child bearing. Only 10% of these would refuse to use the test (Table 7).

The sex of the affected child was female in 62% of respondent families likely to have more children, as opposed to 48% of those unlikely to have more children.

DISCUSSION

Study Design

Our study aimed to poll the attitudes of parents with spina bifida children toward recurrence risks, having more children, and fetal testing for this condition. In pursuit of this aim, we focused on a restricted but well-defined population, and limited the surveys to a few key questions.

We defined our study populations by disease, geography, and time. Each family surveyed had one surviving child with spina bifida living at home. All of the surveyed families, therefore, had shared similar experiences although varying in severity and duration. They all had the same predicted recurrence risk, for which the fetal testing described was applicable. We had no information about whether or when a family had genetic counseling, and whether a family's attitudes and intentions had changed with time.

Geographically, the Yale and Newington Clinics served all of Connecticut, and the Honolulu Clinic served all of Hawaii. Virtually all affected patients in these two states would have been referred to these clinics. The Yale Clinic, at a general hospital with very active maternity and newborn services, accepted most patients directly from its newborn nurseries. The Newington and Honolulu Clinics were referral centers which accepted older patients who had survived immediate neonatal complications. These clinics had somewhat older patient populations (Table 1). We did not attempt to collect data on respondents' ethnic or cultural backgrounds, socioeconomic status, level of education, marital stability, or religion.

Connecticut is a small industrialized New England state with a large Roman Catholic minority. Hawaii is an ethnically heterogeneous, culturally diverse Island state with a mixed agricultural-urban population. Our findings of similarities in attitudes between respondents from these strikingly different populations suggest that our results may be generalizable to a large population of families with spina bifida children elsewhere. The large fraction of non-respondents was probably less favorably inclined toward our survey, but the same non-respondents were also more likely to have been older, disinterested in having more children, and less concerned about fetal diagnosis.

Temporally, the 1974 surveys were conducted at a time when fetal testing for spina bifida was still new and unfamiliar to many physicians,[6] so the respondents were reporting attitudes toward a novel concept. In 1977, fetal testing had become established, and for most of the families in the Newington Clinic it was a repeat of old information (given in the earlier survey) with minor updating of facts about hazards and accuracy. Familiarity with the test had demonstrably enhanced its acceptability by those 1977 respondents who claimed prior knowledge of the procedure. Our four surveys were remarkable for the general similarities in respondents' attitudes, despite differences in family composition, age of affected patient, geography, and time.

We did not attempt to explore the impact of spina bifida on family life[7,8] or general attitudes.[9,10] Our primary goal was to assess the relationship between families' attitudes toward fetal testing and their plans for future children. Therefore, we focused on their subjective impression of the recurrence risk for spina bifida; their acceptance of fetal testing; and their reproductive intentions.

Educational Strategy

We adopted the useful strategy of making knowledge about the test a constant, by providing the brief written explanation. This ensured that a uniform minimum of information was received by each family.

Judgment of the value of this explanation was not a primary goal, but on the one hand, it fulfilled a valuable *service* function in ensuring that all surveyed families become aware of the availability of the test; and on the other hand, we were able to assess its *communication* function as a medium for transmitting fairly complex information.

The explanation was kept brief and simple to ensure that it would be read and understood (Appendix A). We also strove to avoid making it persuasive or directive. The range and quality of the responses gave assurance that it was reasonably well understood by most readers, and that the responses were not merely echoes from a biased explanation. The fact that the 1977 respondents who had no prior familiarity with the procedure were less favorable than those who had known about the test, however, argued that a simple written message by itself was not an effective way to gain acceptability for fetal testing. For effective introduction of novel health-related concepts into a population, a carefully coordinated multifaceted campaign is needed,[11] but within this campaign reinforcement with a simply written explanation may have a cost-effective educational role.

Recurrence Risks

The uniformity of objective information given enabled our study to concentrate on the subjective opinions of respondents. The most meaningful correlation of perceived risk with other variables was that all those who perceived no risk indeed had negligible risk because of infertility or intention to use the test. The large proportion of respondents who felt the recurrence risk was "big" or "huge" clearly demonstrated that the severity or burden of a disorder was a more potent factor than quantitative predictions in a family's perception of the risk of recurrence[12,13] since spina bifida is a low risk-high burden disorder.[14]

PLANS FOR MORE CHILDREN

Attitudes toward reproduction are notoriously treacherous to interpret, and pregnancy is just as likely to arise from impulsive acts as from carefully laid plans.[14] Nonetheless, among our families, the majority in which the affected child was the youngest would appear to be greater than can be attributed to chance alone, and procreative intentions seemed to be influenced by the sex of the affected child.[15] Judging from this, many families were deterred from having more children after the birth of an affected child. Because our surveys were retrospective, this deterrence could have operated long before fetal testing had become a reality. We could not tell whether family attitudes and decisions originated with or without any accurate knowledge about the recurrence risks.[14] The retrospective *reasons* given for not wanting more children in our superficial survey (Table 6) are inadequate indicators of true conscious or unconscious *motives* underlying families' actions.

Even among the "small young families", it was remarkable that less than half the respondents were still fertile. This indicates how powerful the motives against reproduction might be in these families.

The contraceptive practices of these families was not thoroughly studied in this survey, but secular trends are definitely away from unintended toward planned pregnancies, with increasingly effective use of contraceptives to control family plans.[16]

ATTITUDES TOWARD FETAL TESTING

The attitudes toward fetal testing are inextricably associated with attitudes toward abortion, and possibly also attitudes toward euthanasia.[9,11,17] In the 1977 surveys, we found the proportion of respondents agreeing with abortion whenever parent chose was higher than found in the 1970 National Fertility Survey,[18] but similar to the polls conducted through 1975.[19] The proportion approving of abortion for a seriously defective fetus was somewhat lower than in the general 1975 polls. Those respondents who approved of abortion for a seriously abnormal fetus, of course, were, in general, the same ones who approved of fetal testing for neural tube abnormalities and were willing to use the test for future pregnancies.

CONCLUSIONS

The birth of a seriously handicapped child has a profound impact on all aspects of family life.[7] The wisdom of mobilizing intense medical and surgical intervention for the more gravely affected patients has been questioned.[9,20,21] Yet this traumatic experience has not necessarily had a disruptive effect on family integrity.[22,23] More conscientious conveying of genetic risks, and the option of fetal testing to these families will offer them opportunities for having additional, unaffected children, which had not previously been available.

We judge from the responses to our surveys that fetal testing will be generally acceptable to these parents and we speculate that in the future, with timely access to genetic information and to fetal testing, similar families will be far more likely to have additional pregnancies for which they will want the test.

Since about 1 in 600 births is of a child with spina bifida, in the United States with 3 million births per annum, approximately 5,000 children with spina bifida will be born per annum. One-third to one-half of these parents may have future pregnancies and opt for fetal testing. Eventually, from this population, over thirty affected fetuses will be detected for every thousand pregnancies tested Although not included in this survey, parents of anencephalic babies have similar recurrence risks for which the same fetal tests are possible. Their subjective experiences and attitudes may be quite different, but a substantial proportion of these parents will probably also opt for fetal testing.

Until such time as maternal serum alpha-fetoprotein screening becomes widely practiced, which may be inadvisable,[26] parents of children with spina bifida or anencephaly will form a substantial fraction of all couples for whom fetal testing of alpha-fetoprotein can be offered.

In this special-risk population, false-positive test results are much less likely to be a problem than with maternal serum alpha-fetoprotein screening,[24,25] because their probability for true positive results is so much greater.

SUMMARY

Four surveys were conducted among the parents of children attending Spina Bifida Clinics in Connecticut and Hawaii. These parents were informed of their recurrence risks for having a similarly affected child (about 1 in 30), of the availability of fetal diagnosis by ultrasonography and amniocentesis for alpha-fetoprotein concentrations, and of the safety and accuracy of these tests.

The survey objectives were to determine whether these families intended to have more children, whether availability of the test would influence their intentions, and, if a pregnancy occurred, whether a family would use this test.

Results showed generally favorable attitudes toward this test in the 167 respondents.

Most respondents understand the explanation; 76% felt the test was safe for the mother; 68% felt it was reasonably accurate; 78% felt it should be offered for all at risk; 69% would use it for a future pregnancy. Among 57 respondents who probably or possibly might have another pregnancy, 58% would be influenced by the availability of the test and 66% would use the test.

We anticipate that between one-third and one-half of parents of children with spina bifida are likely to request fetal testing in a future pregnancy.

ACKNOWLEDGMENTS

This study would not have been possible without the support and assistance of M. Au and C.C. Emerson, the cooperation of the participating parents, and the kind permissions of Drs. S. Bintliff, F. Flynn, S. Raycroft, D.V. Reddy and J. Venes.

REFERENCES

1. D.J.H. Brock and R.G. Sutcliffe, *Lancet 2*, 197, 1972.
2. A. Milunsky and E. Alpert, *Obstet. Gynecol. 48*, 1, 6, 1976.
3. D.J.H. Brock, *in* Genetic Counseling, H.A. Lubs, F. Dela Cruz (Eds.), Raven Press, New York, p. 225, 1977.
4. NICHD National Registry for Amniocentesis Study Group, *J.A.M.A. 236*, 1471, 1976.
5. Editorial, *Lancet 1*, 907, 1974.
6. Y.E. Hsia, K.K. Bucholz and C. Austein, Genetic Knowledge of Connecticut Obstetricians and Pediatricians: Implications for Continuing Education (see elsewhere this volume).
7. J.H. Walker, M. Thomas and I.T. Russell, *Develop. Med. Child. Neurol. 13*, 462. 1971.
8. E.H. Hare, K.M. Lawrence, H. Paynes and K. Rawnsley, *Brit. Med. J. 2*, 757, 1966.
9. B.M. Freeston, *Develop. Med. Child. Neurol. 13*, 456, 1971.
10. S. Dorner, *ibid. 17*, 765, 1975.
11. E.M. Rogers, Communication Strategies for Family Planning, Free Press, New York, 1973.
12. J.H. Pearn, *J. Med. Genet. 10*, 129, 1973.
13. C.O. Leonard, G.A. Chase and B. Childs, *N. Engl. J. Med. 287,* 433, 1972.
14. Y.E. Hsia, *in* Genetic Counseling, H.A. Lubs, F. dela Cruz (Eds). Raven Press, New York, p. 53, 1977.
15. L.L. Bumpass and C.F. Westoff, The Later Years of Childbearing, Princeton U. Press, Princeton, 1970.
16. C.F. Westoff, *Fam. Plann. Perspect. 8*, 54, 1976.
17. K.M. Laurence, *Develop. Med. Child. Neurol. 16, Suppl. 32*, 117, 1974.
18. E.F. Jones and C.F. Westoff, *in* Demographic and Social Aspects of Population Growth, Vol. I., E.F. Westoff and R. Parke (Eds.), Government Printing Office, Washington, D.C., pp. 569-578, 1972.
19. W.R. Arney and W.H. Trescher, *Fam. Plann. Perspect. 8*, 117, 1976.
20. H.L. Ellis, *Brit. Med. J. 1*, 369, 1974.
21. G.M. Hunt, *Lancet 2,* 1308, 1973.
22. B.J. Tew, H. Payne and K.M. Lawrence, *Develop. Med. Child. Neurol. 16, Suppl. 32*, 95, 1974.
23. P. Martin, *ibid. 17*, 757, 1975.

24. M. Goldberg, Prenatal Screening for Neural Tube Defects: Some Epidemiological Considerations (see elsewhere this volume).
25. J.N. Macri, Maternal Serum Alpha-fetoprotein Screening for Neural Tube Defects: Structure and Organization (see elsewhere this volume).
26. S. Hagard, F. Carter and R.G. Milne, *Brit. J. Prev. Soc. Med. 30*, 40, 1976.

APPENDIX A *

1. Covering letter to parent of the Newington Clinic, 1974. A similar letter accompanied the questionnaires submitted for each survey.

2. Explanation sent to parents in 1977. The 1974 explanation differed only slightly in wording; it cited a 90% accuracy for alpha-fetoprotein, and a miscarriage risk of about 1% for amniocentesis.

3. Questionnaire sent in 1977. The earlier questionnaire differed slightly in sequence, and did not contain questions 2, 4, 10, 11, 13, 14, 15, or 17.

*Modified slightly for use in this volume.

July 1974

Dear Parents:

In June the Newington Children's Hospital "Parents of Spina Bifida Group" invited me to talk about the results of our questionnaire survey. At that time I was able to tell them about the new advances that now offer the possibility of testing for neuro-tube defects such as spina bifida in early pregnancy.

If you were at that meeting you may wish to have this written account of the new tests for your own reference. If you were not at that meeting, this information may be new to you, but, as we promised, we are sending it to you to keep updated with the latest developments. If you have any additional questions about the information on the enclosed explanatory note, please do not hesitate to ask the doctors in your clinic or myself, or the doctors listed on the enclosed account, who are in charge of the prenatal testing program.

For our information we would be most obliged if you could fill out the enclosed questionnaire and mail it back to us within the next two weeks, because this information would be of great value for helping us to determine how much this new potential service might be to parents such as yourselves. We are enclosing two copies so that the husband and wife can each record their own impression and opinion. Of course, if you were at the meeting and have already filled out the questionnaire, there is no need to return another one.

Thank you for your cooperation.

Yours sincerely,

Y. Edward Hsia, M.D.
Associate Professor of Human Genetics and Pediatrics
Director, Genetics Clinic
(Yale University School of Medicine)

YEH:lh
Encl.

PRENATAL TESTING FOR MYELODYSPLASIA AND ANENCEPHALY (MAY 1977)

In the general population, myelodysplasia appears once in every 600 births. Couples who have had one child with myelodysplasia or anencephaly (an extremely severe malformation of the brain) have an increased chance of having another infant with either of these closely related defects. The combined risk for these defects is found to be about 5% or 1 in 20. This may be information that parents would want in planning whether to have more children.

Although doctors are not yet able to prevent or treat myelodysplasia or anencephaly before birth, it has recently become possible to detect these defects during the fourth to fifth months of pregnancy. This is done combining two tests, one called ultrasound scanning, and the other called amniocentesis.

Ultrasound scanning uses echo patterns from sound waves to measure the head size of the fetus in the uterus. An abnormally small fetal head would suggest the presence of anencephaly. Ultrasound scanning is done by passing a sound emitter back and forth over the mother's abdomen, and displaying the echo patterns on a TV screen. The technique has been used for several years, and so far there is no evidence that it causes any harm to the growing fetus or to the mother.

In the second technique, amniocentesis, the doctor inserts a needle (through the mother's abdomen) into the amniotic sac which surrounds the fetus in the uterus. A local anesthetic (like novocaine) is used, and the procedure takes just a few minutes. This test has been in use for the past few years to test for certain chemical abnormalities, and to test for major chromosome defects which can occur in some infants born to older mothers. The test can never guarantee that an infant will be normal, and so is only of use for pregnancies where there is a particular risk which should be ruled in or ruled out. Should the test be abnormal, parents can choose to have a pregnancy terminated.

To test for myelodysplasia, the doctor measures the amount of a special protein present in the amniotic fluid. This protein, called alpha-fetoprotein, is normally made by all fetuses, but if the fetus has myelodysplasia or anencephaly, the amniotic fluid usually contains an increased amount of alpha-fetoprotein.

If amniocentesis shows the alpha-fetoprotein level to be very much higher than normal, then the fetus is very likely to have myelodysplasia or anencephaly. If the alpha-fetoprotein is normal, then the fetus is unlikely to have these defects. The test has not been completely accurate, however, because about 1 in 20 fetuses with myelodysplasia still have a normal level of alpha-fetoprotein. Nonetheless, if the test is normal, the chance that the baby has such an abnormality decreases considerably, from about 1 in 20 to 1 in 400.

There are small risks involved in the amniocentesis procedure itself. The most important is a small chance, about 1 in 250 in expert hands, that it will cause a miscarriage. At many major medical centers where amniocentesis is done, pregnancies have been followed after amniocentesis, and the babies born after the procedure have been examined to look for any unexpected problems. These careful studies have shown that the procedure produces no detectable harm to the infant.

If you wish to learn more about the test, please ask your own obstetrician or physician, or make inquiries of Drs. S. Bintliffe of D.V. Reddy at Kaukeolani Children's Hospital.

Y. Edward Hsia, M.D.
Genetic Counseling Services

QUESTIONNAIRE ABOUT PRENATAL TESTING FOR MYELODYSPLASIA

Please Circle the Answers Which Apply in Your Case

I am the FATHER/MOTHER (please circle) of a child with myelodysplasia.
The age of my SON/DAUGHTER (please circle) is ______ years.
How many brothers and sisters does he/she have?

Ages of brothers	Ages of sisters	Comments†
________	________	________
________	________	________
________	________	________

†Please indicate if adopted, etc.

1. Have you understood the explanation about testing for myelodysplasia that was described in the letter?

   uncertain   all of it   most of it   some of it   little of it   none of it

2. Did you attend the meeting of the "Parents' Group" in March concerning prenatal diagnosis?   yes   no

3. What is your understanding of the risk of myelodysplasia recurring in your family?

   don't know   no risk   small risk   undecided   big risk   huge risk

4. Had you heard about prenatal testing for myelodysplasia before the meeting or before the letter?   yes   no

5. Does the test seem to be reasonably *safe* for the *mother*?

   don't know   very safe   fairly safe   undecided   fairly unsafe   very unsafe

6. Does the test seem to be relatively *safe* for the *baby*?

   don't know   very safe   fairly safe   undecided   fairly unsafe   very unsafe

7. Does the test seem to be reasonably *accurate* for myelodysplasia?

   don't know   very accurate   fairly accurate   undecided   fairly inaccurate   very inaccurate

8. Should this prenatal testing be offered to families at risk?

   yes   uncertain   no

9. Would you use the test if you were going to have another baby?

   yes   uncertain   no

10. Do you agree with abortion whenever parents choose?

    yes   uncertain   no

QUESTIONNAIRE ABOUT PRENATAL TESTING FOR MYELODYSPLASIA (Continued)

11. Do you agree with abortion when the fetus has been found to have a serious abnormality?

    yes uncertain no

12. Are you likely to have another child?

    yes probably possibly unlikely no

13. If unlikely or no, the reason is:
    1. We are satisfied with the present size of our family.
    2. We feel that the risk of having another child with myelodysplasia is too high.
    3. We cannot afford to have any more children.
    4. We are unable to have anymore children.
    5. We feel that we are too old to have any more children.
    6. We want to focus our care and attention on our present child(ren).
    7. Other (please specify) ______________________

14. Are you practicing birth control at the present time?

    regularly occasionally never

15. If yes, please specify method.

16. Has the availability of prenatal diagnosis influenced your decision about having another child?

    yes uncertain no

17. Have you/your wife had amniocentesis?

    yes no

18. If you decide to have another child, will you use the test?

    yes uncertain no

KNOWLEDGE, ATTITUDES, AND ACCEPTANCE OF PRENATAL DIAGNOSIS AMONG WOMEN AND PHYSICIANS IN THE ROCHESTER REGION *

Richard A. Doherty
Klaus J. Roghmann

INTRODUCTION

During the past decade, the possibility of detecting significant fetal chromosomal, biochemical, and structural abnormalities during the second trimester of pregnancy has revolutionized the practice of clinical genetics.[1,2]

Sampling and analysis of amniotic fluid and cultured amniotic fluid cells, ultrasonic (and possibly fetoscopic) visualization of the fetus, analysis of maternal blood for specific fetal products (and possibly for fetal cells), as well as direct fetal blood sampling, have made possible the diagnosis of an increasing variety of fetal abnormalities during the second trimester of pregnancy. Studies documenting safety and reliability of second trimester amniocentesis,[3,4] defining specific indications, and detailing technical results of chromosomal and biochemical analyses of fetal cells and amniotic fluid have recently been reviewed.[1,2,5]

One of the most important fetal abnormalities which can be detected by amniocentesis is trisomy 21 (Down syndrome). The risk of delivering a baby with trisomy 21 is related to the age of the mother at the time of conception, and increases rather rapidly beyond 35 years of age. Cost-benefit analysis has established the economic feasibility of this procedure for women 35 years and older.[6,7] The benefits of detecting fetal chromosomal abnormalities compared to the risks associated with second trimester transabdominal amniocentesis have led to the recommendation that women over 35 years of age should be provided with the option of prenatal screening for trisomy 21.[3,4,5,5a,5b]

A second important group of fetal abnormalities are the neural tube closure defects, especially spina bifida and anencephaly. They can now be detected through measurement of alpha-fetoprotein levels in amniotic fluid.[8]

Families with a history of fetal chromosomal abnormalities, fetal neural tube closure defects, and an increasing number of heritable fetal biochemical disorders can now be assured of absence of the suspected abnormality. The procedures have a high degree of accuracy and reliability and are of low risk to mother and fetus. The clinical objective of prenatal diagnosis is to rule out fetal abnormality for women at increased risk, and thus provide them the opportunity to have

*Supported in part by PHS grant HS 467.

ISBN 0-12-562650-9

healthy children with the same probability as other reproducing couples. This assumes that, should a serious fetal abnormality be detected, parents may consider the option of elective induced abortion.

Although techniques of culture of amniotic fluid cells during the second trimester for cytogenetic and biochemical analyses of fetal abnormality have been available for nearly a decade, only a small fraction of pregnant women at risk have received prenatal diagnostic services. For example, in Massachusetts where prenatal diagnosis has been available on a statewide basis, only 4.1% of pregnant women 35 years and older had prenatal chromosomal studies during 1974.[5] Nadler has estimated that second trimester intrauterine diagnosis is received by less than one percent of the relevant national population.[2]

The major clinical benefit of prenatal diagnosis is parental reassurance concerning absence of certain types of serious fetal abnormality. About 95% of prenatal diagnostic procedures provide no evidence for fetal defects. However, counseling concerning the potential uses of prenatal diagnosis is often coupled with the realization that prenatal screening will prevent birth defects only if used in conjunction with selective abortion. Information concerning the relationship between knowledge of prenatal screening possibilities and attitudes toward abortion under circumstances of probable fetal abnormality is required for analysis of the potential benefits of prenatal screening in terms of possible reduction of incidence of prenatally detectable birth defects.

During the past seven years we have witnessed rapid growth of utilization of prenatal detection counseling and laboratory services in the Finger Lakes Health System Area (Table 1).

TABLE 1

Number of Patients Having Second Trimester Amniocentesis for Prenatal Detection of Birth Defects

1971	1972	1973	1974	1975	1976	1977
2	12	13	22	46	108	(170)*

*Projected estimates.

Currently, approximately 20% of pregnant women 35 years and older in our region, and 30% of pregnant women 40 years and older are provided second trimester prenatal diagnosis counseling and laboratory services. More than 98% of patients are counseled by a genetic associate-physician genetic counselor team prior to amniocentesis. Ultrasound examination immediately precedes amniocentesis, which is performed by one of three obstetricians in our regional medical center. Our success rate in culturing first amniotic fluid samples is $>99\%$ for all diagnoses during the past seven years. There have been no diagnostic errors in a total of more than 350 prenatal diagnoses performed during this seven-year period.

We report a brief history of the establishment of the Rochester Regional

Program for Prenatal Detection of Birth Defects, describe a plan for assessment of regional acceptance and utilization of prenatal diagnosis services, and present preliminary results of the first population survey to evaluate knowledge and attitudes of married women 30 to 45 years of age in our region. These results and the projected surveys which are described should provide the necessary information for assessing needs for counseling and laboratory services in our region, and may enable projections of requirements for prenatal screening services for other areas.

I. DEVELOPMENT OF ROCHESTER REGIONAL PROGRAM FOR PRENATAL DETECTION OF BIRTH DEFECTS

Phase 1 – (1971-77)

Establishment of genetic counseling program and laboratory facilities for provision of regional services for prenatal detection of birth defects, including quality control evaluation procedures. Initiation of routine fee-for-service charges and promotion of third party insurance coverage.

Phase 2 – (1976-79)

Regional assessment of knowledge and attitudes of women and provider physicians in our Health System Area concerning birth defects, genetic counseling, prenatal diagnosis, and elective abortion to identify key recipient, provider, and community variables affecting provision, acceptance, and utilization of prenatal diagnosis counseling and laboratory services. Some key characteristics of the Health System Area are specified in Table 2.

Phase 3 – (1979-)

Regional maximal and minimal projections of needs for personnel and laboratory facilities for future provision of prenatal diagnosis services to interested parents at risk for detectable fetal abnormalities. Evaluation of regional recipient, provider, and community education approaches to assure availability and utilization of prenatal diagnostic services.

TABLE 2

Characteristics of the Finger Lakes Health System Area (1975)

Nine counties: Monroe, Chemung, Livingston, Ontario, Schuyler, Seneca, Steuben, Wayne, Yates	
Total population:	1,254,100
Women of child-bearing age (15-44 years):	267,600
Total live births:	15,834
Birth rate (per 1,000 population):	12.6
	(county range 11.6-15.2)
Total live births to women 35 years and older:	657

II. ASSESSMENT GOALS – ROCHESTER REGIONAL PROGRAM

A. To determine the relative importance of recipient, provider, and community variables which influence provision, access, acceptability, and utilization of genetic counseling and laboratory services relating to prenatal diagnosis of birth defects;

B. On the basis of these observations, to project the demand for prenatal detection services in the Finger Lakes Health System Area for 1980-1985;

C. To evaluate whether key recipient, provider and/or community variables can be influenced by recipient, provider and/or community educational approaches.

The knowledge gained should enable us to increase availability of and access to genetic services in a neutral but supportive health care delivery setting designed to promote the fullest range of reproductive choices to aid interested couples in assuring that each child is born with a reasonable capacity for mental and physical development.

The findings can also be used to estimate possible resultant changes in numbers of children who will be born with birth defects in model target populations under various assumptions.

III. RESEARCH PROGRAM FOR PHASE 2

A sequence of interrelated studies has been designed to assess knowledge and attitudes of patients and health care providers relating to provision, acceptance, and utilization of prenatal diagnostic services.

A. Population Surveys. At intervals of two years, the research program monitors changes in knowledge and attitudes among the main target population; namely, married women in the 30 to 45 year age interval. The first survey was concluded in 1977.

B. Provider Surveys. A register of all physicians providing obstetrical care in the Finger Lakes Health Systems Area has been established. All providers in this region will be surveyed at two-year intervals to collect knowledge and attitudinal data comparable to those obtained for the target population. In addition, their practice patterns, especially regarding genetic counseling and referrals for prenatal diagnostic services, will be analyzed and correlated with medical practice and personal profile variables. The first provider survey will be completed in 1978.

C. Patient Surveys. Follow-up surveys of patients who have received prenatal diagnostic services provide a detailed description of those couples in the target population who actually went through the experience of prenatal diagnosis. The first follow-up survey of one-third of previous patients will be finished in 1978.

D. Student Surveys. Finally, a sequence of surveys is planned to analyze attitudes of current students of the health professions who will be involved in the future provision of genetic counseling and prenatal diagnostic services. The first survey will be conducted in 1979.

IV. THE POPULATION SURVEY, 1977

Planning for services and training of counselors should be based on factors of relevance to acceptance of genetic services by individuals at increased risk. To explore the decision-making process of future patients, our first population survey was conducted in 1977 to ascertain knowledge, values, and expectations concerning prenatal tests among women aged 30 to 45 living in the Health System Area served by the Rochester Regional Program for Prenatal Detection of Birth Defects.

Methods

Questionnaires were mailed during the spring of 1977 to 2,199 women 30 to 45 years of age covered by family contract with the largest health insurance company serving the Rochester area. About 41% responded to the first mailing, another 18% responded to a second mailing four weeks later, and 15% responded to a telephone follow-up interview. The final return of 1,616 questionnaires provided information on 74% of the systematic random sample from the enrollment file. Some key variables of the sample population are presented in Table 3.

TABLE 3

Characteristics of Mail Survey Population Sample

Rochester region counties surveyed: Monroe, Livingston, Ontario, Seneca, Wayne, Yates

2,199 questionnaires mailed to a systematic random sample of the target population:

1,616 (74%), completed questionnaires
94%, married
94%, parous; 88%, two or more offspring
31%, one or more spontaneous or induced abortions
48%, Protestant; 41%, Catholic
Mean highest school grade completed, 13.2

Results of Population Surveyed

Some of the questions asked in the survey are listed in Tables 4 through 7, which include the answer categories provided on the multiple choice questionnaire.

Knowledge of Prenatal Diagnosis of Birth Defects. Eighty-five percent of

TABLE 4

Knowledge of and Sources of Information about Prenatal Diagnosis of Birth Defects

Question 1. Most babies are born healthy, but a few may have birth defects (congenital malformations or abnormalities seen soon after birth). Do you know whether there is now a medical test available to tell *before* a baby is born (prenatal diagnosis) if it will have a birth defect?

Response	N	%
Yes	1,381	(85)
No	227	(14)
No answer	8	(1)

Question 2. How did you learn about this test? (Answer each item.)

	Yes	No	Don't know	No answer
(1) Magazine	49*	23	6	23
(2) Television, radio	46	24	7	23
(3) Newspaper	40	26	7	27
(4) Friends	27	37	6	30
(5) Other	11	33	14	42
(6) My doctor	10	52	4	34

*% of total responses. Total responses = 1,616. Responses have been ordered in terms of decreasing frequencies of Yes answers.

respondents to Question 1 reported knowledge of the availability of medical tests to diagnose fetal birth defects prenatally. There is obviously a general awareness of possibilities for intrauterine detection of birth defects (Table 4). Answers to Question 2 reveal that women reported learning of the prenatal diagnosis test through public media (magazine, television/radio, newspaper) and from friends far more often than through interaction with physicians, from whom only one out of ten respondents had learned of the prenatal diagnosis procedure.

General awareness, however, does not indicate extent or accuracy of knowledge, as is shown by the responses to Questions 3 and 4 (Table 5). Approximately 80% of respondents answered correctly that amniotic fluid would be used for the prenatal test. However, 32% answered incorrectly that maternal blood, and 26% that maternal urine, would be used to detect fetal birth defects. Eight percent replied (again incorrectly) that some other sample would be used.

Further definition of accuracy of knowledge concerning prenatal detection possibilities was obtained by examining answers to Question 4. At present, fetal sex (1), Down syndrome (3), anencephaly (7), spina bifida (8), and Tay-Sachs disease (9) can be reliably determined prenatally. Sickle cell anemia (6) can be diagnosed by analysis of fetal blood, obtained at greater risk, but the approach should still be considered experimental. The other categories of listed abnormalities are not detectable at present. Yet, fetal heart abnormality (2) was the most frequent response (54%). Fetal defect due to German measles (4), which cannot be detected, was chosen as frequently as Down syndrome ("mongolism"), currently perhaps the most common disorder for which prenatal diagnosis is performed, and defect due to German measles (4) was chosen by as many respondents as anencephaly (7) and spina bifida (8) together, which are very frequent indications for second trimester prenatal diagnosis. Only one of five women was aware that Tay-Sachs disease (9) is detectable, and yet, one of eight believed that cystic fibrosis can be diagnosed. Prenatal detection of cystic fibrosis is not yet possible.

Attitudes Concerning Indications For and Physician Interaction Regarding Prenatal Diagnosis. Responses concerning who should have prenatal diagnosis were surprisingly positive, with more positive than negative responses for all the specific categories listed (Table 6). Opinion was evenly divided (41%, Yes; 38%, No) concerning whether women at all ages should have prenatal diagnosis, and there was an increasingly positive response that advanced maternal age is an indication for prenatal diagnosis: age $>$ 35 years (57%); age $>$ 40 years (71%). Four out of five women sampled by this survey believed that a history of a birth defect in the mother's or father's family, or in the immediate family, is an indication for prenatal diagnosis.

Seventy-five percent of the respondents stated that the doctor should discuss prenatal diagnosis test(s) when he thinks it is necessary, and 69% that the doctor should discuss the test(s) whenever the patient asks. More than half of the respondents stated that the doctor should always discuss such tests with patients.

TABLE 5

Knowledge Concerning Amniocentesis and the Types of Fetal Abnormalities Currently Detectable by Second Trimester Prenatal Diagnosis

Question 3. Which sample(s) would be used for such a test? (Answer each item.)

	Yes	No	Don't know	No answer
(1) Amniotic fluid (around fetus)	81*	1	16	2
(2) Mother's blood	32	20	36	12
(3) Mother's urine	26	23	38	13
(4) Something else	8	17	50	25

*% of total responses. Total responses = 1,616. Responses have been ordered in terms of decreasing frequencies of Yes answers.

Question 4. Can each of the following be detected in the baby (fetus) before birth? (Answer each item.)

	Yes	No	Don't know	No answer
(1) Sex of the baby	64*	13	21	2
(2) Heart abnormality	54	5	39	2
(3) Down syndrome ("mongolism")	53	7	38	2
(4) Defect due to German measles	53	8	37	2
(5) Mental retardation	36	16	46	2
(6) Sickle cell anemia	31	10	56	3
(7) Brain defect (anencephaly)	30	9	58	3
(8) Spinal defect (spina bifida)	23	11	63	3
(9) Tay-Sachs disease	19	6	73	2
(10) Cystic fibrosis	12	15	70	3
(11) Cancer	8	24	65	3
(12) Cleft lip and/or palate	6	29	62	3

*% of total responses. Total responses = 1,616. Responses have been ordered in terms of decreasing frequencies of Yes answers.

TABLE 6

Attitudes Toward Utilization and Provision of Prenatal Diagnosis

Question 5. In your view, *who* should have prenatal diagnosis? (Answer each item.)

	Yes	No	Don't know	No answer
Women who have:				
(1) Baby with birth defect	82*	2	3	13
(2) History of birth defect in family	81	2	4	13
(3) History of birth defect in husband's family	78	3	5	14
(4) Age > 40 years	71	6	6	17
(5) Age > 35 years	57	15	11	17
(6) All ages	41	38	10	11
(7) Other	14	19	21	46

*% of total responses. Total responses = 1,616. Responses have been ordered in terms of decreasing frequencies of Yes answers.

Question 6. Do you think doctors who care for women during pregnancy should discuss such tests with the patient? (Answer each item.)

	Yes	No	Don't know	No answer
(1) When doctor thinks necessary	75*	4	1	20
(2) Whenever the patient asks	69	5	1	25
(3) Always	57	25	7	11

*% of total responses. Total responses = 1,616. Responses have been ordered in terms of decreasing frequencies of Yes answers.

TABLE 7

Attitudes Toward Availability and Uses of Elective Abortion

Question 7. Do you think a pregnant woman should be able to obtain a *legal* abortion under any of the following circumstances? (Answer each item.)

	Yes	No	Don't know	No answer
(1) Woman's life or health endangered	91*	7	1	1
(2) Pregnancy result of rape	82	15	2	1
(3) Strong chance serious birth defect	81	15	2	2
(4) Not married – doesn't want baby	48	48	2	2
(5) Family cannot afford another child	41	55	2	2
(6) Has children – does not want more	40	57	1	2
(7) Couple does not want child now	30	66	2	2
(8) Couple does not want child – sex	8	89	1	2

*% of total responses. Total responses = 1,616. Responses have been ordered in terms of decreasing frequencies of Yes answers.

Attitudes Concerning Availability of Legal Elective Abortion Under Various Conditions. Table 7 is a summary of the responses concerning absolute and relative acceptability of legal elective abortion under various circumstances. Nine of ten who responded agreed that endangerment of a woman's life or health is an acceptable reason for induced abortion. Serious fetal birth defect and pregnancy resulting from rape are equivalently acceptable indications to four out of five women who responded. Respondents were evenly divided concerning the appropriateness of abortion for pregnancy out-of-wedlock, and more women opposed than supported the use of induced abortion for terminating unplanned or unwanted pregnancies of married women. Only one in twelve women, however, answered that sex selection is an acceptable indication for elective induced abortion.

DISCUSSION

This study documents that the existence of prenatal diagnostic procedures is widely perceived among married women 30-45 years of age in our region. The acceptance of these new tests is surprisingly high. Implications of our findings are probably not limited to one metropolitan area in Upstate New York. In the fall of 1976, a national opinion survey was conducted by household interview using a probability sample of 1,679 adult Americans of both sexes.[9] More than 80% of the respondents thought that women should have access to prenatal diagnostic services. If the test revealed that a woman's baby would be born with serious defects requiring life-long care, 23% answered that she should definitely have an abortion, and 50% said she should have an abortion if she wants to. Only 21% of the respondents were opposed to abortion under such circumstances. In our study of married women 30 to 45 years of age, only 15% of respondents opposed abortion for fetal abnormality. Our more extensive regional sample results correspond very closely to those reported for the national survey, suggesting that our findings may be representative for the nation at large.

In contrast to the general awareness of prenatal diagnostic services and their widespread acceptance, knowledge concerning specific abnormalities which can be reliably detected was low and often erroneous. Though respondents readily acknowledged that they did not know the answers to some questions, it is uncertain how often they relied on educated guesses. Thus, there is need for provision of more detailed information than is currently available through mass media.

Further analysis is needed to assess what effect better information would have on acceptance rates. An analysis of probable efficacy of educational approaches has been made,[10] and we conclude that educational efforts will raise the acceptance of the new technique. The underlying preventive health objective is to reduce the numbers of children born with serious birth defects. Only if parents opt for selective abortion, however, will this goal be approached. To the extent that reproductive behavior is based on informed, rational decision making, education and counseling may have an effect.

Further research is also needed on the influence of personal experience on specific decision making. There may be a greater willingness to accept innovative medical services in the abstract, or as far as others are concerned, than when a couple, or an individual, becomes personally involved and has to make a decision. In such circumstances, other factors may emerge and affect the decision-making process.

A more detailed analysis of our previous data, and continuing surveys of health professionals involved in provision of services, as outlined above, will be needed to clarify the role of various factors affecting provision and utilization of prenatal diagnostic services. Such knowledge will help us in preparation of larger-scale genetic services to all who may request them.

REFERENCES

1. A. Milunsky, *in* The Prevention of Genetic Disease and Mental Retardation, A. Milunsky (Ed.), W.B. Saunders Company, Philadelphia, pp. 221-263, 1975.
2. H.L. Nadler, *Adv. in Ped. 22*, 1-81, 1976.
3. NICHD National Registry for Amniocentesis Study Group: Midtrimester Amniocentesis for Prenatal Diagnosis: Safety and Accuracy, *J.A.M.A. 236*, 1471, 1976.
4. N.E. Simpson, L. Dallaire, J.R. Miller, L. Siminovich, J.L. Hamerton, J. Miller and C. McKeen, *Can. Med. Assoc. J. 115*, 739, 1976.
5. A. Milunsky, *N. Engl. J. Med. 295 (7)*, 377, 1976. 5a. Cooper, T., *Pub. Hlth. Reports 91*, 116, 1976. 5b. A.C.O.G. Technical Bulletin No. 39, May, 1976.
6. S. Hagard and F.A. Carter, *Brit. Med. J. 1*, 753, 1976.
7. R. Conley and A. Milunsky, *in* The Prevention of Genetic Disease and Mental Retardation, A. Milunsky (Ed.), W.B. Saunders Company, Philadelphia, 442-455, 1975.
8. D.J.H. Brock, Progress in Medical Genetics, Vol III, Biochemical and Cytological Methods in the Diagnosis of Neural Tube Defects, W.B. Saunders Company, Philadelphia, pp. 1-37, 1977.
9. Policy Research Inc., A Comprehensive Study of the Ethical, Legal and Social Implications of Advances in Biomedical and Behavioral Research and Technology – National Opinion Survey, Baltimore, 1977.
10. R.R. Sell, K.J. Roghmann and R.A. Doherty (submitted for publication).

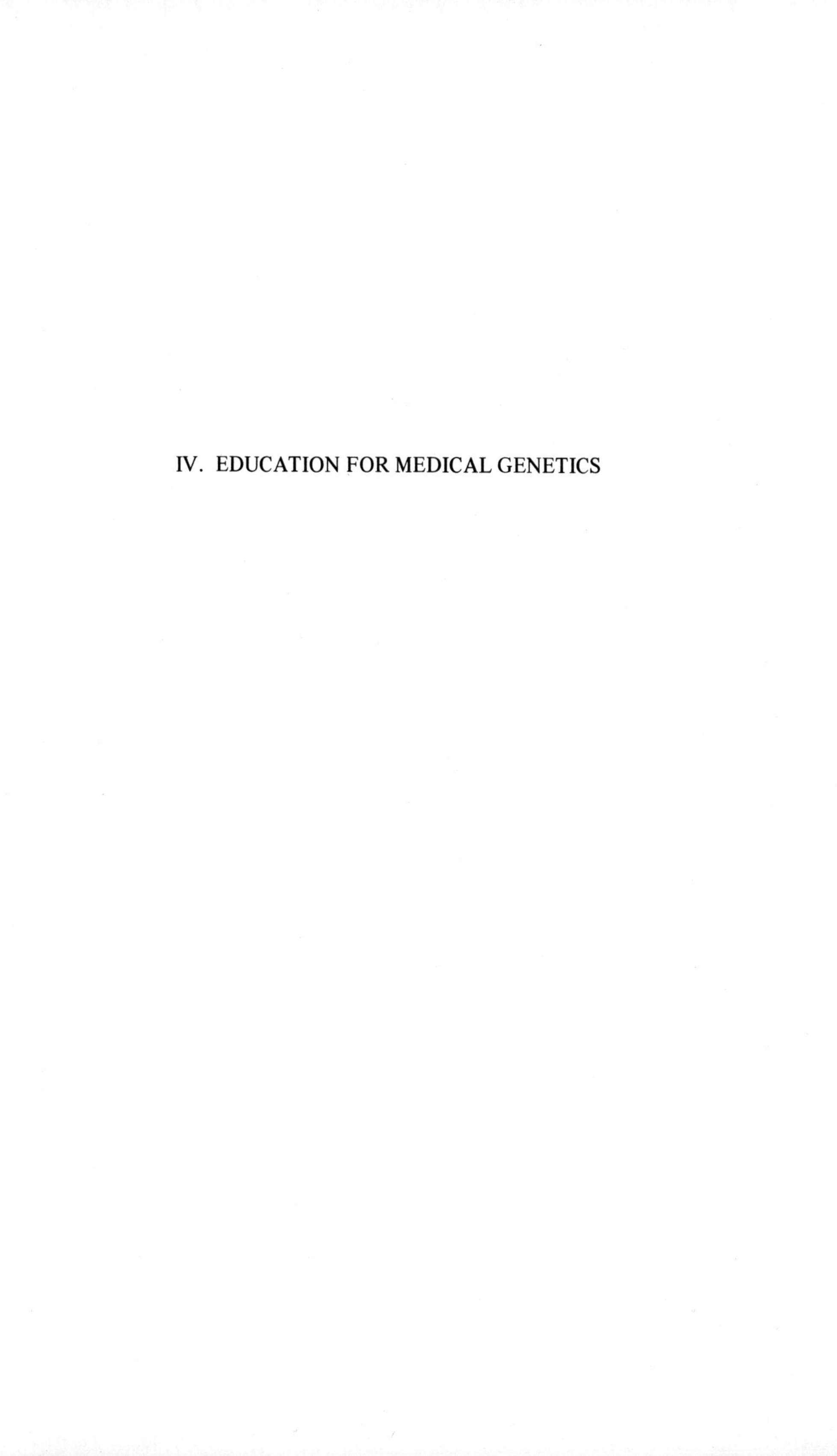

IV. EDUCATION FOR MEDICAL GENETICS

HUMAN GENETICS EDUCATION IN THE HIGH SCHOOL: A WORKING EXPERIENCE*

Carol L. Clow
Mindy Schok
Charles R. Scriver
Dorothy E. Scriver

Nicolaus Copernicus formulated his ideas about the nature of the physical universe over four centuries ago. Kepler, Galileo, Newton and others then produced the data which abolished the Ptolemeic universe. Students are now taught the revised doctrine about the physical world as a matter of course. During the past century new doctrine pertaining to our view of the biological world has been promulgated; the place of man in the universe has been interpreted. Yet students are not taught biology and genetics as a matter of course. Accordingly they do not always learn about themselves. Our report which follows is about high school students and their teachers, their knowledge of human genetics and biology, and their attitudes toward these subjects. Our report is also about the text books used by students and teachers.

BACKGROUND OF PROJECT

One of us (Dorothy E. Scriver) graduated recently from high school. One of us (Mindy Schok) retired recently from the teaching of biology in high school. These credentials influence the perspective of our report. The two remaining authors have several domains of experience relevant to the material at hand; they include:

(1) a direct experience with 50,000 families through genetic screening programs which lead to an awareness of public knowledge and attitudes;
(2) participation in the Quebec Network of Genetic Medicine;[1]
(3) living in a region where science broadcasting and science news has received public recognition and approval;
(4) participation in seminars for science writers on human genetics to improve public awareness.

Our specific association with a large regional school board, its students and its teachers began when we initated Tay-Sachs carrier screening in the high schools

*This study was supported jointly by the Quebec Network of Genetic Medicine, the Medical Research Council, and the P.S.B.G.M.

ISBN 0-12-562650-9

TABLE 1

Human Biology and Genetics in High School Biology Texts Available to Teachers Under the Protestant School Board of Greater Montreal

Text (and Authors)	Date	Pages	% of Contents Genetics	% of Contents Human Biology
Modern Biology* (Otto and Towle)	1975	824	9.2	15.1
Human Physiology* (Morrison *et al.*)	1972	470	6	82
BSCS: Green	1973	725	6	3
Yellow	1968	756	9	8
Blue	1973	523*	19.5**	14.4**
Biology: Intro. to Life (Nason and Goldstein)	1969	750	11	17
Biological Science (Gregory and Goldman)	1971	714	6	19
Foundations of Biology (McElroy *et al.*)	1968	724	11	22
Biology and Man (Swanson *et al.*)	1975	614	10.7	30.6
Average		677	9.8	23.4 (16.1)***

*Recommended by the Board to meet curriculum requirements.
**Excludes laboratory curriculum.
***Percent excluding the textbook *Human Physiology*.

in 1973.[2,3] This exposure led to in-service seminars for biology teachers during the academic years 1974-1976; and to a course in human genetics, which we gave at the request of teachers in the region during the winter term of 1977 in the Masters in Education Program at Concordia University in Montreal.

THE SURVEYS

1. Survey of Text Books

Methods: The survey of text books, performed in 1975 and 1977, was limited to nine books, all published in North America. These texts are recommended by the PSBGM (Protestant School Board of Greater Montreal) for use in the schools. Two texts are used in particular to meet the needs of the prescribed curriculum. They are: Otto and Towle, *Modern Biology*; Morrison *et al., Human Physiology*. The index, table of contents, and relevant text material of each book was examined, the number of pages devoted to *human* biology and genetics recorded, and the percent of total text material represented by this material calculated.

The relative importance of human genetics in the sections on genetics in the two recommended texts was calculated by counting all examples used in the text, tables and illustrations and noting those which specified human examples; results are expressed as a percentage of the total number of examples.

Results: Human biology and genetics are not important components of most high school biology texts (Table 1). Only one text (*Human Physiology*) has a strong emphasis on human biology – in keeping with its title. Examples from human experience are used less than half the time to illustrate genetic themes and topics in the two recommended texts (Table 2). An amusing comment on the non-human bias in the texts was found in the very first monochrome illustration for the section on genetics in *Human Physiology*; it shows the chromosomes of drosophila! Modern pictures of human chromosomes with banding patterns are readily available. Why were human chromosomes not illustrated when they are more relevant to the reader of *Human Physiology*?

2. Survey of Students

Methods: The survey of students was carried out in March, 1975, with a multiple-choice instrument (138 questions) which solicited selective demographic information, and knowledge and attitudes about topics in human genetics. The questionnaire was administered to 930 students in grades 9, 10, and 11 in 16 different schools. All students were enrolled in the biology curriculum. They represent 44 percent of those taking biology and 11 percent of all students in the schools surveyed. One period of class time was assigned for completion of the survey; answers were entered on mark-sense cards, compiled by computer and then transferred to computer tape for further comparative analysis.

Results: The sex ratio of respondents was 0.991 (M:F). The age range was 14 to 18 years; 74.8% of students were 16 and 17 years of age. There was a

TABLE 2

Text Book Examples Relating to Human Experience Used to Illustrate Genetic Themes

Text	Chapter	Number of Examples*		% From Human Experience
		Human	Total	
Morrison *et al.*: *Human Physiology*	33. Genetics	11	32	34.4
	34. Nucleic Acids; Human Genetics	13	19	68.4
	TOTAL	24	51	47.2
Otto and Towle: *Modern Biology*	9. Principles of Heredity	3	18	16.6
	10. The Genetic Material	3	34	8.8
	11. Genes in Human Populations	21	26	80.6
	12. Applied Genetics	0	16	0
	TOTAL	27	94	28.7

*Includes material in text, as well as that cited in tables and charts and shown in illustrations.

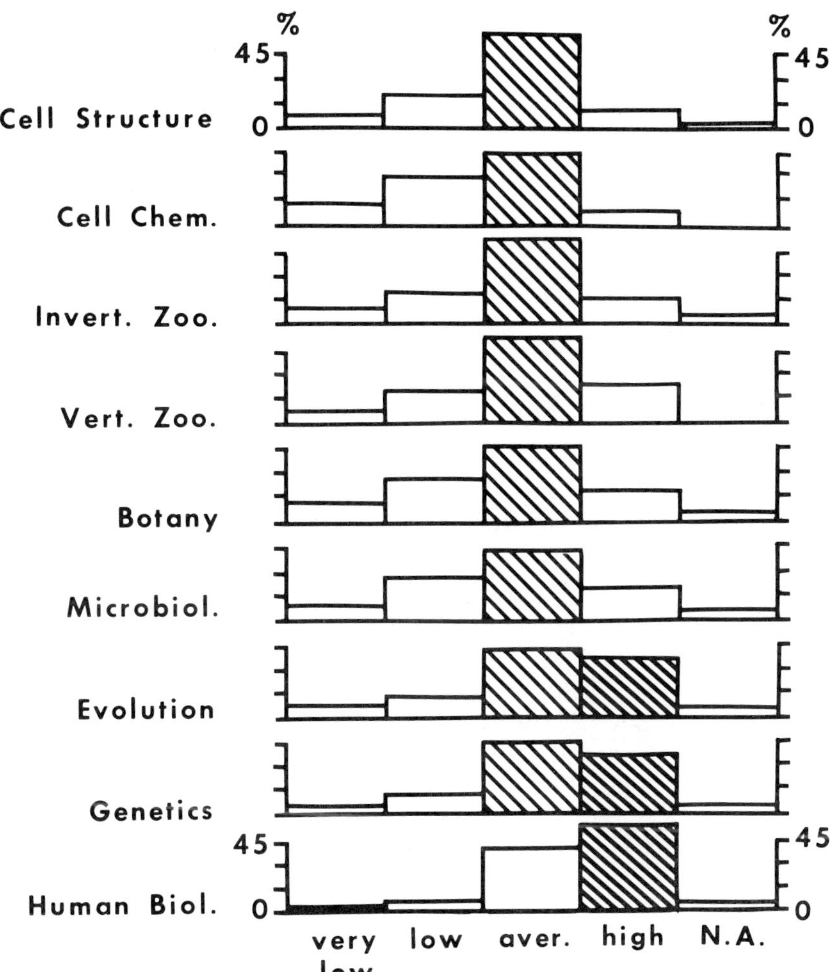

Fig. 1. Character of student interest in nine subject areas in the high school biology curriculum. Height of each bar indicates % of students selecting one of the choices ("very poor"; "poor"; "average"; "high"; and "no answer"). Note increased interest in evolution and genetics and particular interest in human biology.

preponderance of Protestant respondents (45.3%), but Greek-Orthodox (10.6%), Jewish (28.3%), and Roman Catholic (4.6%) religious affiliations were also represented. Caucasians represented 78.8% of the total survey population; the remainder were: Negro, 6.5%; Oriental, 9.1%; "Other", 5.6%. The social class of the student's families were: middle class (60%), upper middle (29.9%); lower middle (6.5%); lower (4%); and upper (3.2%). These findings indicate that the survey is reasonably representative of anglophone, North American, junior and senior high school students.

Almost half (48.8%) of the students presently taking a biology course do not intend to continue with further education in the subject. This implies that they will have little formal opportunity to learn more about human genetics. Accordingly, the high school is the place to explain the relevance of human genetics to citizens.

There are additional impediments to the transmittal of genetics information which could influence the self-knowledge and lifestyle of citizens. In our school system, only 26 percent of all students will have taken a biology course by the time they leave high school. While the frequency is apparently even lower in other school systems in Quebec province, we are aware that it is higher in other regions of North America.

The information considered essential to an understanding of human biology and genetics must be incorporated into the standard syllabus which stipulates what material a teacher is required to cover in regular class time. There are several indications that the basic course material is crucial to the development of an accurate, pertinent knowledge of genetics. Sixty-four percent of respondents have done no additional reading in genetics outside the school curriculum, and 57.4% do not use any biology reference material. Only 19.6% of students do extra reading in genetics and biology.

Only about 10% of the biology curriculum is allotted to genetics in the PSBGM program. With corrections for holidays, examination time, etc., we estimate that 11.4 hours are currently available to teach genetics. One-fifth (22.8%) of respondents claimed less than 5 hours of instruction in genetics while another 39.8% had received 5-10 hours. In total, 62.6% of our students recall having less than 10 hours of "genetics" in high school.

When asked whether they had performed laboratory experiments as well, 48.7% of students had never done so and 94.7% had done fewer than five. The laboratory studies in question use the common models: onion-tip meiosis on prepared slides; probability demonstrations with coins and corn kernals; mating in paramecium and other species; blood typing.

With regard to their declared interest in the major topic areas covered in the biology curriculum (Fig. 1), 51.7% of students have a "high interest" in human biology, as opposed to "very poor", "poor" and "average" interest; 35.8% indicate a high interest in genetics, and 34.5% have an equivalent interest in evolution. None of the six remaining subject areas (*e.g.*, cell structure and chemistry, zoology, botany or microbiology) evoked comparable interest. Three-quarters of the students (73.5%) stated they "would have liked to learn more about human genetics than they did".

The student survey included 35 questions designed to test knowledge of genetics and heredity. For these "knowledge" questions, the range of correct response was from 14.0% to 87.8% per question; the average for the 35 questions was 59%. Despite a declared interest in genetics and an acceptable performance on some of the knowledge questions, it is obvious that students lack knowledge in several areas of prime importance. Basic to the study of genetics is a firm understanding of the concepts of genes, chromosomes, fertilization, sex determination, and probability; yet it is precisely those concepts that we found to be vaguely, incompletely, or incorrectly understood.

Students are confused about the difference between a gene and a chromosome. When asked to define a gene, 64.4% of all the respondents offered the correct answer ("a unit of heredity") but another 25.9% chose "a unit made up of many chromosomes". This finding suggests that many students do not understand the relationship between genes and chromosomes. In reply to the question: "How many genes is it estimated that we each have?", 48.3% of all respondents selected the option "46". Our students apparently confuse or equate a gene with a chromosome.

Students understand simple probability; 81.1% gave the correct response to a question involving the chance of a certain number being thrown while playing dice. But when considering sexual reproduction and Mendel's laws of gene segregation and assortment they have a fuzzy view of the facts. For example, we stated that a couple had four daughters; we then asked: "What is the genetic probability that their next child will be a son?"; only 59.5 of respondents gave the correct response. Two other questions indicated that students fail to apply the concepts of probability to autosomal recessive inheritance. Told that for each pregnancy a man and wife had a one in four chance of having a child with a specific genetic disease, and that they already had three normal children, they were asked what was the chance that their next child would have the disease; only 47.2% of the respondents offered the correct answer.

The second question, designed to check the validity of the first, stated: "Mr. and Mrs. Jones are carriers for an autosomal recessive condition. What is the chance at each pregnancy that their child will have the disease?" Only 38.1% answered correctly. The poorer performance on the second question may also indicate that the term "autosomal recessive" is not as well understood as an anecdotal definition.

Students also lack a firm grasp of one of the basic facts of human reproduction. Only 51.3% responded correctly to the true-or-false statement: "The father determines the sex of the child". The performance on this question is compatible with random selection of the answer and it leads us to wonder whether students have an informed perception of sexual reproduction and the chromosomal basis of heredity.

Questions were posed to test familiarity with the concept of host-environment interaction and the concept of heritability in the interpretation of metrical characteristics. Most respondents (83.2%) believe that intelligence is influenced both by environment and heredity. Most students (78%) are aware that dermatoglyphic patterns have high heritability. For the more subtle question concerning height, about half (47.7%) of the students believe it is determined by heredity alone, while about half (47.5%) believe heredity and environment together determine this quantitative character. These findings suggest that a discussion of the quantitative differences in dermatoglyphics between twins, non-twins, and the two hands of a single individual, or a discussion of polygenic inheritance as the basis for understanding the frequency distribution of standing heights in a classroom population could be used to illuminate the concept of heritability of human characteristics. We believe that these topics offer advantages over a discussion of intelligence where there is so much speculation concerning the reliability of the primary data.

One of our major concerns is that students do not learn of the applied aspects of genetics which touch their own lives. They are assimilating information from texts which are deficient in this context (Table 2); and teachers are often unfamiliar with human examples which illustrate applied genetics. Our survey revealed, for example, that students are underinformed both about genetic screening ongoing in their own community and newsworthy ethnic diseases relating to themselves. Many of the questions in this area, dealing with human applications of genetic principles, elicited the highest percentages of "don't know" responses.

Students do know that an apparently normal phenotype does not exclude the occurrence of a variant genotype; 87.8% said the following statement was true: "A person may transmit to his offspring characteristics which he himself does not show". Yet, the students were less perceptive that this probability could encompass themselves. We asked: "Do you think that there is a possibilty that you are a carrier of one or more defective genes?"; only 42.1% or respondents said "yes". This response may indicate that most students do not accept the fact of heterozygosity with risk; or it may imply that the concept of genetic diversity among persons is not well understood. The respondents may also have reacted to the perjorative term "defective" in the question, whereas "variant" or "unusual" might have had a different value for the respondent.

Knowledge questions concerning ethnic genetic disease produced interesting replies. Within the particular religious and racial groups participating in the survey, we found that a relatively high percentage of students were aware that certain diseases are more prevalent in their group than in others. Among the Jewish respondents, 88.3% knew that Tay-Sachs disease affects Ashkenazi Jews predominantly; 62.1% of all Negro respondents related sickle cell anemia predominantly to Blacks; 76.0% of all Greek respondents knew that thalassemia selectively affects Greeks; 52.6% of all Caucasian respondents knew that cystic fibrosis is a prevalent disease among North American Whites.

However, a high percentage of members of the specific groups, having identified "their" disease, did not know the significant medical characteristics associated with it. The poor correct-response rate from students identifying themselves with specific high-risk groups indicates that specific knowledge of the relevant genetic condition is poor. For example, only 24.2% of Jewish respondents knew that Tay-Sachs was a "disease in which the nervous system degenerates" (vs. 19.6% correct response from the total survey population) and only 43.1% of Negro respondents knew that "red cells don't work properly due to their altered shape" in sickle cell anemia (vs. 62.7% correct response from the total survey). When one examines only those respondents who indicated, in answer to the appropriate question, that a particular genetic disease was present in their (extended) family, there is still a dearth of knowledge about the specific problem. Only 14 (53.8%) of the 26 respondents claiming familial experience with Tay-Sachs disease knew that it affects Ashkenazi Jews predominantly; and only 5 of the same respondents recognized Tay-Sachs as a disease causing degeneration of the nervous system. Similarly, only 60% of the 25 respondents claiming familial experience with thalassemia, only 61% of the 87 claiming experience with sickle cell anemia, and only 48% of the 29 students in contact with cystic fibrosis knew the appropriate ethnic distribution of the relevant disease. The qualifying characteristic of the pertinent diseases was known to less than half of those claiming familial experience. These findings either imply improper answers to the original question: "Is there anyone in your family. . . who has had. . . disease x, y, etc.?" or they indicate an inverse correlation between "experience" and knowledge.

The survey contained 26 questions which probed attitudes and opinions on a variety of genetic topics. When asked whether genetic screening for hereditary conditions is important to society, 78.2% of students agreed. Students also believe in the importance of genetic research (80.7% in favor). Questions about the possible effects of "genetic engineering" reveal an overall positive attitude; students feel it will bring about more good than bad in society. The trend toward derogatory media coverage of applied genetics has not had much impact on our students – a matter of interest since they indicate that the press is a major source of their knowledge of genetics.

Because abortion is a major social issue today, we asked the students whether abortion should be available to parents following prenatal diagnosis of various conditions. Most respondents are in agreement with termination of pregnancy for the Tay-Sachs fetus (79.3%) and the fetus with Down syndrome (72.2%). Only 10.8% considered it appropriate to use prenatal diagnosis and abortion for selection of sex in offspring. In this matter of sex selection, students are more conservative than the genetic counselors surveyed by Fraser and Pressor;[4] among the latter, 21% could recommend amniocentesis and abortion for sex selection.

3. Survey of Teachers

Methods: The survey of biology teachers was performed in March 1975. Thirty-three teachers involved in the biology curriculum were asked to fill out a 38-part questionnaire; all replied.

Results: The age range of those responding was 27-55 yrs. (mean, 36 yrs.). Males outnumbered females 3:1. Seventy percent of the teachers had majored in biology. Two-thirds took their biology course(s) in the 1960's; two-thirds of the total group had taken refresher courses after 1970. One-third of the group expressed a strong preference to teach science subjects in addition to biology.

The group of teachers devoted 14% of their teaching hours in the biology curriculum to topics in human biology. Genetics received only 7% of their effort. These allotments of time correspond to the allotment of material in the text books; they imply that the text book determines the material taught in class. The majority of teachers (80%) felt the class time devoted to human biology and genetics was insufficient. Only 45% of teachers were satisfied with the prescribed texts; BSCS texts were utilized and preferred as back-up sources.

Our contacts with teachers during in-service education seminars and the course in human genetics corroborated the experience of one of us (MS) that lack of familiarity with human examples is the major deterrent to the use of them to illustrate genetic themes in the classroom.

DISCUSSION

When is the best time to introduce human genetics into the curriculum? The students themselves hold a clear opinion on this topic. In our survey they indicated the high school, as opposed to elementary or post-secondary education, as the appropriate time to encounter detailed instruction/education in human genetics. In their opinion the experience should begin in junior high school.

What is the meaning of this preference? Perhaps it indicates that the elementary school, which all students have experienced, is too early to learn a subject as difficult and controversial as genetics. There are many ethical issues in the applied aspects of human genetics and grade school students are not likely to cope with them effectively. On the other hand, some of the evidence for inter-individual variation and an appreciation of biological individuality could probably be introduced without an interposition of value judgements in the late primary grades or in the first year of high school To delay genetics teaching until the post-secondary level will deprive over half the population (in our region) of knowledge that is an integral part of their lives. What is surprising to us is the fact that human biology and human genetics are not requirements for graduation from high school and indeed are not considered a prerequisite to being an informed citizen with some understanding of the vehicle which will negotiate the remaining years of life.

What can be done to improve genetics instruction/education in the schools? Our personal experience indicates several options.

1. The Text Books: Teachers are dependent on the material at hand for their teaching strategies in the classroom. Our survey revealed that most teachers rely on the text books at hand and particularly on those recommended by the School

Board. Accordingly a change in curriculum perspective will require a change in the text books. The introduction of human orientation in the illustration of basic themes will be more satisfying to students and teachers and it will be relevant. To this end the Biological Sciences Curriculum Study (BSCS) is likely to be an effective agent, with its interest in change and in development of a biology curriculum;[5] and with its commitment to the assessment of future needs in human genetics education and to the development of guidelines for meeting these needs.[6] Guidelines written in mid-1977 specify tactics in the middle school and upper high school curriculum which have the potential to improve student knowledge and awareness. We are aware that the Scopes trial took place not long ago in enlightened America[7] and that even today regional school boards may oppose curriculum change and may insist upon equal time for other views of man's place in the physical world.[8] That should not deter change when change is indicated.

2. Teacher Training: Most teachers of biology are unfamiliar with human genetics and in particular with the details that illuminate, in an interesting and relevant manner, the principle themes of genetics. In our experience participation of human and medical geneticists, in the continuing education and in-service training of teachers is welcome. From such interaction in our own experience we learned of the teachers needs while the teachers obtained material from us for use in the classroom. We believe that human and medical geneticists and local school boards could improve the level of mutual interaction to the benefit of the curriculum.

We have also prepared a resource book of modules comprising text, diagrams, slides and references which provide material on topics often raised by students in the classrooms or needed by the teachers; amniocentesis, thalassemia, sickle cell disease, genetic screening, polygenic inheritance, Down syndrome and hemophilia are among the topics in our "resource kit". Half the teachers provided with the first edition of the modules have been able to use it regularly and have found it to be useful.

3. Increase in Awareness of Needs: In order to extend the awareness of the problems and needs in genetics instruction/education – which we know to be quite general and not limited to our region – we have submitted a modified version of the present report to the *American Biology Teacher.*[9]

4. Physician Participation: Our interest in genetics education originated to a certain extent with our experience in Tay-Sachs heterozygote screening of high school students and of adults. The stimulus for continuing and extending our domain of involvement is our belief that better informed citizens will utilize medical services more effectively. About 30 percent of the disease burden in the pediatric age group originates in mutation, congenital malformations and multifactorial (genetic plus environmental) events.[10] About 12 percent of adult-onset disease is of like origin.[11] Accordingly there is cause to improve citizen awareness of the origins of their own illnesses. Measures to reduce or prevent the occurrence of "genetic" disease will be more effective when informed citizens can understand the rationale for such measures.

The Academy of Pediatrics has recently formed a Committee on Genetics; one of its charges is to improve physician education with respect to genetics. In turn, pediatricians as potential members of school boards, as constituents, as parents and as physicians to school children can assist in the upgrading of genetics instruction/education in the schools. The chairman of the Academy's Committee on School Health has recently recommended improved genetics education in the school curriculum.[12]

5. A National Agenda: Whereas the aforementioned proposals are useful tactics, the campaign is likely to fail without an overriding strategy. That strategy should originate in a national agenda where science is important and where the vital relation of genetics to human affairs is clearly perceived. We have no such national agenda. Science is too much in the control of the bookkeepers and illiteracy in the affairs of science abounds. Everyone is a legatee of Copernican and Darwinian insights; and yet we are slow to inform ourselves of our rightful inheritance.

SUMMARY

A survey of 930 high school students (11 percent of those attending the junior and senior grades and 44 percent of those taking biology courses) reveals a strong preference for more and earlier teaching of *human* biology and (human) genetics. A survey of current classroom texts reveals they are deficient in one or both areas and less than half their pedagogical material in genetics is drawn from human experience. The students have inadequate knowledge of basic principles; the application of these principles to themselves, their families and their communities is poorly perceived. On the other hand, attitudes to principles and practice are very positive. A survey of teachers reveals they have not been prepared to meet the challenge of teaching genetics, although they have a strong preference to do so. A major opportunity and need exists to inform citizens of their "biological rights" and of their genetic identity through curriculum reform.

ACKNOWLEDGMENTS

The enthusiastic support of Dr. John Simms, past Chairman of the Protestant School Board of Greater Montreal and of its members and staff is warmly acknowledged. The exceptional cooperation of many teachers and students in the classrooms made these surveys possible. In particular, we acknowledge the interest and advice of the following teachers: Morrie Bakerman, Margaret Capes, Margo MacDonald, Don Norman and Renwick Spence. Ellen Beck and Shirley Blaichman, during a summer research project supported by bursaries from the Faculty of Medicine of McGill University, helped to design the student survey. Lynn Prevost and Huguette Ishmael handled many other details in this work. The example and guidance of Dr. Barton Childs, Johns Hopkins University Medical School, is evident throughout our project. We are grateful to Manert Kennedy and Faith Hickman of BSCS for their encouragement in the preparation of this report.

REFERENCES

1. C.L. Clow, F.C. Fraser, C. Laberge and C.R. Scriver, *Prog. Med. Genet. 9*, 162, 1973.
2. E. Beck, S. Blaichman, C.R. Scriver and C.L. Clow, *N. Engl. J. Med. 291*, 1166, 1974.
3. C.L. Clow and C.R. Scriver, *Pediatrics 59*, 86, 1977.
4. F.C. Fraser and C. Pressor, *in* Genetic Counseling, H.A. Lubs and F. de la Cruz (Eds.), Raven Press, New York, p. 109, 1977.
5. W.V. Mayer, *B.S.C.S. Newsletter No. 64*, 4, 1976.
6. Biological Sciences Curriculum Study. Guidelines for educational priorities and curricular innovations in the areas of human genetics, genetic diseases and birth defects. A Needs Assessment Project. BSCS/National Foundation-March of Dimes. Boulder, Colorado, 1977.
7. J.V. Grabiner and P.D. Miller, *Science 185*, 832, 1974.
8. N. Wade, *Science 178*, 724, 1972.
9. C.R. Scriver, D.E. Scriver, C.L. Clow and M. Schok, *Amer. Biol. Teacher* (in press).
10. C.R. Scriver, J.L. Neal, R. Saginur and A. Clow, *C.M.A.J. 108*, 111, 1973.
11. B. Childs, S.M. Miller and A.G. Bearn, *in* Mutagenic Effects of Environmental Contamination, H.E. Sutton and M.I. Harris (Eds.), Academic Press, New York, p. 3, 1972.
12. D.E. Cook, Chmn., Comm. on School Health, Amer. Acad. Ped., Personal Communication, 1977.

MASTERS LEVEL TRAINING PROGRAMS FOR GENETIC COUNSELORS: AN EIGHT YEAR REPORT*

Joan H. Marks

The need to assess the current role of Genetic Associates or genetic counselors with non-M.D. training is particularly appropriate in 1977 in view of the rapidly expanding demand for genetic counseling services and the cognizance of this demand evidenced in such developments as the approaching National Institutes of Health hearings on the implementation of the National Genetics Diseases Act and the recent decision of the American Society of Human Genetics to consider formation of an accrediting organization for all the members of the clinical genetics team.

My charge is to review our experience at Sarah Lawrence College with our Human Genetics Program, begun in 1969, which was the first program in the United States to train genetic counselors at the allied health level.[1] In addition, I will relate our training program to the five other programs which have been established in the past five years to provide a broader perspective for considering the training needs and roles of the Genetic Associate. I believe the medical profession, as well as the consumer, has accepted the need and the efficacy of genetic counseling by non-physicians.[2,3,4,5] The presently established training programs, in order of their development are: Sarah Lawrence College, Rutgers University, the University of California at Berkeley and Irvine, The University of Colorado at Denver, and the newest, the University of Wisconsin. This last program, while not yet a registered program, is, nonetheless, training Genetic Associates. I will consider these programs with respect to the following: (1) the number of students currently in training, (2) the curricula, (3) the number of graduates, (4) where and how the graduates function in health services, and (5) a profile of the activities of graduates from the Sarah Lawrence College program since its initiation eight years ago.

Table 1 indicates the current enrollment in masters programs training genetic

---

*Supported in part by grants from the Division of Associated Health Professions, Bureau of Health Manpower, Health Resources Administration, Public Health Service, Department of Health, Education and Welfare, Grant number 5D12 AH 00792-03; The National Foundation-March of Dimes; the Babcock Foundation; and the J.M. Foundation.

ISBN 0-12-562650-9

TABLE 1

1977-1978 Enrollment in M.S. Programs

University of California	
Berkeley	16
Irvine	5
University of Colorado	7
Rutgers University	15
Sarah Lawrence College	52
University of Wisconsin	10
Total	105

TABLE 2

Curricular Areas in M.S. Programs in Human Genetics

Curricular Areas
Biochemistry
Human Development and/or Human Physiology
Mendelian and Molecular Genetics
Medical Genetics
Human Cytogenetics
Genetic Counseling Techniques
Clinical Genetics Practicum

counselors. While there are great differences in the methods by which each program selects its students, there are certain similarities. All programs require an undergraduate degree, with some coursework in at least biology or chemistry. Some programs consider the life experience of mature applicants, often associated with earlier career training in the health field, to be a significant asset. Some programs allow for part-time study over a three year period, while the Rutgers program is of one year's duration. All programs accept both men and women. The overwhelming majority of students seeking training as Genetic Associates, however, are women. From our experience at Sarah Lawrence, most people who now seek training in human genetics have taken undergraduate courses in genetics and have been intrigued with the implications of genetic disease from both a public health and psychological point of view. Recognizing the magnitude of the public health challenge, they feel confident it necessitates the development of services to meet this need. In other words, students are willing to enter these training programs recognizing that job security in this field is inadequate. While no data are available on the number of students motivated to seek such training, I have the impression that all six programs receive a minimum of three to four applicants for each available place. In summary, we have numerous young people hoping to serve as genetic counselors in clinical service programs, and the number of people seeking this training is growing.

The stated purpose of the six programs training Genetic Associates is to provide professionals competent to serve existing and potential community needs for genetic services in both counseling and related areas in clinical genetics. While curricular differences certainly exist among all the programs, all programs offer course work in most of the areas in Table 2.

The 1977-1978 Sarah Lawrence College curriculum is described in more detail in Table 3. The 500 hours of fieldwork training is made possible by the diverse clinical opportunities available at the 17 hospitals where students train in the greater New York metropolitan area.

Let us now turn to the question of how this training has been put to use. Information about all 195 graduates of masters programs for Genetic Associates between 1971-1977 was obtained from each of the five programs to have awarded degrees. Rutgers and Sarah Lawrence have trained the majority of these graduates.

Table 5 presents data on the employment patterns of Genetic Associates and also includes information about graduates who are not serving in the field of clinical genetics. The first category, Clinical Genetics and Genetic Counseling, includes individuals serving as counselors whose primary function is patient-oriented. The second category, Research and Teaching, Laboratory and Clinical, would include graduates working in the area of genetics but without direct patient contact. These two categories of graduates total 135 individuals. This indicates that 69.2% of graduates from masters programs in human genetics are currently utilizing their training in the delivery of genetic services.

The data of graduates who have sought further training after receiving an M.S.

TABLE 3

1977 Curriculum
Human Genetics Program – Sarah Lawrence College

Prerequisite Undergraduate Courses:	
Biology	Probability and Statistics
Developmental Biology	Chemistry
Two Year Curriculum	
Mendelian and Molecular Genetics	1 Semester
or	
Seminar in Human Genetics	1 Semester
Human Physiology and Anatomy	2 Semesters
Laboratory Techniques in Human Cytogenetics and Human Biochemical Genetics	1 Semester
Introduction to Medicine	½ Semester
Biochemistry	1 Semester
Issues in Clinical Genetics Seminar	3 Semesters
Seminar in Techniques of Genetic Counseling	2 Semesters
Advanced Medical Genetics	2 Semesters
Fieldwork and Supervised Clinical Training	10 Credits (500 hours)

TABLE 4

M.S. Graduates in Human Genetics 1971-1977

Berkeley	15
Colorado	4
Irvine	7
Rutgers	69
Sarah Lawrence	100
	195

TABLE 5

How are Graduates Using Their Training?

	Number
Clinical Genetics/Genetic Counseling	
Berkeley	5
Colorado	2
Irvine	3
Rutgers	39
Sarah Lawrence	67
	116
Research/Teaching, Laboratory and Clinical	
Berkeley	3
Colorado	1
Irvine	1
Rutgers	2
Sarah Lawrence	12
	19
Further Graduate Study	
Berkeley	2
Colorado	1
Rutgers	17
Sarah Lawrence	6
	26
Seeking Employment in Clinical Genetics	
Berkeley	3
Irvine	3
Rutgers	8
Sarah Lawrence	11
	25
Employed in Non-Genetics Field or Not Seeking Employment	9

is interesting. While career goals inevitably change for some students, we at Sarah Lawrence are anxious not to dilute our effectiveness by encouraging graduates to seek further advanced training, thereby preventing their entry into clinical genetics. To avoid this, careful screening of applicants allows students to make realistic career choices. The Rutgers program, however, considers masters training in human genetics to be an appropriate educational effort for those who seek medical, dental, or doctoral degrees. For this reason, you will note that about 25% of their graduates have entered programs for advanced degrees.

To document further the history of this new health career, I have studied closely what graduates of the Sarah Lawrence program do once they become members of a genetic counseling team. To do this, a questionnaire was mailed in August 1977 to each employer of a graduate who was known to be working in clinical genetics or genetics-related work. An 86% response was achieved. If we assume that the Sarah Lawrence College graduates are fairly representative of the field as a whole, then we have a profile of what Genetic Associates are doing around the country. The 55 Genetic Associates on whom this profile is based are employed in 12 states and in Israel and represent 82% of all Sarah Lawrence graduates in clinical work.

The clinical responsibilities assigned to these graduates are detailed in Table 6. You will note that the physicians supervising these 55 Genetic Associates tell us that 24 of them are responsible for primary genetic counseling. This information may be challenged or questioned by those geneticists who believe primary counseling should be exclusively the domain of the physician. Our data reveals, however, that in practice a sizable number of geneticists are confident that primary and follow-up counseling can be handled by non-physicians once a diagnosis has been made and provided there is close and adequate physician supervision of the overall program of care. I would draw your attention to two areas in clinical genetics where Genetic Associates increasingly serve an important role; namely, follow-up counseling, where 93.6% of this group function, and in pre-amniocentesis counseling, where 74.5% are utilized.

Because amniocentesis is not a well-known procedure and the concept of penetrating the abdomen and uterus is highly anxiety-provoking to most pregnant women, a thorough explanation of the procedure itself is essential. Experience has shown that women who receive only a cursory description are apt to refuse the procedure out of unfounded fear. To reach an informed decision, women must understand the severity of the defects that may be uncovered and they must have a clear idea of what information will *not* be disclosed by the test. It is especially important to inform women prior to amniocentesis that there may be difficulty obtaining the proper fluid or that the culture may fail to grow. Prior knowledge of these possibilities will help dispel the idea that the fetus is abnormal should these problems arise.

The questionnaire sought data on the degree of independence accorded Genetic Associates in their clinical work. Their supervisors were asked to rate independence according to the categories, “considerable, a moderate amount, almost

TABLE 6

Clinical Responsibilities Assigned to Sarah Lawrence College Genetic Associates

	Number	Percent*
Intake	45	81.8
Family History	54	98.2
Pedigree	53	96.4
Searching the Literature for Incidence Figures	39	70.9
Clinic Coordination	38	69.0
Coordination of Community Screening Programs	22	40.0
Formulation of Diagnosis	14	25.5
Primary Counseling	24	43.6
Follow-up Counseling	46	83.6
Pre-Amniocentesis Counseling	41	74.5
Library Research in Preparation of Research Manuscripts	44	80.0
Teaching	46	83.6
Laboratory	6	10.9

*100% equals 55 Associates.

TABLE 7

Sarah Lawrence College Genetic Associates Offer Instruction About Genetic Counseling to the Following Groups:

	Number	Percent*
Medical House Staff	24	43.6
Medical Students	23	41.8
Continuing Education Courses for Physicians	22	40.0
Other Health Professionals	43	78.2
Consumers	39	70.9

*100% equals 55 Associates.

none" and "not applicable". The replies indicate that 63.6% felt considerable responsibility accompanied the position of Genetic Associate, and 36.4% thought it to be a moderately independent position.

Another area of responsibility accorded 78.2% of genetic counselors is particularly interesting; that is, teaching other health professionals genetic concepts and acquainting them with the indications for a genetic counseling referral. Table 7 indicates a breakdown of particular groups served by Genetic Associates in this educational capacity.

Several publications in recent years have directed attention to the need for massive public education efforts to inform the American people of the availability and the necessity of preventive services in genetics.[6,7] The National Genetic Diseases Act[8] includes the provision that the development and dissemination of informational and educational materials on genetic diseases be an integral part of any comprehensive program to deal with genetic disease on a national scale. The extensive use of Genetic Associates' time in such educational efforts indicates that these health professionals are presently serving in this capacity: 78.2% are teaching health professionals, particularly nurses, and 70.9% are regularly engaged in educational efforts with consumers. This educational function could, and probably will, expand as services develop throughout the country. Perhaps training programs for genetic counselors need to assume greater responsibility for preparing their students to be effective public educators. At Sarah Lawrence our efforts in this area have been sporadic.

The unanimously positive response to the following question prompts me to share this information. Respondents were asked if the clinic responsibilities assigned to the Genetic Associate allow physician time to be spent more productively: 92.3% of the physician-supervisors responded "yes"; and many said "absolutely", "very definitely", or "of course". These same people told us that their unit has employed a Genetic Associate for periods that ranged from seven years to two months. A surprising number, 33 of 55, referred to positions of at least two years duration.

Increasingly, Genetics Associates' salaries are paid by the hospital. In the group covered by this survey, 11 positions, or 20%, were funded in this way; 33, or 59.9%, were funded by grants, both government and private. The salary range for Genetic Associates is $10,000 – $21,000. While genetic counseling is a reimbursable service in some areas, it is not reimbursable in many instances. Some hospitals have begun to charge on an hourly basis for genetic counseling perfomed by Genetic Associates. Clearly, an effort must be made to educate and encourage third party payers to consider genetic counseling an essential element of clinical genetic care.

While reimbursement of genetic counseling by non-physicians at the same rate accorded physicians may enhance the professional acceptance of Genetic Associates, it does not create a cost-effective rationale for increasing the ranks of Genetic Associates in the health care system.[9] In the long run, this may be a self-defeating development for those whose goal is to extend preventive services in genetics to the broadest segment of society.

Although genetic counseling is usually considered to be a service of the out-patient department, it is interesting to note the number of Genetic Associates serving in-hospital patients as well. Our information reveals that 43, or 78.2%, of the Genetic Associates serve patients on the obstetrical, pediatric, neurological, neonatal, and medical services. Perhaps the only service conspicuously absent might be the orthopedic!

A final question directed at suggestions for improving the training of Genetic Associates elicited a few interesting thoughts. Several suggested that Genetic Associates be taught to do venipuncture, that even more intensive training in counseling skills be offered, and that organizational skills relative to administering genetics clinics be taught along with instruction in the art of follow-up letter writing. Perhaps the wisest suggestion of all was to maintain diversity of training!

In summary, masters level training for Genetic Associates, or genetic counselors, has been offered for eight years and has trained 195 persons, of whom 136 are presently serving as members of clinical genetics services throughout the United States and in Israel. We know that the 55 graduates from Sarah Lawrence, about whom we have in-depth information, are making a strong professional contribution to the field of clinical genetics in terms of patient care and educating diverse groups of individuals about inherited disease and preventive care. The present number of graduate programs training genetic counselors have the capacity to train nearly 50 persons per year. While any expansion of preventive genetic services on a national scale will quickly absorb these counselors, the present rate of growth in the field seems well matched to the number of trainees.

REFERENCES

1. J.H. Marks and M.L. Richter, *Am. J. Publ. Hlth. 66*, 388, 1976.
2. Nat. Res. Coun. Genetic Screening: Programs, Principles, and Research, Washington, D.C., Nat. Acad. Science, 1975.
3. A. Milunsky (Ed.), Prevention of Genetic Disease and Mental Retardation, W.B. Saunders, pp. 64-87, 1975.
4. V.M. Riccardi, The Genetic Approach to Human Disease, Oxford Univ. Press, New York, pp. 225-229, 1977.
5. C.L. Clow, F.C. Fraser, C. Laberge and C.R. Scriver, *in* Progress in Medical Genetics, Vol. 9, A.G. Steinberg and A.G. Bearn (Eds.), Grune & Stratton, Inc., New York, pp. 159-213, 1973.
6. R.P. Cox, E.W. Reich and J.B. Cox, *in* Trends and Teaching in Clinical Genetics, J.H. Marks (Ed.), *Birth Defects: Orig. Art. Ser. Vol XIII, 6*, Alan R. Liss, New York, pp. 155-165, 1977.

7. Commission for the Control of Huntington's Disease and Its Consequences, Vol. I, Summary Report, Washington, D.C., October 17, 1977.
8. The National Genetic Diseases Act, P.L. 94-278, Title IV.
9. C.E. Lewis, R. Fein, D. Mechanic, A Right to Health, the Problem of Access to Primary Medical Care, John Wiley, New York, 111-126, 1976.

GENETIC KNOWLEDGE OF PEDIATRICIANS AND OBSTETRICIANS (CONNECTICUT, 1975, 1977): IMPLICATIONS FOR CONTINUING EDUCATION *

Y. Edward Hsia
Katherine K. Bucholz
Cheryl A. Austein

INTRODUCTION

Under the theme of education in genetics, our study is an assessment of the knowledge, attitudes, and learning preferences of primary physicians.

Primary physicians are in a pivotal position for determining the access of their patients to medical genetics services. Their recognition of patients' genetic enquiries must necessarily be based upon the extent of their own genetic knowledge.[1,2] Practitioners' performance is exceedingly difficult to measure, is not assured by the posession of knowledge, but cannot be adequate in the absence of knowledge.[3] Since experience and training appear to be key determinants of medical performance,[4] assessment of knowledge should be compared with practitioners' backgrounds.

We therefore compared five fundamental factors related to genetic performance: primary physicians' training and experience; their knowledge; their attitudes toward a clinical genetic problem; their opinions about the relevance of genetics to their professional responsibilities; and their continuing education preferences. Our objectives were to obtain descriptive definitions of these factors, so that prescriptive measures can be proposed to enhance their genetic knowledge. We believe our findings have important implications for the planning of continuing education strategies for genetics.

METHODS

We focused on circumscribed target populations, in the expectation that the validity of our findings may then be generalizable to a greater population of

*Supported in part by a special grant from the Connecticut Chapter of The Sons of Italy, by NIH Grant GM 20124-04 and by the National Foundation-March of Dimes Medical Service Grant C-143.

ISBN 0-12-562650-9

primary physicians.

The two target populations selected were the universal subsets of all pediatricians and all obstetricians in Connecticut. These two groups are both trained medical specialists with professional standards set by their own Certification Boards. In Connecticut, a small, moderately affluent, industrial New England state, these specialists, rather than the traditional family practitioners, serve as the primary physicians[5] for most mothers and children. The Connecticut State Health Department Licensing Division registers all pediatricians and obstetricians by specialty, and so we were able to avoid any bias of sampling by surveying every pediatrician and every obstetrician in our target population.

These populations have had professional interaction with our medical genetics services at Yale for the past decade, and we hoped they would be responsive to our enquiries. We sought to optimize the response rate by obtaining the endorsements of their respective State professional organizations, their academic and community leaders, and the Offices of Continuing Education at the major medical centers in the State.

We used self-administered questionnaires, pre-tested on geneticists and other physicians, under protocols approved by the Human Investigation Committee at Yale.

Pediatric Survey

For the pediatricians, the survey was conducted in August 1975, immediately before the first Personal Assessment of Continuing Education (PACE) examinations conducted by the American Academy of Pediatrics. The questionnaire (Appendix A) contained 19 FACT questions about neonatal screening, prenatal diagnosis, and indications for chromosome testing; and seven REASON questions about recurrence risks for some common Mendelian disorders, such as cystic fibrosis; so-called polygenic malformations, such as Fallot's tetralogy; and conditions where new mutations have to be considered, such as achondroplasia. A second section asked how they would deal with a young couple whose child had trisomy 21.

Demographic information was requested about their professional training, type and size of practice. The questionnaire also asked which areas of genetics they deemed important for their practice, and their learning preferences both in general pediatrics and in genetics. Interviews with 44 respondents and 11 non-respondents explored their attitudes and preferences in greater depth.

Obstetric Survey

For the obstetricians, the survey was conducted in May 1977 (Appendix B). Their FACT questions covered topics on chromosome tests for women, genetic diseases in mothers, effects of maternal genetic disease on the fetus, and teratological agents in pregnancy. The same questions on fetal diagnosis were used as for the pediatricians' survey. The obstetric REASON questions had more simplified wording, but covered the same concepts. The same questions on fetal diagnosis were used as for the pediatricians' survey. The obstetric REASON questions had more simplified wording, but covered the same concepts. The other sections were similar, but included questions on the number of births, therapeutic abortions, and mid-trimester amniocenteses they had had in their practices in 1976.

Scoring

Scoring for the genetic questions awarded one point for each correct question. More sophisticated scoring systems did not alter the interpretations or implications of our findings. For their preferred learning sources, respondents were asked to rank their top four choices in order. Four points were given for top choice, down to one point for fourth choice.

As an additional incentive, all respondents were invited to request explanatory notes that we had prepared for the objective genetic questions. This furthered two ulterior purposes of these surveys, which were to heighten the awareness and increase the knowledge of these practitioners about genetic problems their patients might have.

RESULTS

Response Rate and Demographic Characteristics

Analyzable responses were obtained from 218 of 374 pediatricians (58% response rate), and 122 of 317 obstetricians (38% response rate), after excluding all on the Licensing Division lists who had expired, retired, or were not in clinical practice, and eliminating all incomplete responses (Table 1). We also received responses to our first survey from 52 of 112 pediatric residents in the six pediatric training programs in Connecticut.

Because the Licensing Division had key demographic data on non-respondents, we were able to determine that there were no significant differences in sex, time and place of training, or type of practice between respondents and non-respondents. The only significant differences were in Board-Certification. Among the pediatricians, 82% of respondents were Board-Certified, versus 67% of non-respondents, and among obstetricians, 86% were Board-Certified versus 68%. A difference between the two groups was that the obstetricians had more older graduates. The proportion who responded in each decade of training, however was representative for both surveys.

One-third of the responding pediatricians had subspecialty training in various areas, 33% were in solo practice, 41% in group partnerships, 15% hospital-based (13% had full time academic appointments), and the others ran clinics, worked part-time, etc. The obstetricians had longer residency training (4-6 years versus 3-4 years), 7% had subspecialty training, 40% were in solo practice, and 60% were in group partnerships. Those in solo practice tended to be older and to

TABLE 1

Selected Demographic Data on the Surveyed Populations

	Pediatricians		Obstetricians	
	Total	Respondents	Total	Respondents
	374	218	317	122
Decade of graduation:				
Before 1940	34	17	13	6
1940-1949	73	43	109	28
1950-1959	105	66	100	38
1960-1969	152	87	85	46
1970-	10	5	10	4
Residents:	118	52		
Foreign medical graduates:	63	39	45	19
Board certified:	282	178	238	105
Men:	312	192	298	115
Women:	62	26	19	7

have graduated earlier.

Attempts to characterize the size of the pediatricians' practices were unsuccessful. Even in the interviews, most had sparse data on the number of patients they served. Many could recall patients with genetic problems in the interviews, especially when prompted, but could give no valid estimate of the proportion of patients with genetic problems in their practices.

Obstetric practices could be more precisely characterized by the number of births supervised per annum. By this criterion, the respondents claimed responsibility for 18,000 births, which was approximately 50% of the births in Connecticut in 1976. The number of therapeutic abortions per annum varied from some respondents who had none to 17 respondents who had more than 500 each. Severty-two percent claimed to have had patients who had undergone amniocentesis.

Respondents' Scores

The knowledge questions were divided into FACT questions, about recent advances in clinical genetics likely to be relevant to these practitioners, and REASON questions on basic genetic principles, using clinical problems which might occur in their practices.

Summaries of respondents' scores are presented in Tables 2-6.

Answers to these objective questions showed analyzable differences between those questions which were well-answered and those which were less well-answered, and also between respondents who had answered well and those who had answered less well (Tables 2-6). No respondent had all correct answers, and no one had no correct answers. The pediatric FACT question on thyroid screening and the obstetric FACT question on breast cancer were excluded from analysis, as were the two prediatric REASON questions on Down syndrome, because poor responses raised doubts as to their clarity or validity. (Inclusion of these would not have altered the thrust of our findings.)

In the pediatric questions on neonatal screening (Table 2), there was a correlation with time of development of the screening tests. The highest scores were for phenylketonuria (PKU), a test in use in Connecticut for the past ten years; lower scores for galactosemia, in use for five years; and lowest scores for hypothyroidism, not yet in use then in Connecticut, although publicized in the current literature.[6]

On indications for chromosome testing, pediatricians scored best on those where fewer had indicated "don't know", and least well on rarer conditions where many respondents erroneously expected chromosome tests to be informative. Obstetricians indicated "don't know" more frequently on chromosome testing. Again apparent was the tendency to expect this test to be informative in less familiar conditions.

The only area where almost identical questions were used in the two surveys was on fetal diagnosis (Table 3). The correct answers to questions about trisomy 21, Tay-Sachs, and myelomeningocele, as well as the incorrect answers on PKU,

TABLE 2

Responses to Pediatric Fact Questions About Neonatal Screening Tests And Chromosome Testing

Tests Possible on Drop of Dried Blood	Percent Correct Answers
Phenylketonuria	99%
Hemophilia*	81%
Galactosemia	64%
Athyreotic cretinism**	20%

*Not possible
**Excluded from analysis

Chromosome Testing Indicated	Percent Correct Answers
Ambiguous genitalia	93%
Multiple malformations	90%
Suspected cystic fibrosis*	89%
Suspected mucopolysaccharidosis*	74%
Delayed puberty	86%

*Not indicated

TABLE 3

Responses to Pediatric and Obstetric Fact Questions About Fetal Diagnosis

	Percent Correct Answers	
Fetal Testing Routinely Possible	Pediatric	Obstetric
Achondroplasia*	53%	21%
(Cleft lip and palate*)	(77%)	–
Cystic fibrosis	62%	38%
Diabetes mellitus*	87%	76%
Down syndrome, Trisomy 21	95%	99%
Fallot's tetralogy*	87%	64%
Myelomeningocele	52%	91%
Phenylketonuria*	55%	47%
(Sickle cell anemia*)	(63%)	–
Tay-Sachs disease	83%	91%

*Not possible

(The questions about cleft lip and palate and about sickle cell anemia were not posed to the obstetricians.)

TABLE 4

Responses to Obstetric Fact Questions About Chromosome Testing And Hazards of Pregnancy

Chromosome Testing Indicated		Percent Correct Answers
Primary amenorrhea		77%
Possible Duchenne carrier*		28%
Mother of child with spina bifida*		58%
Multiple abortions		73%
*Not indicated		
Obstetric Hazards to Mother		
Diabetes mellitus		89%
Marfan syndrome		35%
Phenylketonuria*		64%
Sickle cell disease		94%
*No obstetric hazard to mother		
Fetal Hazards	**Maternal Exposure**	
Malformations	Operating Room personnel	72%
Withdrawal symptoms	Alcoholism*	52%
Abortion indicated	Rubella exposure of immune mother*	76%
Fetal loss, not malformations	Lysergic acid (LSD)	32%

*Not major hazard (alcoholism causes fetal loss and malformations; rubella exposure is safe for immune mother).

TABLE 5

Responses to Pediatric Reason Questions

Recurrence Risk for Future Children of Parents	Percent Correct Responses
Fallot's tetralogy, greater risk with second affected child	54%
Duchenne muscular dystrophy, greater risk with second affected child	33%
Sickle cell disease, equal risk with one or two affected children	66%
Sickle cell disease, greater risk with affected child, no risk with only affected mother	78%
Achondroplasia, greater risk with affected parent than with affected child	26%

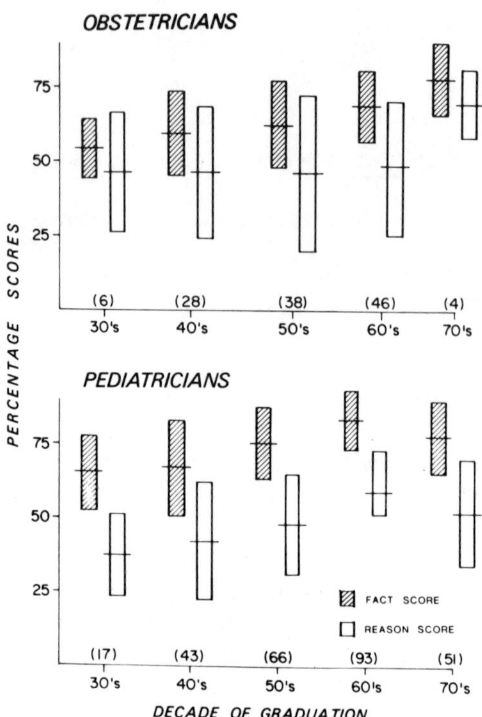

Fig. 1. FACT and REASON Scores of Respondents. Obstetricians' scores are in the upper graph and pediatricians' in the lower graph. The bars represent mean ± 1 standard deviation of respondents' FACT (striped) and REASON (open) scores plotted by decade of graduation. The numbers in parentheses are the number of respondents in each category.

cystic fibrosis and achondroplasia, again demonstrated the tendency to expect rare genetic disorders to be testable, and well-established tests were better recognized than more recent albeit well-publicized tests.[7] Obstetricians scored better on the testable conditions, perhaps, in part, because of the greater relevance of these tests to their clinical responsibilities, but possibly also because the pediatric survey was conducted 20 months earlier than the obstetric survey, when there may have been less familiarity with these tests.

The REASON questions (Tables 5, 6) showed better familiarity with inheritance of sickle cell disease than of multifactorial disorders; the concept of new mutations for the X-linked disorders was poorly answered; for achondroplasia, the wording of the obstetrician's question may have been too obvious.

When the scores were compared with the demographic characteristics of respondents, the only significant findings were all related to chronological factors such as age, time in practice, etc. Since all these factors were obviously interrelated, analyses are presented only for scores by decade of graduation from medical school (Fig. 1).

There was a clear association of FACT scores with time for both obstetricians and pediatricians, but the REASON scores showed this trend only for pediatricians. The data for graduates in the 1970's are not significant; for the obstetricians because there were too few respondents; and for the pediatricians because virtually all the respondents were still house officers who may have represented a different population from Connecticut practitioners.

Opinions and Attitudes

Respondents' opinions are tabulated (Tables 7, 8); their judgement of importance of areas of genetics are presented graphically (Fig. 2), and their learning references, scored according to ranking, are also presented graphically (Fig. 3).

In questions about the attitudes of these specialists toward informing their patients (Tables 7, 8), the majority of each group felt they themselves should be responsible for informing parents about the diagnosis, recurrence risks, and the option of fetal testing. The pediatricians were more unanimous about their own responsibility for the diagnosis and the obstetricians about their own responsibility for fetal testing.

Importance of Areas of Genetics

The ratings of areas of genetics showed differences between the two groups (Fig. 2). Fetal diagnosis was easily the most important area for obstetricians, but was the least important for most pediatricians. Another noteworthy finding was that pediatricians gave high ratings both to inheritance patterns and to congenital malformations, although they had scored much lower on analysis of inheritance. Rating of gynecologic genetic disease was only asked of obstetricians, who rated it

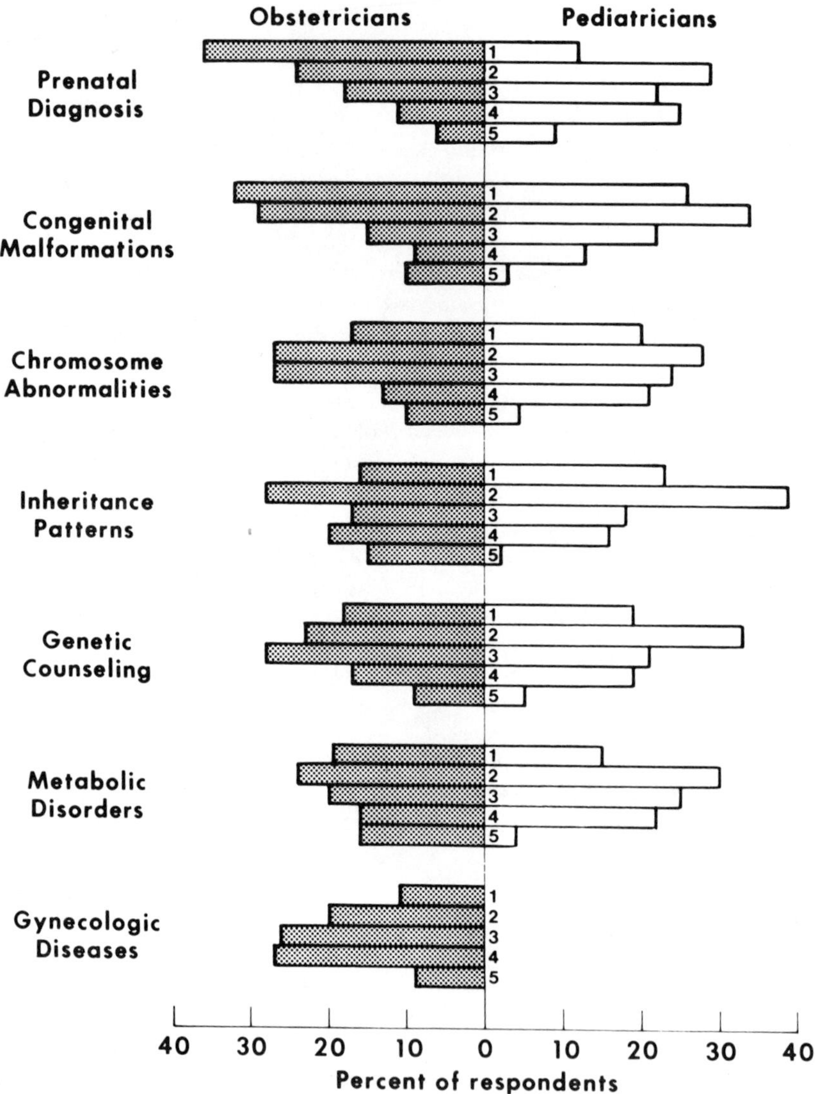

Fig. 2. Areas of Genetics of Importance to Respondents. For each area of genetics, the bars represent ratings (1= very important, 2 = important, 3 = somewhat important, 4 = slightly important, 5 = not important) by obstetricians (hatched bars) and pediatricians (open bars). The areas are listed in the sequence of importance as rated by obstetricians.

TABLE 6

Responses to Obstetric Reason Questions

Recurrence Risk for Future Children to Parents	Percent Correct Responses
One child with Fallot's tetralogy increases risk	41%
Hemophilic fathers cannot pass it to son	58%
Mother of a child with Duchenne muscular dystrophy need not be a carrier	15%
The number of children with sickle cell disease does not affect the recurrence risk	41%
A child with achondroplasia could have normal-statured parents	74%
The risk of Down syndrome for a 20 year old mother is less than 1 in 1,000	97%
The risk of Down syndrome for a 40 year old mother is about 1 in 100	82%
A normal amniocentesis test result does not assure a normal baby	94%

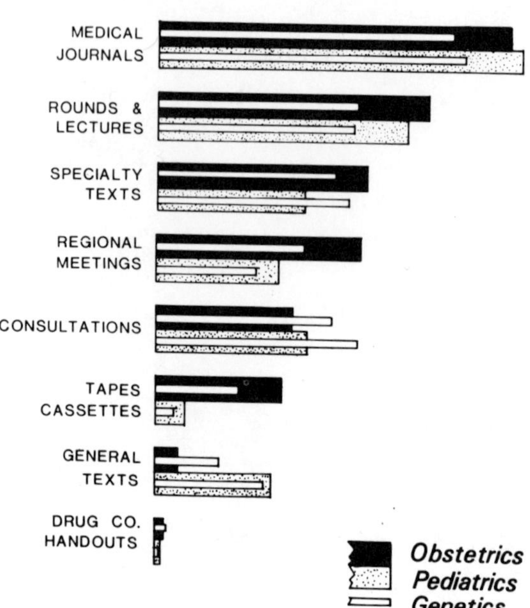

Fig. 3. Learning Preferences of Respondents. The thick bars represent obstetricians' (solid) and pediatricians' (dotted) ranking of continuing education modalities for their own general specialty. The superimposed narrow (open) bars represent respondents' ranking of continuing education modalities for genetics. The learning modalities are listed in the sequence of obstetricians' preferences.

TABLE 7

Pediatricians' Opinions

91%	would approve of fetal diagnosis.
95%	would test chromosomes of an infant with typical features of Down syndrome. (56% would test both parents as well.)
82%	estimated they informed most of their families with genetic problems about risks of recurrence.
44%	rarely discuss a genetic problem with a family.
90%	would tell the parents within the first week that an infant with Down syndrome was not normal.
94%	felt the pediatrician should first explain about the nature of Down syndrome. (None felt it should be the obstetrician.)
62%	felt the pediatrician should first explain about the recurrence risk for Down syndrome. (30% felt the geneticist should first explain it.)

TABLE 8

Obstetricians' Opinions

91% would suggest neonatal diagnosis for a woman who has had a child with Down syndrome, trisomy 21.

81% would recommend the option of fetal testing for sex to a hemophilia carrier who desired unaffected children.

91% would recommend heterozygote testing for Tay-Sachs to couples at risk.

Who should first explain about Down syndrome to parents of an affected baby?

The obstetrician	24%
The pediatrician	53%
Both together	10%

Who should first explain about recurrence risk and fetal diagnosis to parents of a baby with Down syndrome?

The obstetrician	67%
The pediatrician	3%
The geneticist	19%

disappointingly low. These ratings failed to show clear correlations with overall knowledge scores or with scores in specific areas of genetics.

Learning Preferences

The preferred learning patterns for genetics, or for general pediatrics and general obstetrics, were remarkably similar for the higher ranked options, except that genetic consultations were ranked higher than general consultations by both groups, and use of specialty texts for genetics was ranked high by pediatricians. Among the lower-ranked preferences, obstetricians claimed to have access to better tape cassette material (there were several favorable comments to this effect by obstetric respondents), but they appeared to place little reliance on general texts except, apparently, to brush up on their basic genetics. There was no clear correlation of learning preferences with knowledge scores, or with decade of graduation.

DISCUSSION

Study Design: Population

The choices of study population were based both on targets of opportunity and upon minimizing the inevitability of incomplete responses. We chose to define universal populations of specific practitioners in Connecticut rather than attempt to sample a respresentative fraction of a larger population. Since the proportion with Board-Certification for both obstetricians and pediatricians exceeded the national average,[8] we judged it extremely unlikely that the genetic knowledge of our target populations was less than that of physicians in general. Furthermore, within our populations, those who responded were unlikely to have known less than the non-respondents.[9] Therefore, it is reasonable to assume that our respondents' scores represented a best possible view of Connecticut physicians and of practitioners in general.

Our respondents' scores, opinions, and attitudes, being determined partly by their experiences, are not altogether generalizable. In Connecticut, these practitioners are in close proximity to major medical centers, have had frequent opportunities to attend rounds and lectures sponsored by the Regional Medical Program, and had ready access to two medical genetic centers for consultations and case referrals. Since this concentration of medical and educational resources is found mainly near large metropolitan areas, the experience of Connecticut practitioners can be expected to have enriched their exposure to advances in medical genetics, compared with many practitioners elsewhere.

Instrument

Our questionnaires, designed to be brief and simple, were intended merely to reveal areas of genetics where continuing education input was indicated. The results cannot be construed to be a measure of the actual genetic knowledge of the respondents, which must have been more extensive than can be tested by our instrument. Furthermore, it would not be valid to compare or contrast the overall scores of our two studies, because they used differing questions, addressed to two different specialist populations, and were conducted at different times. Our intent was to analyze each group's performance scores in terms of its own training and attitudes.

IMPLICATIONS

How much genetic knowledge should primary physicians have? Should they be able to diagnose, treat, and counsel about all genetic diseases? Will it suffice for them to check the literature or consult a geneticist whenever a genetic problem arises?

Optimal knowledge must lie between these extremes, because a primary physician must have enough knowledge to recognize a problem as genetic and should have enough familiarity with genetic principles to be able to use the literature wisely, or to consult with a geneticist intelligently.

Basic principles, as used in problem-solving, was tested by our REASON questions, and the imperfect scores of our respondents raise doubts about the effectiveness of formal medical education in imparting a command of these principles to practitioners. The lack of convincing improvement in REASON scores by more recent graduates, who had less time to forget what should have been better teaching, indicates a need for review of basic principles in continuing education. The high rating of patterns of inheritance by pediatric respondents is a commendable recognition of this need.

Recent advances in genetics was tested by our FACT questions. Indications for chromosome testing related to information established for one or two decades, whereas newborn screening, fetal diagnosis, and fetal hazards explored more recent advances, despite an overwhelming claim of reliance on medical journals.

How should continuing education address the genetic needs of practitioners? We feel the strategy would be to use well-recognized educational approaches applied in the context or practitioners' stated opinions and preferences. Repeated exposure,[10] using a variety of educational modalities, is most likely to suceed when the material is perceived to be relevant.[11] Retention of this material will be maximally reinforced with personal experience.[12]

Therefore, in areas of genetics perceived to be important, the challenge will be to provide both review and new information via journals and specialty texts, reinforced by rounds and consultations on patients presenting in the community. For areas deemed unimportant, however, the task of awakening interest is the more difficult one of changing attitudes by convincing practitioners that knowledge in the area is relevant to their clinical responsibilities.

Another important but difficult attitudinal problem would seem to be in the sharing of clinical responsibilities for the family. Apart from a few respondents, there was a distinct lack of any sense of shared responsibilities between the obstetricians and pediatricians. These two specialty groups, both in privotal positions for providing care to mothers and children, did not work together. In fact, in the interviews, many pediatricians disassociated themselves from any obligation to explain about fetal testing, while complaining that their obstetric colleagues were not fulfilling this obligation. Few respondents in either specialty indicated they saw families together with the other specialist.

Ideally, planned education programs, focusing on the needs of these practitioners, should have interactive feedback from participants about the value and effectiveness of the programs.[13] Criteria for judging the efficiency of educating primary physicians in genetics should focus on the care given to patients with genetic problems by primary physicians,[14] and on the teamwork developed by primary physicians with medical geneticists.[15]

ACKNOWLEDGMENTS

These studies would not have been possible without the endorsements of the Hezekiah Beardsley Society and the Connecticut Section of the American College of Obstetricians and Gynecologists, the Offices of Continuing Medical Education at the University of Connecticut and Yale University, the support and guidance of Drs. S.S. Mick, S.P. Korper, and Ms. E. Cohen, and the cooperation of all our colleagues who responded to our questionnaires.

REFERENCES

1. B. Childs, *Amer. J. Human Genet. 26*, 120, 1974.
2. B. Childs, *in* Trends and Teaching in Clinical Genetics, Birth Defects: Original Article Series, XIII, No. 6, Alan R.Liss, New York, p. 131, 1977.
3. R.H. Brook, *N. Engl. J. Med. 296*, 170, 1977.
4. E.H. Wagner, R.A. Greenberg, P.B. Imrey, C.A. Williams, S.H. Wolfe, and M.A. Ibrahim, *N. Engl. J. Med. 294*, 871, 1976.
5. J.R. Willson and D.M. Burkons, *Amer. J. Obstet. Gynecol. 126*, 627, 1976.
6. J.H. Dussault, P. Coulombe, C. Laberge, J. Letarte, H. Guyda and K. Khoury, *J. Pediatr. 86*, 670, 1975.
7. A. Milunsky and E. Alpert, *J. Pediat. 84*, 889, 1974.
8. Profile of Medical Practice 1975-1976, American Medical Association, Chicago, 1976.
9. R. Rosenthal and R.L. Rosnow, The Volunteer Subject, Wiley and Sons, New York, 1975.
10. R.N. Rodell, L.R. Gary and K. Keller, *J. Med. Educ. 50*, 888, 1975.
11. A.J. Scott, *N. Engl. J. Med. 295*, 444, 1976.
12. L. Gordis, B. Childs and M.G. Roseman, *Amer. J. Publ. Health 67*, 469, 1977.
13. F.L. Bowler, P.L. Brading, F.D. Burg, A.J. Finestone and J.P. Hubbard, *J.A.M.A. 237*, 1346, 1977.
14. T. Kushnick, *J.A.M.A. 235*, 623, 1976.
15. D.D. Rutstein, W. Berenberg, T.C. Chalmers, C.G. Child, A.P. Fishman and E.B. Perrin, *N. Engl. Med. 294*, 582, 1976.

APPENDIX A *

PEDIATRICIANS' SURVEY QUESTIONNAIRE
AND
EXPLANATORY NOTES ABOUT THE FACTUAL QUESTIONS

*Modified slightly for use in this volume.

QUESTIONNAIRE FOR CONNECTICUT PEDIATRICIANS ABOUT MEDICAL GENETICS

Instructions: Please *circle* the choice that you consider corresponds to the best answer. Please feel free to add any comments. A stamped envelope is provided for returning the questionnaire. If you wish to receive brief explanatory notes about the factual questions, please return your request in the second stamped envelope. Thank you for your cooperation.

I. QUESTIONS ABOUT GENETICS

A. Screening Tests

1. *Can* mass screening tests on a drop of dried blood be used to test the following disorders in the newborn population?

	Yes	No	Don't know
Phenylketonuria	1	2	3
Athyreotic cretinism	1	2	3
Hemophilia	1	2	3
Galactosemia	1	2	3

B. Prenatal Diagnosis

2. Are tests *routinely* used in Genetics Centers for diagnosing the following conditions *of the fetus* in mid-pregnancy? (By "routinely used", we mean established procedures performed regularly)

	Yes	No	Don't know
Achondroplasia	1	2	3
Cleft lip and palate	1	2	3
Cystic fibrosis	1	2	3
Diabetes mellitus	1	2	3
Down syndrome, Trisomy 21	1	2	3
Fallot's tetralogy	1	2	3
Myelomeningocele	1	2	3
Phenylketonuria	1	2	3
Sickle cell anemia	1	2	3
Tay-Sachs disease	1	2	3

C. Chromosome Tests

1. Are chromosome tests *indicated* for the following clinical situations?

Newborn infant with ambiguous genitalia	1	2	3
Newborn infant with multiple malformations	1	2	3
Child suspected to have cystic fibrosis	1	2	3
Child suspected to have mucopolysaccharidosis	1	2	3
Delayed puberty in a 17 year old girl	1	2	3

D. Recurrence Risks

For each of the following family situations, is the risk of recurrence of the condition in *future children* greater in family A or in family B?

	Greater risk in:	A or	B	Comparable	Don't know
4.	A: Fallot's tetralogy affecting *only one child* or B: This condition affecting *two* siblings	1	2	3	4
5.	A: Duchenne muscular dystrophy affecting *only one child* or B: This condition affecting *two* siblings	1	2	3	4
6.	A: Sickle cell SS disease affecting *only one child* or B. This condition affecting *two* siblings	1	2	3	4
7.	A: Sickle cell SS disease affecting *only one child* or B: Sickle cell SS disease affecting *only a mother* (father AA)	1	2	3	4
8.	A: Achondroplasia affecting *only one child* or B: This condition affecting *only a father*	1	2	3	4
9.	(Risk for Down syndrome): A: A 25 year old mother whose child has trisomy 21, Down syndrome, or B: A 40 year old mother whose child was normal	1	2	3	4
10.	In a family with one child affected by trisomy 21, Down syndrome, and another child affected by meningomyelocele, which condition has the greater recurrence risk: A: Trisomy 21, Down syndrome or B: Meningomyelocele	1	2	3	4

II. QUESTIONS ABOUT YOUR GENETIC PRACTICES

Please circle the response that most closely corresponds to your practice. There are no "correct" answers.

11. If a family of yours may be in a position to use prenatal diagnostic tests, what would you do *before* the mother becomes pregnant?
    a. Would you approve of the test?
        1. Yes.
        2. No, I would not approve because I feel the test is dangerous.
        3. No, I would not approve because I feel the test is inaccurate.
        4. No, I would not approve because I am against abortion.
        5. Other (please specify) ____________________
    b. Would you introduce the topic of testing as an option for the mother?
        1. Yes.
        2. No.
    c. Regardless of who introduced the topic of the tests, if it is brought up, would you:
        1. discuss the possibility of the test with the mother?
        2. refer her to an obstetrician directly?
        3. refer her to a geneticist directly?
        4. other (please specify____________________

If you had an infant with typical features of Down syndrome, born to a 30 year old mother, would you:

1. have the chromosome test done on the infant?
2. have the chromosome test done on the infant and both parents?
3. consider the chromosome test unnecessary?
4. consider the chromosome test the obstetrician's responsibility?
5. other (please specify) ____________________

Please mark on the following line the approximate proportion of your *families* with a serious genetic condition. (By this, we mean one that threatens the life expectancy or physical or mental well-being of the affected individual.)

1% 5% 10% 25% 40%
......./........./.........../........................../............................./..............
0 50%

Approximately what proportion of your *families* with serious genetic conditions do you inform about the nature and predicted recurrence risk for the condition? The proportion I inform *personally* is:

1. all of these families
2. most of these families
3. about half of these families
4. a few of these families
5. none of these families

How frequently in your practice are you likely to discuss a genetic problem with:

	daily	weekly	monthly	rarely	never
a parent	1	2	3	4	5
a colleague	1	2	3	4	5
a geneticist	1	2	3	4	5

III. QUESTIONS ABOUT YOUR OPINION

Assuming that the specialists are well-informed and there are no extenuating family circumstances, please circle the best *single* response for the following.

If an infant with Down syndrome but no cardiac or gastrointestinal complications is born to 20 year old parents, and found to have trisomy 21 by chromosome testing,

a. when, in your opinion, should the parents be told that this infant is not normal?
   1. within the first week after the birth of the child
   2. within the first month after the birth of the child
   3. later than the first month after the birth of the child

b. who should offer the first explanation to the parents about the nature of Down syndrome and their infant's future?
   1. the pediatrician
   2. the obstetrician
   3. the genetic counselor
   4. other (please specify) ______

c. who should offer the first explanation to the parents about the risk of having another child with Down syndrome and the option of prenatal diagnosis?
   1. the pediatrician
   2. the obstetrician
   3. the genetic counselor
   4. other (please specify) ______

IV. QUESTIONS ABOUT YOU AND YOUR PRACTICE

Age ______

Sex M___ F___

Training

Year you graduated from medical school ______

Medical school ______

Are you board certified? Yes ___ No, board eligible ___ No ___

Have you had subspecialty training? Yes (please identify) ______

No ___

Proportion of time practicing subspecialty ______%

Proportion of time practicing general pediatrics ______%

100%

Years of internship and residency training ______________

Years of fellowship training ______________

Practice

Years in practice after training ______________

Type of practice Solo_ Partnership__Group__(Number in group:__)

Hospital based___House staff__Other (please specify)______________

Approximate number of families in your practice __________

To how many hospitals do you have admitting privileges? __________

Do you have: a full time faculty appointment? __________

a part time faculty appointment? __________

neither _______ (check one, please)

How often do you teach:

	weekly	monthly	occasionally	rarely
House staff	1	2	3	4
Medical students	1	2	3	4
Other health personnel (please identify) ______________	1	2	3	4
Non-health personnel	1	2	3	4

Continuing Education

Please rank in order of importance the *4* most important resources you use to keep up with advances in pediatrics and genetics. (1 = most important, 2 = next most important, etc.)

Pediatrics

_ General texts
_ Specialty texts
_ Medical journals
_ Consultations with colleagues
_ Pharmaceutical company information
_ Rounds and seminars
_ Regional and national conferences
_ Other (please specify)

Genetics

_ General texts
_ Specialty texts
_ Medical journals
_ Consultations with colleagues
_ Pharmaceutical company information
_ Rounds and seminars
_ Regional and national conferences
_ Other (please specify)

How important are the following areas of genetics for your practice?

	Very important	Impor-tant	Somewhat important	Slightly important	Not important
Inheritance patterns	1	2	3	4	5
Congenital malformations	1	2	3	4	5
Chromosomes	1	2	3	4	5
Metabolic diseases	1	2	3	4	5
Prenatal diagnosis	1	2	3	4	5
Genetic counseling	1	2	3	4	5

EXPLANATORY NOTES

Dear Doctor:

Thank you for responding to our questionnaire. The questionnaire was designed to ask about important aspects and concepts of genetics rather than to evaluate individual performance.

The following are brief explanations about the factual questions. If you disagree with the explanations, please do not hesitate to contact me to discuss the matter.

Sincerely,

Y. Edward Hsia, M.D.
Associate Professor of Human Genetics
and Pediatrics

EXPLANATIONS TO FACTUAL QUESTIONS ABOUT GENETICS

A. Screening Tests

Which disorder *can* be detected on a drop of blood in newborn screening tests?

a. Phenylketonuria, affecting 1 in every 15,000 infants, is an autosomal recessive condition. It is regularly being tested for in Connecticut, but the test is most reliable after the fifth day, so the Department of Health and the Hezekiah Beardsley Society are recommending that *all* infants be tested on discharge from hospital *and* at the first office visit, which for general pediatric reasons should best be in the second week. Once diagnosed, patients can be protected from major brain damage by a carefully regulated low phenylalanine diet if it is started in the first few weeks of life.[1,2,7]

b. Athyreotic cretinism, a non-genetic disease, *can* be tested for, although the test has just been developed. One in every 7,000 infants may be hypothyroid at birth, so this test could detect 6 to 12 infants per year in Connecticut and enable replacement treatment to be started early. (Dussalt *et al., J. Pediat. 86*, 670, 1975.)

c. Hemophilia, an X-linked recessive condition, due to deficiency of coagulation factor VIII, cannot be detected on dried blood, but can be detected on fresh plasma. This condition affects about 1 in every 5,000 males.[1,2,7]

d. Galactosemia, an autosomal recessive condition, is being tested for in Connecticut. This condition, affecting only 1 in every 100,000 infants, causes neonatal jaundice, cataracts, gastrointestinal upset, and can be lethal or cause brain damage unless galactose is *promptly* excluded from the diet.[1,2,7]

B. Prenatal Diagnosis

Which conditions can be *routinely* tested for in the fetus in mid-pregnancy?

Amniotic fluid can be safely obtained at the 14th to 16th week of pregnancy for chemical analysis. Another useful test in mid-pregnancy is diagnostic ultrasonography for fetal head size. Fetoscopy, by means of an optical device in a needle inserted into the uterus, is still a research tool with great promise, but has not yet been proven to be safe, and is technically not yet reliable enough for visualizing congenital malformations. (J.C. Hobbins, M.J. Mahoney, *N. Engl. J. Med. 290*, 1065, 1975.)

a. Achondroplasia cannot be detected in mid-pregnancy, although x-rays in late pregnancy might show diagnostic bone changes. This would serve no useful purpose.

b. Cleft lip and palate cannot yet be visualized during pregnancy.

c. Cystic fibrosis cannot be reliably detected yet, although there are many tantalizing biochemical clues to its true biochemical nature, and a prenatal diagnostic test may be just around the corner. In people of Western European origin, about 1 in 20 is a carrier, and about 1 in 1,600 births is a child with cystic fibrosis.[2]

d. Diabetes mellitus has up to a 20% probability of affecting the infant if there is a strongly positive family history for juvenile diabetes, but the condition is *not* detectable in the fetus. Other fetal risks for diabetic mothers include miscarriages, congenital malformations, prematurity, and the IDM hypoglycemia syndrome.[1,3]

e. Down syndrome, trisomy 21, and all other chromosomal anomalies can be detected, including fetal chromosomal sex.[2,7]

f. Fallot's tetralogy and other congenital heart lesions cannot be detected yet, although there is promise that ultrasonography might detect the thickness, structure, and movements of the heart chambers in the near future.[1,3,7]

g. Meningomyelocele and anencephaly are associated with abnormally elevated alpha-fetoprotein in the amniotic fluid. This test has only been available for about three years, but is now offered routinely by genetics centers. It has at least 95% accuracy for these CNS malformations and may be abnormal in some other malformation syndromes too. Maternal blood alpha-fetoprotein has also been measurably abnormal in at least some pregnancies when the fetus has a CNS malformation; this could become a basis for screening all pregnancies for these conditions, which have a population incidence of about 1 in 600.[1,7] (H.L. Nadler, *Pediatrics 55*, 751, 1975.)

h. Phenylketonuria cannot be detected because the abnormal enzyme is only present in the liver, and is probably not active even in normal fetuses until late in gestation.

i. Sickle cell anemia can theoretically be detected by obtaining a drop of fetal blood from a placental blood vessel via fetoscopy. This has actually been successfully done, but only as an experimental procedure, and is not routinely available.[7] (J.C. Hobbins, M.J. Mahoney, *Lancet 2*, 107, 1975.)

j. Tay-Sachs disease, most of the lysosomal storage diseases such as the lipidoses and mucopolysaccharidoses, and several inborn errors of metabolism such as galactosemia and maple syrup urine disease are caused by enzyme deficiencies which can be detected in cultured amniotic cells. Each one of the tests is difficult and is carried out only in a few research laboratories, but every genetic center can arrange to have the appropriate test done in a pregnancy if indicated. The carrier rate for Tay-Sachs in Ashkenazim is 1 in 30. The Jewish community in Connecticut has a community screening program to detect carriers. Then, when two parents are both carriers, prenatal testing can be offered for their pregnancies.[5,7]

C. Chromosome Tests

When are chromosome tests indicated? In general, the test is indicated to confirm or exclude suspicion of a known chromosomal syndrome, or when multiple malformations and mental retardation suggest the possibility of an unrecognized chromosome abnormality. Chromosome abnormalities arise from errors of cell division and often are non-hereditary, but *unbalanced* translocations may be inherited from a parent who has a *balanced* translocation. Identification of the cause of the abnormalities as chromosomal will help define the prognosis, may alleviate any unreasoned parental guilt feelings, and could offer predictions and prenatal testing for future pregnancies.[3,4,7]

a. An infant with ambiguous genitalia should have chromosomes obtained without delay (unless it is known, for instance, that the child has congenital adrenal hyperplasia by family history). Chromosomal sex is much more *reliable* than a buccal smear, especially in the newborn infant, and should be one of the key considerations for sex designation of the infant.[2]

b. Any child with multiple malformations that suggest a chromosomal syndrome, or which do not obviously fit a known malformation syndrome, should have chromosome testing.

c. A child suspected to have cystic fibrosis should have testing of the meconium at birth for plasma proteins, or a reliable sweat chloride test at any age. The chromosomes show no detectable abnormality in this condition, which is caused by a single gene, far too small to be seen under the microscope.[2]

d. The mucopolysaccharidoses may show characteristic x-ray changes in the skull, hands, ribs, or spine, and may have abnormal glycoproteins in the urine, but will not show any detectable abnormalities by chromosome analysis. Special centers can provide tissue culture and enzyme tests to define the precise type of mucopolysaccharidosis, which may help in prognosis, genetic counseling, and prenatal testing.[2,5,7]

e. Delayed puberty in a 17 year old girl, even if there are no physical stigmata, could be due to chromosomal abnormalities such as testicular feminization or Turner syndrome. Chromosome testing is indicated as being more reliable than the buccal smear, and is of value for diagnosis, treatment, prognosis, and genetic counseling.[2]

D. Is the Recurrence Risk Greater in Family A or Family B?

4. Fallot's tetralogy, like most congenital heart lesions, is thought to be caused by a combination of multiple factors unless the heart lesion is part of a chromosome anomaly syndrome, or a multiple malformation syndrome, or unless it was caused by exogenous agents, such as rubella. The incidence of congenital heart lesions is about 1 in 200 of all births. If parents have had one affected child (or a parent is affected), the multiple factors evidently have already been operating unfavorably, so experience has shown that the recurrence risk is increased over 10-fold, to 2%-5%. After a family has had two affected children, the unfavorable factors are evidently even more potent, and the recurrence risk is even higher, about 10%-15%. Therefore, the greater the number of siblings affected, the worse the risk. The same observations apply if a parent is affected.[1] (greater in B)

5. Duchenne muscular dystrophy is an X-linked recessive condition, affecting about one boy in every 6,000. (A rarer autosomal myopathy has similar clinical features, but perhaps can be differentiated. (Gardner-Medwin, *J. Neuro. Sci. 13*, 459, 1971.) Since affected boys virtually never survive to reproduce, the high incidence must be maintained by new mutations. If one boy is affected, the mathematical probability, ignoring family history and maternal creatine phosphokinase, is 1 in 3 that the boy has a fresh *mutation* and 2 in 3 that the mother is a carrier; therefore, the risk for a second son is 33%. In this type of problem, the more normal sons a mother has, the less likely she is to be a carrier unless her brother or a second son is affected. If two brothers are affected, the odds are remote that they each represent a fresh mutation, so the mother is virtually certainly a carrier, with a 50% probability that any future sons will also be affected. Hence the risk is greater in family B with two affected sons. (A.E.H. Emery, *J. Neuro. Sci. 8*, 579, 1969.)

   In either case, the family may wish to know about the true probability of having another affected son, plus the option they would have of prenatal identification of fetal sex, to select for birth of only female offspring. Maternal relatives may also need to be informed about their risks.[6] (greater in B)

6. Sickle cell disease has an autosomal recessive pattern of transmission, like most inherited diseases affecting hemoglobin protein or enzyme proteins. Both parents have to be carriers (AS) for a child to have SS disease. Each child of the same parents then has a 25% risk of having SS disease, regardless of how many siblings have been affected.[6,7] (comparable, A = B)

7. If a mother has SS disease, she may have obstetric problems including: complications of urinary tract infections, and increased risk during induction of anesthesia. If the father has hemoglobin AA, then every child of that couple will inherit hemoglobin A from one parent and S from the other and be a carrier (AS) but will not have SS disease. Hence, family B has no

risk of a child having the disease.[6] (greater in A)

8. Classical achondroplasia has an incidence of about 1 in 100,00. It is an autosomal *dominant* condition, so an affected parent (family B) has a 50% risk for each child to be affected. If only a child is affected, however, and both parents are clinically normal (family A), the child must have a fresh *mutation* and the parents would face no risk of the condition reappearing. The child is genetically affected though, and will risk transmitting achondroplasia to his or her offspring. The differential diagnosis of achondroplasia includes diastrophic dwarfism, an autosomal *recessive* condition, so a correct diagnosis must precede genetic prediction of recurrence risks.[1–6] (greater in B)
9. The common form of Down syndrome, trisomy 21, represents 97% of such patients. The incidence is 1 in 600 for all births, but is only about 1 in 2,000 for a mother aged 25, and rises steeply with maternal age to about 1 in 300 at age 35, and to about 1 in 100 at age 40, regardless of number of normal children. After the birth of an affected child, however, there is evidence that additional factors other than maternal age may have been operating, and these factors cause the recurrence risk to be about 1 in 100 regardless of maternal age. (comparable, A = B)

   Three percent of Down syndrome patients have translocations. About one-third of these are familial with unbalanced translocations. Some family members would be balanced translocation carriers. So chromosome testing of the patient may indicate whether testing is needed for parents and their relatives.

   Patients at risk for having a child with a chromosomal abnormality such as Down syndrome may wish to learn about the availability of prenatal diagnostic tests. Then they can decide whether they want to use the test in a pregnancy.
10. Because trisomy 21 (family A) has a recurrence risk of about 1 in 100, and meningomyelocele (family B) has a multifactorial pattern of inheritance with a recurrence risk of about 1 in 20 or 30 after one affected child (including the risk for anencephaly and vice versa), the multifactorial condition has the higher recurrence risk.[1,2,3,6,7] (greater in B)

REFERENCES

1. An interesting and useful compendium of many genetic articles from Hospital Practice, edited by V.A. McKusick and R. Claiborne, is Medical Genetics (Hospital Practice Publishing, New York, 1973).
2. The second edition of L. Gardner's Endocrine and Genetic Disease of Childhood (Saunders, Philadelphia, 1975), is soon to be released.
3. An outstanding monograph on Congenital Malformations by J. Warkany (Yearbook Publishers, Chicago, 1971) will remain the definitive work for a long

time.

4. The best of the atlases is Atlas of Mental Retardation by L. Holmes, H.W. Moser, S. Halldorssom, C. Mack, S.S. Pant, and B. Matzilevich (MacMillan, New York, 1972).
5. The key reference catalog for all single gene diseases is V.A. McKusick's Mendelian Inheritance in Man (4th edition, Johns Hopkins University Press, Baltimore, 1975).
6. A good basic textbook is Genetics in Medicine by J.S. Thompson and M.W. Thompson (2nd edition, Saunders, Philadelphia, 1973).
7. Prenatal diagnosis is advancing and changing so rapidly that any book would be outdated. One recent authoritative review is in A. Milunsky's The Prevention of Genetic Disease and Mental Retardation (Saunders, Philadelphia, 1975). This book also has chapters on screening, treatment, etc.

APPENDIX B*

OBSTETRICIANS' SURVEY
INTRODUCTORY LETTER, QUESTIONNAIRE, AND EXPLANATORY NOTES ABOUT THE FACTUAL QUESTIONS

*Modified slightly for use in this volume.

February 1977

Dear Doctor:

Enclosed, please find a copy of a "Questionnaire for Connecticut Obstetricians About Medical Genetics". As you know, medical genetics has become highly relevant to obstetric practice because of the recent advances in heterozygote detection and in prenatal diagnosis of many genetic disorders. Your patients are being deluged with genetic "facts and fancies" by the mass media and are turning to you for information and guidance.

In order to assess how best to provide genetic information to the practicing obstetrician, please respond to these questions, which ask what you know about genetics, what you feel is important about genetics in your practice, and how you want genetics to be presented in continuing education.

Through this questionnaire, we hope to assess your needs as an obstetrician and as a primary care physician for a large proportion of women of childbearing age.

The Connecticut Chapters of ACOG and of Board Certified Obstetricians and Gynecologists, and the Departments of Obstetrics and Gynecology at the Universities of Connecticut and Yale have all endorsed this project as being of potential benefit to practicing obstetricians.

Please return your questionnaire before March 1. If you wish to receive answers and brief explanatory notes to the factual questions, we will be happy to send these to you after receipt of your questionnaire. In order to preserve your anonymity, please fill out the separate enclosed card for the explanatory notes. Your questionnaire responses will be examined only by coded number, and every precaution will be taken to preserve your confidentiality as we analyze the data. Finally, please feel free to comment on the questionnaire.

Thank you for your cooperation.

Sincerely,

Y. Edward Hsia, M.D.
Associate Clinical Professor of Human Genetics and Pediatrics
Director, Genetic Consultation Service

Cheryl F. Austein, M. Ph.
Associate in Research

Yale University School of Medicine

Enclosures

QUESTIONNAIRE FOR CONNECTICUT OBSTETRICIANS ABOUT MEDICAL GENETICS

INSTRUCTIONS: Please circle the choice that you consider corresponds to the best answer. Please feel free to add any comments.

A stamped envelope is provided for returning the questionnaire. If you wish to receive brief explanatory notes about the factual questions, please return the enclosed card. Thank you for your cooperation.

I. GENETIC INFORMATION

A. CHROMOSOME TESTS

Are chromosome tests of the *woman* indicated for the following clinical situations?

	Yes	No	Don't know
1. For a 20 year old woman who presents with a history of primary amenorrhea	1	2	3
2. For a 25 year old primipara who has two brothers with Duchenne muscular dystrophy	1	2	3
3. For a 30 year old woman who has had a child with spina bifida and hydrocephaly	1	2	3
4. For a 25 year old woman who has had 4 first trimester spontaneous abortions with no apparent obstetric or gynecologic cause	1	2	3

B. MATERNAL RISK

For which of the following medical conditions is pregnancy liable to cause serious maternal complications?

	Yes	No	Don't know
5. Diabetes mellitus	1	2	3
6. Marfan syndrome	1	2	3
7. Phenylketonuria (PKU)	1	2	3
8. Sickle cell anemia (HbSS)	1	2	3

C. GENETIC DISEASES IN GYNECOLOGY

	Yes	No	Don't know
9. Sisters of young women with bilateral breast cancer may have a 50-50 risk of developing breast cancer	1	2	3

D. PRENATAL DIAGNOSIS

Are established tests available in major medical centers for diagnosing the following conditions of the *fetus* in mid-pregnancy?

	Yes	No	Don't know
10. Achondroplasia	1	2	3
11. Cystic fibrosis	1	2	3
12. Diabetes mellitus	1	2	3
13. Fallot's tetralogy	1	2	3
14. Myelomeningocele	1	2	3
15. Phenylketonuria	1	2	3
16. Tay-Sachs disease	1	2	3
17. Trisomy 21, Down syndrome	1	2	3

E. FETAL RISK

	Agree	Disagree	Don't know
18. Pregnant women working in operating rooms have an increased risk of malformations affecting their babies.	1	2	3
19. If a mother is a chronic alcoholic, the major risk to her infant is one of serious withdrawal symptoms in the first week of life.	1	2	3
20. A woman has been exposed to rubella in the 8th week of pregnancy. If IgG rubella antibodies are found in her blood 5 days later, this is an indication for a therapeutic abortion.	1	2	3
21. Lysergic acid (LSD) is associated with increased fetal loss, but not increased limb malformations.	1	2	3

F. RISKS TO FETUS

	Agree	Disagree	Don't know
22. The birth of one child with Fallot's tetralogy increases the risk of this condition recurring in future offspring.	1	2	3
23. A man with hemophilia can never pass this condition on to his son.	1	2	3
24. A woman who has had one son with Duchenne (X-linked) muscular dystrophy need not be a carrier for this condition.	1	2	3

	Agree	Disagree	Don't know
25. The birth of two children with sickle cell disease (HbSS) does not alter the risks for future children of these parents.	1	2	3
26. A child with achondroplasia could not have normal-statured parents.	1	2	3

27. The risk of Down syndrome for the first born child of a 20 year old woman is: (please circle)
    more than 1 in 10 about 1 in 100 less than 1 in 1,000
28. The risk of Down syndrome for the first born child of a 40 year old woman is: (please circle)
    more than 1 in 10 about 1 in 100 less than 1 in 1,000

II. YOUR OPINION

Assuming that there are no extenuating family circumstances, please circle best *single* response for the following. There are no correct answers.

29. If a woman has had one child with Down syndrome, trisomy 21, would you suggest prenatal diagnosis for her?
    a. Yes.
    b. No, because I feel the test is not indicated.
    c. No, because I feel that the test is dangerous.
    d. No, because I feel that the test is inaccurate.
    e. No, because I am against abortion.
    f. Other ________________ (please specify)
30. Would you raise the subject of the test as an option to the mother?
    a. Yes.
    b. No.
31. Regardless of who introduced the subject of the test, would you:
    a. discuss the test with the mother?
    b. refer her to another obstetrician without discussing it?
    c. refer her to a geneticist without discussing it?
    d. other ________________ (please specify)
32. If a woman is known to be a carrier for hemophilia (she has a 50-50 risk of having an affected son) and desired unaffected children, would you recommend as an option:
    a. not having any children
    b. a prenatal chromosome test to determine the sex of a fetus during pregnancy
    c. having children without prenatal testing
    d. would make no recommendation
    e. other ________________ (please specify)

33. Would you recommend heterozygote screening for a couple at risk for Tay-Sachs disease?
    a. yes
    b. no, because ______________________ (please specify)
34. Who should offer the first explanation to the parents of a child with Down syndrome about the nature of the condition and their infant's future?
    a. the obstetrician
    b. the pediatrician
    c. the genetic counselor
    d. other ______________________ (please specify)
35. Who should offer the first explanation to the parents about the risk of having another child with Down syndrome and the option of prenatal diagnosis?
    a. the obstetrician
    b. the pediatrician
    c. the genetic counselor
    d. other ______________________ (please specify)

III. DEMOGRAPHIC DATA

(This information is for statistical analysis and will be kept confidential.)

36. Age _____
37. Sex: Male _ Female _
38. Year you graduated from medical school______________________________
39. Name of medical school ______________________________
40 Hospital and state of residency training ______________________________
41. Are you board certified? Yes _ No _
42. Have you had subspecialty training? Yes_ No __
43. Years of internship and residency training ______________________________
44. Years in practice after training ______________________________

IV. YOUR PRACTICE

(This information is for statistical analysis and will be kept confidential.)

45. Type of practice: __ Solo ___ Partnership ___Group (_No. in group)
    __ Hospital based ___ House staff____ Other ___________ (specify)
46. To how many hospitals do you have admitting privileges? __________
47. Approximate number of patients in your practice: _______________
48. Approximate number of deliveries in 1976: ___________________
49. Number of patients who had amniocentesis for genetic reasons (not for Rh or maturity) in 1976: ______________________________
50. Number of therapeutic abortions for genetic reasons in 1976: ________
51. Total number of therapeutic abortions in 1976: _________________

V. TEACHING

52. How often do you teach obstetrics or reproductive health to:

	weekly	monthly	occasion-ally	never
House staff	1	2	3	4
Medical students	1	2	3	4
Other health personnel (please specify)	1	2	3	4
Non-health individuals	1	2	3	4

53. How frequently in your practice are you likely to discuss a genetic problem with:

	daily	weekly	monthly	rarely	never
a parent	1	2	3	4	5
a colleague	1	2	3	4	5
a geneticist	1	2	3	4	5

VI. CONTINUING EDUCATION

Please rank in order of importance the *4* most important resources you use to keep up with advances in each category of obstetrics/gynecology and genetics. (1 = most important, 2 = next most important, etc.)

OBSTETRICS/GYNECOLOGY

___ General texts
___ Specialty texts
___ Medical journals
___ Consultations with colleagues
___ Pharmaceutical company information
___ Rounds and seminars
___ Regional and national conferences
___ Tapes
___ Other ________________________________ (please specify)

GENETICS

___ General texts
___ Specialty texts
___ Medical journals
___ Consultations with colleagues
___ Pharmaceutical company information
___ Rounds and seminars
___ Regional and national conferences
___ Tapes
___ Other ________________________________ (please specify)

How important are the following areas of genetics in your practice?

	very important	important	somewhat important	slightly important	not important
Inheritance patterns	1	2	3	4	5
Congenital malformations	1	2	3	4	5
Chromosomes	1	2	3	4	5
Metabolic diseases	1	2	3	4	5
Prenatal diagnosis	1	2	3	4	5
Genetic counseling	1	2	3	4	5
Genetic diseases of women	1	2	3	4	5

ANSWERS TO GENETIC QUESTIONNAIRE FOR OBSTETRICIANS

Dear Doctor:

Thank you for your response and interest. What follows is a general explanation of the answers to the factual questions in the questionnaire. We realize some of the answers are a matter of opinion, but trust that our answers will, nonetheless, be informative. We regret we cannot give any information on your individual performance, as we have preserved confidentiality by processing the responses without identification of the respondents.

I. GENETIC INFORMATION

A. *Chromosome Tests:* These are technically sophisticated tests, just as dependent on specialist interpretation as are x-rays or histopathology reports. These tests are used generally for determination of chromosomal sex and for abnormalities of chromosomal number or structure, or both.

"ARE CHROMOSOME TESTS OF THE WOMAN INDICATED IN THE FOLLOWING CLINICAL SITUATIONS?"

1. For a 20 year old woman with primary amenorrhea, the answer is "yes". (Danforth, p. 39, 743. Novak, p. 362, 364.)

   Abnormalities of the sex chromosomes, or abnormal genital development in an XY individual, can both produce primary amenorrhea. About 10% of women with primary amenorrhea may have Turner syndrome, due to an abnormality of X-chromosome structure or number; the commonest is absence of one X chromosome, 45,X. A buccal smear for Barr body heterochromatin alone is of limited value because of the possibilities of chromosome structural rearrangements or of mosaicism. Most patients with Turner syndrome have short stature, and may have other physical stigmata, but a diagnosis should be confirmed or excluded by chromosome tests in all patients with primary amenorrhea (Gardner).

   Patients with a testicular feminization syndrome have the male chromosome constitution, 46,XY. They have an X-linked gene causing end-organ unresponsiveness to testosterone. These patients have absent uteri, and may have maternal sisters with primary amenorrhea (Gardner).

2. For the sister of two brothers with Duchenne muscular dystrophy (which is an X-linked recessive disorder) the answer is "no".

   Chromosomes are irrelevant to the question of whether she is or is not a genetic carrier because genes cannot be seen microscopically.

3. For the mother of a child with spina bifida and hydrocephaly, the answer is "no".

   There is no chromosomal abnormality of either the parents or a patient with this disorder.

4. For a 25 year old woman with multiple spontaneous abortions with no apparent gynecologic cause, the answer is "yes". (Danforth, p. 42, 337. Novak, p. 335.)

   Either the woman with multiple abortions, or her husband, may have a 2% to 10% probability of having a chromosomal anomaly, a balanced translocation. The patient herself is clinically normal, but she would have a much higher risk of miscarrying, or of having a liveborn child with a serious malformation syndrome due to maldistribution of chromosomes in her ova (*N. Engl. J. Med. 293*, 844, 1975).

B. *Maternal Risk:* When the mother has an inherited disease, such as a myopathy, or a nephropathy, pregnancy can be associated with serious complications to herself. For instance, in neurofibromatosis, the nodules can increase drastically in size and number during pregnancy. In the Ehlers-Danlos syndromes (hyperelasticity of the skin, lax joint ligaments, and poor scar formation), there is reportedly a risk both of uterine atony and of uterine rupture in pregnancy (McKusick, 1972). Obstetricians cannot be expected to have first-hand experience with rare genetic diseases, but they should be aware, in general, that a genetic disease may increase the risk of maternal morbidity or even mortality. (The response "do not know" is more creditable than an incorrect response.)

   "FOR WHICH OF THE FOLLOWING MEDICAL CONDITIONS IS PREG–NANCY LIABLE TO CAUSE SERIOUS MATERNAL COMPLICATIONS?"

5. Diabetes mellitus is well recognized to increase the risks of pregnancy for the mother, so the answer is "yes". The management of a diabetic pregnancy can be extremely complicated (Danforth, p. 462; Burrow).

6. Marfan's syndrome has life-threatening complications of the cardiovascular system which are aggravated by pregnancy, so the answer is "yes".

   This is an autosomal dominant condition producing long body habitus and arachnodactyly, associated with scoliosis, dislocation of the ocular lenses, medial degeneration of the elastic arteries, and prolapse of the mitral valves. During pregnancy and the puerperium, there are dangers of dissecting aneurysm, but the size of this risk is not well defined (McKusick, 1972). Nonetheless, affected patients, if forewarned, may prefer to avoid pregnancy (*Obstet. Gynecol. 47*, 358, 1976).

7. Phenylketonuria (PKU) in the mother may damage the fetal brain, but has no known risk to the mother herself during pregnancy, so the answer is "no".

   The risk of brain damage from this inherited metabolic disease persists from birth only for the first few years of life, during which time a regulated diet may be vital for preserving a patient's intellect. The mature brain, however, is no longer susceptible to metabolic damage by PKU (Gardner).

8. Sickle cell disease (HbSS) in the mother gravely compromises her ability to endure the physiological stresses of pregnancy, so the answer is "yes" (Danforth, p. 472).

   She suffers from the complications of chronic anemia; reduced resistance to pneumococcal, salmonellar and other infections; impaired renal concentration ability; and is susceptible to the hazards of hypoxia and sickling crises (Burrow).

C. *Genetic Disease in Gynecology:*

Many serious genetic diseases can present initially to the gynecologist, or have important gynecological complications. Inherited coagulopathies such as von Willebrand's disease are complicated by menorrhagia; genetic abnormalities affecting the sex hormones produce malformations of the reproductive organs and external genitalia; other inherited hormone deficiencies may retard sexual maturation; abnormalities of the sex chromosomes may affect menstruation or fertility (Gardner).

9. For a young lady with a family history of premenstrual carcinoma of the breast affecting mother or sisters, especially if there have been multiple primaries, there is a high probability of a single dominant gene for carcinoma of the breast segregating in her family, so the answer is "yes".

   The risk of breast cancer is increased two-to three-fold if one close relative had premenstrual breast cancer, and up to nine-fold if it was bilateral (*J. Nat. Cancer Inst. 48*, 1029, 1972). Furthermore, there is convincing evidence of familial aggregation of cancer of the breast (or breast and ovary) following autosomal dominant patterns of inheritance (*Arch. Surg. 111*, 126, 1976).

D. *Prenatal Diagnosis:*

Fetal diagnosis in the second trimester is possible by non-invasive ultrasonography for placental location, head size, and very gross malformations. By needle aspiration, amniotic fluid can be obtained for chemical analysis, or amniotic cells can be cultured for chromosome analysis, ultrastructure, and metabolic studies. In experienced centers, amniocentesis has a hazard of fetal loss of less than 1 in 200 (*J.A.M.A. 235*, 1471, 1976). The usual indications are advanced maternal age; previous child with known autosomal chromosome abnormality; previous child with anencephaly or spina bifida; and known risk for an inherited biochemical disorder detectable in amniotic cells (Danforth, p. 696; Novak, p. 80). Fetoscopy, for fetal inspection, and fetal blood analyses for the hemoglobinopathies, are still experimental.

"ARE ESTABLISHED TESTS AVAILABLE IN MAJOR MEDICAL CENTERS FOR DIAGNOSING THE FOLLOWING CONDITIONS OF THE FETUS IN MID-PREGNANCY?"

10. For achondroplasia, the answer is "no".

    It is possible to demonstrate bony disproportions in late pregnancy radiographically, and it might become possible to measure limb shortening in mid-pregnancy by ultrasonography, but no test has been established yet. The incidence of new mutations for achondroplasia is about 1 in 100,000; the risk for a child of an affected parent is 50%. Maternal achondroplasia will complicate the pregnancy (Danforth. p. 487; McKusick, 1972).

11. For cystic fibrosis, the answer is "no".

    Many tests have been devised but no single test has been proven to be reliable up to the present (Gardner). This disease affects 1 in 1,600 births to parents of Western European descent, and has a recurrence risk of 25% for a sibling of an affected child.

12. For diabetes mellitus, the answer is "no".

    There is no test for whether the fetus will become diabetic. There is a genetic component in the etiology of diabetes, so if one of the woman's parents or siblings or children has juvenile onset insulin-requiring diabetes mellitus, her risk of developing diabetes mellitus is increased many-fold over the general population (*Lancet 1*, 589, 1977). Good diabetic control will decrease maternal complications, and may also reduce the hazards to the fetus of miscarriage, prematurity, stillbirth, immaturity (IDM), and congenital malformations.

13. For Fallot's tetralogy, the answer is "no".

    It may become possible, however, to detect major heart malformations in mid-pregnancy by ultrasound as the technique is refined.

14. For myelomeningocele or spina bifida, the answer is "yes".

    After the birth of one affected child, the recurrence risk is for both anencephaly and spina bifida, the combined risk being about 1 in 20. Over 95% of fetuses with major CNS malformations are associated with marked elevation of amniotic alpha-fetoprotein in mid-pregnancy (*Amer. J. Obst. Gyn. 122*, 313, 1975; *Obstet. Gynecol. 48*, 1, 6, 1976). This protein is also elevated in some other rare malformation syndromes. Ultrasound measurements of fetal head diameters can be useful for anencephaly, but not spina bifida.

    Maternal serum alpha-fetoprotein is detectably elevated in about two-thirds of pregnancies with major fetal CNS malformations, and screening of all mothers for the 1 in 500 or so abnormal pregnancies has been attempted in Britain (*Lancet 2*, 923, 1973).

15. For phenylketonuria, the answer is "no".

    The deficient enzyme, phenylalanine hydroxylase is a hepatic enzyme. Some recent claims that trace amounts of this enzyme are detectable in cultured cells have not yet been confirmed for amniotic cells (Gardner).

16. For Tay-Sachs disease, the answer is "yes".

    In the Ashkenazi Jewish population from Eastern Europe, about 1 in 30 individuals are carriers for Tay-Sachs. By measurements for the defective enzyme, hexosaminidase A, most carriers are found to have partial deficiency. For any couple who are both carriers, the risk of Tay-Sachs in a child is 25%. Amniotic cell hexosaminidase A is an accurate test for diagnosing Tay-Sachs in a fetus (Milunsky).

17. For trisomy 21, Down syndrome, the answer is "yes".

    Amniotic cells can be cultured for chromosomal analysis, which will show any chromosomal abnormality, and also the genetic sex of the fetus.

E. *Fetal Risk:*

Other than inherited disabilities, exogenous factors can threaten a conception or fetus. Some of these, such as thalidomide and rubella, are potent teratogens. Many other agents, such as diagnostic radiography, many drugs and hormones (including birth control pills) appear to be weaker teratogens (Danforth, p. 300, 428). Any pregnancy would be less hazardous or worrisome if all potential teratogens were avoided, but inevitably some mothers are exposed, and more data is needed on the actual harmfulness of each agent. (Heinonen *et al.*).

18. Pregnant women working in operating rooms do have an increased risk of congenitally malformed babies, so the answer is "yes".

    The risk for malformations seems to be increased two-fold for mothers and 25% for fathers working with anesthetic gases. The risk is less if the woman avoids exposure on becoming pregnant, but the risk for hospital personnel, in general, is double the population risk for congenital malformations (*Anesthesiology 41*, 341, 1974).

19. For a mother who is a chronic alcoholic, neonatal withdrawal symptoms are not the major risk, so the answer is "no".

    Alcoholic mothers have much higher rates for abortion, prematurity, stillbirths, and growth failure, but also have increased risks for the recently recognized fetal alcohol syndrome of malformations (*J.A.M.A. 235*, 1458, 1976; *Ann. N.Y. Acad. Sci. 273*, 115, 1976, May). Obviously, these mothers are candidates for malnutrition, poor antenatal care and other less complex problems, but this specific teratogenic effect of alcohol on fetal growth and development is another major risk.

20. For a woman exposed to rubella, IgG rubella antibodies would *not* become elevated in five days, hence, she must have been infected previously, and this finding is *not* an indication for abortion, so the answer is "no".

21. For lysergic acid (LSD), there is excellent evidence for increased abortions, and no convincing evidence for causing limb malformations in live births, so the answer is "yes". (Danforth, p. 429; *Science 172*, 431, 1971.)

F. *Risks to the Fetus:*

Recurrence risks for many disorders are well defined and predictable, following classical Mendelian inheritance patterns (autosomal, X-linked; dominant, recessive). Other disorders, such as spina bifida and anencephaly, have a definite but small genetic component, often with an additional environmental contribution (*e.g.*, folates and the fetus, *Lancet 1*, 462, 1977). These are multifactorial conditions, generally, with a 3% to 5% risk if a parent, brother, or sister is affected, and an 8% to 15% risk if two close relatives are affected. For a condition which has an unequal sex distribution such as spina bifida or congenital dislocation of the hips with preponderance of females, the risk is greater for affected individuals of the less affected sex (Thompson; *J. Med. Genet. 11*, 374, 1974).

22. The birth of one child with Fallot's tetralogy does increase the risk for future offspring, so the answer is "agree".

    This syndrome, like most congenital heart lesions (not secondary, *e.g.*, to Down syndrome) is multifactorial in etiology, and the greater the number of immediate relatives affected, the greater the risk for future offspring (Thompson; *Lancet 2*, 692, 1975).

23. A man with hemophilia can never pass this condition to his son, so the answer is "agree".

    This is an X-linked condition; since a man passes his Y chromosome to a son, and his single X-chromosome to a daughter, all of his daughters will become carriers, and none of his sons will be affected (Thompson).

24. A woman who has one son with Duchenne muscular dystrophy (DMD) need not be a carrier, so the answer is "agree".

    The reason is that, at least in theory, a new mutation might have occurred in her son. If assumptions are made that there is an equal likelihood of a mutation occurring in any X-chromosome, and that the disease incidence is not changing, then it can be calculated that there is one chance in three that she is not a carrier (Thompson). Serum creatine phosphokinase measurements will detect some carriers, and may determine whether she is a carrier, but no test is yet available to guarantee that she is *not* a carrier.

25. The birth of a second child with sickle cell disease (HbSS) does not increase the risks for future children of these parents, so the answer is "agree".

    The inheritance pattern is autosomal recessive, so the risk to carrier parents remains 25% regardless of the number of affected or unaffected children already born (Thompson).

26. A child with achondroplasia could have normal-statured parents, so the answer is "disagree".

    This is an autosomal dominant condition, with 50% risk to offspring of an affected parent, but many affected patients never have children, so the incidence of this condition in the population is sustained by new mutations. In fact, the majority of people with achondroplasia are born to normal-statured parents, and represent new mutations (McKusick, 1972).

27. The risk of Down syndrome for the first-born child of a 20 year old mother is "less than 1 in 1,000".

    Regardless of birth order, the risk is about 1 in 2,000 for a 20 year old mother. Once she has had an affected child, however, her risk for having another similarly affected child is about 1 in 100, unless the child has a chromosome translocation and she is a translocation carrier, when her risk could be higher (Gardner).

    There is no evidence for a higher risk in teenage mothers.

28. The risk of Down syndrome for the first-born child of a 40 year old mother is about "1 in 100".

    The risk for chromosome abnormalities rises steeply with maternal age after 30. Between age 35 and 40 the risk is about 1 in 300; by age 45 it is 1 in 35 (*Lancet 2*, 1198, 1976).

REFERENCES

I. Obstetric and Gynecologic References Cited

1. G.N. Burrow and T.F. Ferris, Medical Complications During Pregnancy, Saunders, Philadelphia, 1975.
2. D.N. Danforth (Ed.), Textbook of Obstetrics and Gynecology, Second Edition, Harper and Row, New York, 1971.
3. E.R. Novak, G.S. Jones and H.W. Jones, Gynecology, Ninth Edition, Williams and Wilkins, Baltimore, 1975.

II. Useful Genetic References

4. P. Bondy, L.E. Rosenberg, (Eds.), Duncan's Diseases of Metabolism, Seventh

Edition, Saunders, Philadelphia, 1974.
5. L. Gardner (Ed.), Endocrine and Genetic Disease of Childhood and Adolescence, Second Edition, Saunders, Philadelphia, 1976.
6. O.P. Heinonan, D. Slone and S. Shapiro (Eds.), Birth Defects and Drugs in Pregnancy, Publishing Sciences, Littleton, Mass., 1977.
7. V.A. McKusick, Heritable Disorders of Connective Tissue, Fourth Edition, Mosley, St. Louis, 1972.
8. V.A. McKusick, Mendelian Inheritance in Man: Catalogues of Autosomal Dominant, Autosomal Recessive, and X-Linked Phenotypes, Fourth Edition, Hopkins, Baltimore, 1975.
9. A. Milunsky, The Prenatal Diagnosis of Hereditary Disorders, C.C. Thomas, Springfield, 1973.
10. J.S. Thompson and M.W. Thompson, Genetics in Medicine, Second Edition, Saunders, Philadelphia, 1973.

POSTDOCTORAL EDUCATION AND TRAINING IN MEDICAL GENETICS*

A.G. Motulsky

Until recently the field of medical genetics was mainly concerned with research and most medical geneticists entered the field with a strong research bias. Research activities covered many areas; *i.e.*, biochemical genetics, cytogenetics, somatic cell genetics, clinical genetics, immunogenetics, statistical genetics and behavioral genetics. The research was usually laboratory-based or laboratory-oriented. With the development of clinical genetics in the last few years, much more clinical research without direct laboratory involvement is being carried out.

The last few years have also seen an expansion of clinical genetic services such as genetic counseling, genetic screening, and prenatal diagnosis. A few medical geneticists now spend their entire effort on service activities. However, unlike most other medical specialties where the majority of professionals are practicing and do not perform research, most genetic counselors are research oriented.[1] Genetic counseling and other genetic service activities are rarely carried out as a full-time occupation. Genetic service activities are usually performed in university medical centers and occasionally in health department clinics. Outreach clinics in smaller communities – usually under university auspices – are becoming more frequent.[2]

The majority of genetic activities in medical schools are now being carried out by pediatricians in departments of pediatrics.[3] Physicians with training in medicine, obstetrics and gynecology, and pathology represent other specialties involved in medical genetics.[1,3] Only 10% of genetic counselors with doctoral degrees are Ph.D.'s.[1] Some research in medical genetics is also carried out in a few basic science departments.

The range of diagnoses currently encountered in clinics involved in the delivery of genetic services is wide but is often biased by local expertise and interest. Mendelian diseases and chromosomal aberrations are frequently seen. All types of birth defects are handled. Patients with mental retardation are worked up in many clinics. The common psychiatric disorders with genetic etiology such as schizophrenia and affective disorders are rarely referred to genetic clinics. Few adult diseases with multifactorial inheritance are seen by medical geneticists. Exotic and externally visible disorders of the pediatric age group are more likely

*Supported by grant GM 15253 from the National Institutes of Health.

ISBN 0-12-562650-9

to be referred than more common diseases even if of clear genetic etiology. Intrauterine diagnosis is becoming increasingly popular and is widely – although not yet maximally – employed to rule out Down syndrome in older mothers. Screening programs for phenylketonuria and other rare metabolic diseases, for sickle cell trait, and for Tay-Sachs disease require genetic services. Special clinics such as those for cleft lip and cleft palate, for cystic fibrosis, and for the muscular dystrophies use genetic consultations less frequently than might be advisable for their patients.

Training programs must consider the realities of current work loads but need to consider newly developing service patterns. For instance, it is likely that programs for the detection of neural tube defects based on α-fetoprotein elevations of *all* maternal bloods may be widely introduced. Since completely new techniques may be discovered, precise long range predictions are impossible.

It is certain, however, that the demand for genetic counseling will increase. The role of genetic factors in many diseases is becoming better known among physicians and the general public. With small families, parents would like to have as much information as possible about health and disease of their planned offspring. It has been estimated that 2% of the 3.5 million births/year in the United States (or 70,000 parents) could benefit from genetic counseling.[4] The backlog of cases not having received counseling in the past needs to be added to this figure. However, as the indications for genetic counseling are widened, the recurrence risks decline. Fewer Mendelian diseases with high recurrence risks will be seen and more birth defects and cytogenetic aberrations with relatively low recurrence risks are encountered. An increasing service load among the currently research-oriented genetic counselors will lead to lessened research efforts unless more personnel become available or patterns of counseling change radically with much more extensive use of nondoctoral genetic associates.

More medical geneticists are becoming practice-oriented. The development of medical genetics as a practice specialty, however, is counterbalanced by difficulties in obtaining payments for genetic services. Practically all medical geneticists – even those who spend almost all their time on service activities – work under institutional auspices and are paid by medical schools, hospitals, private or governmental third party providers, state health departments, March of Dimes service programs, and only partially by patients. A private practice specialty of medical genetics does not exist. A considerable amount of genetic services is paid for by "bootlegged" funds earmarked for other purposes including research and teaching.

Expansion of genetic services therefore is not likely to proceed as rapidly as foreseen by a projection of public needs unless federal government or third party sources will subsidize these services more widely in the future than appears likely at this time. Sly[4] has estimated that 100 medical genetics centers – able to handle complex medical genetics problems – would be required nationally in the U.S., and would cost a minimum of about 25 million dollars/year (1974 estimate). An additional 10 million dollars/year would be needed, according to his estimates, for 300 less specialized facilities to handle all genetic service needs.

Training Programs

With this background of current activities, some pattern of training in human and medical genetics can be described.

A. Training of full-time researchers in human and medical genetics

Training for full-time research and teaching careers without clinical involvement will mostly attract Ph.D.'s. This group is essential for maintaining the momentum of innovative research in human genetics. There will be two rather different groups of trainees: laboratory-oriented geneticists on the one hand and statistically-oriented geneticists on the other. The total number of laboratory-oriented research geneticists which can be employed will be somewhat dependent upon the level of research support in our field. According to Sly[4] each of the 100 tertiary referral genetic units should employ one statistical human geneticist. A significant amount of the statistical work in this group may become service-oriented if computer assessment of genetic risks will be utilized more frequently.

A large number of Ph.D.'s are being trained in general genetics. Only a few of such trainees obtain exposure to human problems. More attention to attracting highly talented basic scientists to human genetics problems will have a high yield in research results.[5] Creation of more departments of medical genetics in medical schools would aid in providing appropriate outlets for Ph.D. human geneticists who have difficulties finding employment in genetic units of clinical departments such as pediatrics.

Another group of Ph.D. trainees in human genetics is currently trained in neither specific laboratory involvement nor in sophisticated quantitative genetics. Such persons will mostly locate in teaching positions in colleges where students need instruction in human genetics. Moreover, increasing interest in human genetics is counterbalanced by demographically explained lower student populations and fewer college teaching opportunities.

B. Training of physicians for academic careers in medical genetics.

Since most genetic units are in pediatric departments, most trainees are physicians with previous pediatric training. It is likely that the wider use of intrauterine diagnostic methods will attract more academic obstetrician/gynecologists to medical genetics. Ideally, all academic medical geneticists should be educated to develop expertise in investigation, teaching, and clinical work of medical genetics. A minimum 2-3 years clinical work after the M.D. degree and 2-3 years in a medical genetics unit is required. Some of these trainees will have acquired a Ph.D. degree in combined M.D.-Ph.D. programs and may require less postdoctoral *research* experience if their Ph.D. was obtained in a human genetics unit. If their Ph.D. was granted in another basic science, a minimum of two years exposure to medical genetics appears necessary.

Advanced course work in human genetics, biochemistry, immunology, and statistics is required. While postdoctoral fellows with a medical degree often audit these courses, enrollment for credit should be encouraged. Contact with geneticists who are experimentally oriented is to be encouraged. Larger training units where such contacts are possible have an advantage over smaller units.

Training in clinical genetics involves participation in genetics out-patient clinics and in-patient ward rounds where genetic diagnosis and genetic counseling are carried out and where problems of intrauterine diagnosis are considered. Trainees should be responsible for genetic and medical workup of cases, should survey the pertinent literature in detail and give recommendations for genetic counseling and management. Experience in providing consultative services should always be included in the program. Exposure to dysmorphology, clinical cytogenetics, *human* teratology, and syndrome recognition is essential. Genetic counseling should be an integral part of the training program.

The clinical program should expose trainees to a wide spectrum of genetic disorders and enable them to deal expertly with most genetic diseases. Consultation with appropriate specialists and acquaintance with reference literature in the various medical specialties should be part of their training. Good training in literature surveys is particularly important since the medical geneticist often deals with rare diseases.

Clinical exposure should be more intensive than extensive. Trainees should be taught the methods by which genetically relevant information is obtained, how diagnoses are made, how genetic risks are assessed, and how genetic counseling is given. "Snowing" trainees with a superabundance of clinical cases at the expense of research should be avoided. The emphasis on training is to create productive clinical investigators. While research training (see below) and clinical exposure is usually carried out at the same time, it may often be necessary to separate periods of clinical training from research efforts. The equivalent of a minimum of 25% of continuing efforts over a period of two years would be an appropriate allotment of clinical training in the academic pathway.

Skills in teaching need to be developed by journal club and seminar presentations as well as by outside lectures in medical genetics to various medical and lay groups. Communication skills to deal with a variety of medical personnel need to be developed.

Each trainee should be involved in at least one research project in depth. While such a project can be a clinical project, laboratory projects preferably should be selected. The most innovative solutions to problems in medical genetics will genetics will come from laboratory studies. The trainee needs to identify with a subfield of medical genetics where he has mastered the laboratory techniques and is not dependent upon other scientists for his results. The young physician-researcher should make use of his medical training in selecting projects not likely to be picked by a nonmedical researcher. In human genetics, animal work is less crucial than in many other areas of medical research, and a project requiring work with patients and/or human subjects, their cells or body fluids is mandatory. Involvement in the many logistical and ethical problems of investigations with human patients, normal human subjects, and their respective families is an important aspect of training future "clinical" investigators in medical genetics.

B. Training physicians for careers in medical genetics services

The need for professionals in medical genetics service makes this group of ever-increasing importance. Rational use of personnel to fulfill service demands in medical genetics may be best met by full-time professional personnel and not by medical geneticists who only spend some of their time on service activities.[4] The content of clinical training was described earlier in the recommendation for the academic group. Training for service careers in medical genetics should stress more extensive exposure to clinical cases of all sorts.

The clinical geneticist needs to acquire an excellent background in dysmorphology, embryology, syndromology, and cytogenetics as well as in all facets of genetic counseling and of other genetic services. Exposure to basic courses in genetics, statistics, and embryology is to be encouraged. Unlike most other practitioners, the service oriented clinical geneticist needs to search the literature much more frequently. Involvement in a clinical research project is desirable but not essential.

Physicians trained in this manner will be able to function in pediatric departments, genetic service units in public health departments and hospitals, and as pediatricians in large practice groups where they would act as subspecialists in birth defects and genetic diseases.

Much attention to cost-effectiveness must be given. Much wider use of genetic associates in pedigree taking, routine counseling, and post-counseling follow-up should be encouraged in establishing the ideal genetic practice teams of the future. Such new patterns of practice require particular attention in designing training programs for service-oriented medical genetics.

Medical Geneticists in Pediatrics and Other Medical Specialties

While most positions for physicians with training in medical genetics are available in pediatrics, genetic concepts and practices impinge on most fields of internal medicine (such as hematology, cardiology, gastroenterology, allergy, endocrinology, nephrology), as well as on dermatology, neurology, psychiatry, ophthalmology, and obstetrics and gynecology. Service demands, however, most frequently originate from pediatrics, and with expanding needs for intrauterine diagnosis will also come from obstetrics/gynecology. The scope for research using genetic concepts is immense in most fields of medicine. It is therefore important that a flow of trainees from specialties other than pediatrics be attracted to in-depth training in medical genetics. Understanding of many diseases with multifactorial genetic etiology will require genetic approaches. A dearth of clinical investigators in fields other than pediatrics will make for a slowing in the solution of many problems which demand genetic concepts. Ph.D. geneticists will be unlikely to provide the necessary liaison with physicians in the various clinical sciences. Medical genetics may not fulfill its promises if it fails to attract physicians other than pediatricians. Therefore strong efforts need to be exerted to attract young academic physicians in fields such as neurology, psychiatry, dermatology, ophthalmology, and in all fields of internal medicine to training in medical genetics.

Human Geneticists with Ph.D. Degrees

About 70 Ph.D.'s are being trained in various aspects of human genetics in medical schools and major hospital affiliated institutions.[3] Their training is largely research oriented[3] and their research is likely to be carried out in units affiliated with medical schools. However, a fairly large number of this group will devote most of their efforts to full-time service laboratory activities such as in cytogenetics or in biochemical genetics.There are probably not enough academic jobs in universities or colleges away from medical schools to provide teaching and research appointments for this group. Research in medical genetics in nonmedical college environments often will be difficult because of lack of facilities and lack of access to patients with genetic disease.

Training of Ph.D. geneticists in genetic counseling is not carried out widely. Education of Ph.D.'s for counseling requires more time than similar training for physicians who have been schooled in interviewing and dealing with patients and their problems. While nonmedically trained Ph.D.'s can and do function as counselors after a diagnosis has been made, the nature of their training and the absence of a medical background make it difficult for them to function optimally. Assessment of risks in genetic counseling rarely requires the genetic knowledge acquired in most Ph.D. training programs. Most genetic service activities therefore are best carried out by physician-geneticists in conjunction with paraprofessionals (genetic associates) who require less training than the Ph.D. degree. While occasionally Ph.D.'s will function well in patient-related genetic service activities, the training of large numbers of Ph.D. geneticists for these functions is not recommended except for those individuals who will have responsibility for cytogenetic and similar laboratories.

Numbers

A minimum of 80 M.D. and about 70 Ph.D. fellows enter medical genetics training fellowships each year.[3] The specially designated (Weinberger) training program in medical genetics of the National Institute of General Medical Sciences (NIGMS) trained 86 individuals (23 M.D.'s , 4 M.D.-Ph.D.'s, and 59 Ph.D.'s) in various aspects of human and medical genetics between 1974-1977.* Currently, about 25 fellowship slots per year are provided in various medical genetics training grants.* A few additional fellows are supported by individual fellowships. Because of problems in taxonomy it is difficult to obtain an exact number of personnel trained in medical genetics from the various institutes of the National Institutes of Health. No official figures except for the data of Levine *et al.*[3] cited

*Personal communication, D. Miller, NIGMS.

here are available for the total number of medical genetics fellowships and training slots, including those not supported by sources other than the NIH.

Recommendations regarding the number of trainees will depend upon many uncertainties such as the pace of introduction of new genetic units, the level of support of research in medical genetics, the passage of the National Genetics Disease Act and the amount of money allotted to the Act, the role of third party insurers in paying for genetic service, the possible advent of national health insurance, the role of genetics associates, and the exact distribution of the work load of the various professionals involved in genetic services. Will the current model of a fairly large number of profesionals spending part of their efforts on genetic service activities continue or will there be more full time professionals?

A report of the genetics training committee of the National Institute of General Medical Sciences in 1971 recommended that 1,211 geneticists be available by 1988 for positions in medical and dental schools, in health departments, for prenatal diagnosis, and for genetic counseling.* This estimate was based on a recommendation that every genetic unit at a medical school consist of (a) one M.D. medical geneticist-pediatrician, (b) one M.D. medical geneticist-internist, (c) one medical geneticist in another medical specialty, (d) one Ph.D. population or statistical geneticist, (e) one M.D. or Ph.D. cytogeneticist, (f) one Ph.D. molecular biologist. In addition, the estimate assumed a 20% expansion of medical faculties between 1970 and 1990. It was also assumed that 300,000 amniocenteses would be performed per year; *i.e.,* that about 8% of all pregnancies coming to term would be monitored. This figure is probably too high.

If about 150 M.D.'s and Ph.D.'s continue to enter genetics training programs per year[3] and the average training requires two years, about 750 (1,500/2) additional professionals would be available in another 10 years in 1988 – the target date for the NIGMS report. Judging from current numbers in training, almost 50% of these 750 would be Ph.D.'s, yet there is a greater need for M.D. geneticists. If Ph.D.'s will serve more frequently in various service functions, their current training is not appropriate. If the currently active medical geneticists and those trained in the last few years are added to the 750 who will be trained, the target figure of 1,211 professionals in 1988, as given in the NIGMS report, is likely to be exceeded. It is essential that a representative body such as a committee of the American Society of Human Genetics carefully monitor the training situation since an oversupply could easily occur in view of the uncertainties regarding future expansion of services.

Standards and Accreditation

No uniform standards in training programs exist. The NIH sponsored pro-

*Unpublished document from NIGMS by D. Miller.

grams, whether for training grants or individual fellowships, are peer-reviewed and generally are of high quality. There are no standards for more clinically oriented training programs. Faculty members have widely differing expertise in different training units. The American Society of Human Genetics is in the process of organizing a committee to set standards for accreditation in the various activities which are carried out as genetic services. Training standards undoubtedly will be included.

Medical Genetics in Competition Against Other Forms of Health Expenditure

The very steep rate of growth in medical expenditures over the last few years has caused much alarm. Strong efforts are being developed by a variety of national bodies to decrease health expenditures. Any proposed new programs therefore are critically scrutinized regarding their cost and benefits and whether the proposed funds are spent wisely and judiciously.

Criteria other than mere economic ones must often be used to justify health related programs. In analogy with other new health services, the cost of genetic services is likely to escalate as has happened with all other health related programs. We in medical genetics are asking for support of genetic needs at a difficult time. The medical genetics community therefore needs to marshal carefully the very best evidence to document the social, medical and psychological benefits likely to be provided by our activities.

Summary

The current scene of training in human and medical genetics has been surveyed. Three types of training programs for human geneticists are recommended: (1) training for research geneticists (largely Ph.D.), (2) training of physicians for service careers in clinical genetics, and (3) training of academic physicians (and occasionally Ph.D.) geneticists involved in clinical work, teaching, and research. The problems associated with these various programs and of training Ph.D.'s in medical genetics are discussed. The "pediatricization" of medical genetics may prevent the field from fulfilling the promise for *all* of medicine. The economic difficulties of launching an expansion of existing service and training programs during a time of financial stringency are pointed out.

Numerical estimates of current trainees are imprecise. Future estimates are difficult since they depend upon unpredictable trends affecting the growth of genetic services such as state and federal support, the possible advent of national health insurance, and many other factors. Current training trends probably will provide a sufficient number of personnel although there may be tendencies to train too large a number of Ph.D.'s in medical genetics. The standards of many clinical training programs are not monitored and quality differs considerably. Coordination of future patterns of practice with paraprofessional genetic associates needs to be considered in the design of training programs.

REFERENCES

1. J.R. Sorenson and A.C. Culbert, *in* Genetic Counseling, H.A. Lubs and F. de la Cruz (Eds.), Raven Press, New York, pp. 131-156, 1977.
2. L.G. Jackson and M.A. Barr, *in* Genetic Counseling, H.A. Lubs and F. de la Cruz (Eds.), Raven Press, New York, pp. 83-91, 1977.
3. M.D. Levine, J.M. Gursky and D.L. Rimoin, *in* Genetic Counseling, H.A. Lubs and F. de la Cruz (Eds.), Raven Press, New York, pp. 349-368, 1977.
4. W.S. Sly, *in* Genetic Counseling, H.A. Lubs and F. de la Cruz (Eds.), Raven Press, New York, pp. 535-550, 1977.
5. A.G. Motulsky, *Am. J. Hum. Genet. 30*, 123, 1978.

FUTURE EDUCATIONAL NEEDS IN GENETICS

Barton Childs

One purpose of this conference is to examine how genetic services are being made available to the public and how best to do so. It is well known that horses brought to water may not drink, so part of the conference is devoted to considering how to make the public aware of these opportunities and how to persuade them of their value. The aim of these services is mainly preventive and supportive rather than therapeutic. Both therapeutic and preventive medicine require a collaborative relation between the doctor and patient, but while the spur of pain or the fear of death prompts an attitude of supplication or surrender in the presence of illness, the absence of these inspirations may engender indifference to preventive measures. Our problem, then, is how to induce, if not the same urgency as that appropriate for sickness, at least an attitude of readiness for action whenever a convincing argument for action can be made.

One way to this goal is through education – everyone would agree to that – but what education, and for whom? The latter question is more easily answered than the former; the need for education is general and embraces both the medical profession and the public. Indeed, if the armentarium of preventive medicine were now abundant, we would have serious difficulty in using it widely because doctors must dispense it, and adults who carry responsibilities for themselves and their children must accept it, and neither has any well-developed tradition for it. But since there is so little now that can be done, there is time for experiments with education for both agencies appropriate for each. And the nature, content, amount, and most important, the method of the education are all open for experiment.

Experience tells us that not much can be expected of attempts simply to apprise the public of preventive opportunities, so some effort should be made to make human biology, with its relation to health and disease, available to all beginning in elementary school This will require two fundamental changes in thinking: (1) the recognition by the public of just how deeply science is ingrained in all our lives; and (2) a shift by educators from disciplinary teaching to the creation of awareness that the biology being taught in school is connected with living. It is surprising that this connection is so frequently and so well accom-

*This work was supported in part by NIH grant, HD 00486.

ISBN 0-12-562650-9

plished in vocational schools, but so little in conventional classroom teaching. Indeed, the latter may "promote ways of learning and thinking which often run counter to those nurtured in practical daily activities".[1] The lack of such a connection is perhaps most salient in schools where health education is taught altogether out of the context of courses in biology being given elsewhere in the same school. But it may be in just such schools that this awareness can be best achieved if these two subjects can be seen by both faculty and students to have some common ground.

Health Education

Health education has now entered the secondary school curriculum in earnest. Once it was the property of the department of athletics where attitudes of cleanliness, moderation, and continence were encouraged; virtues which teenagers characteristically found derisory, whether out of over-experience or under-experience, or greeted with indifference.

For its method, health education has drawn mainly on the disciplines of epidemiology and behavioral science; for its content, on hygiene, public health practices, and general and preventive medicine. It consists of attempts to demonstrate the wisdom of avoiding conditions hazardous to health, especially those in which individual choice can be exercised. Much of what health educators actually do is with people who have disease and need to learn to live with it, but their preferred goal is preventive, and unfortunately, success in the latter has measured up neither to hope nor to expectation. Curiously, health educators have paid little attention to genetics, a discipline plainly central to their efforts since it gives a very pointed individual meaning to preventive medicine. For example, it has been demonstrated that those people who perceive their own susceptibility to some serious disease are the most likely to avail themselves of relevant services.[2] The experience with Tay-Sachs screening bears witness to this idea, revealing that people with reason to believe they might be carriers are the most likely to appear for testing.[3] And it has been shown that the probability of use of anmiocentesis by women over 35 is directly related to educational experience.[4] So it is an immediate educational mission to persuade health educators to adopt a genetic point of view from which to see and teach their subject.

Elementary and High School Biology

General science is now widely taught in elementary schools, and in the United States perhaps 80% of high school students have a course in biology. But in the past these courses contained little human biology and even less human genetics, and, in general, biology has not been seen by the writers of books as related to questions of health which arise in daily life. In a survey of 128 books or series devoted to biology, Hurd traced the changing fortunes of human genetics from 1900 to the present.[5] Until recently there was little genetics in these books, and even less attention was given to the human condition, although eugenics claimed some space up to the 1940's. After 1950, although genetics is given more space, there is not much reference to its application to man and even less recognition that the genes have much to do with disease. Indeed, Hurd concludes that most textbook writers have regarded references to disease as out of place. But very recently, mainly during this decade, biology teachers have begun to emphasize the biology of man, taking examples from human experience to illuminate the principles of genetics, and the social implications of the uses of genetic knowledge, as in counseling and screening, have begun to surface here and there in some books. But these are still exceptional.

The importance of text books, especially in high school biology, is underlined in a survey of 1,000 teachers which revealed that what is taught in the classroom is what is in the books.[6] And what is not taught in the classroom has been shown in two recent studies not to be in the minds of the students. One survey of 930 high school students in Quebec revealed that the students' knowledge of the genetic principles was wanting and that the social applications of those principles were poorly perceived.[7] A second study of about 1,000 students widely distributed over the United States revealed a similar ignorance of the relation of genetics to health and disease; the students did not lack for opinions or a lively interest, they lacked knowledge.[6]

So it is apparent that these biology courses are disciplinary and miss what might be a primary mission – to prepare children for life. The position is better in college where more attention is given to the biology of man, including human and medical genetics, and some schools even have a major in human biology. But not everyone goes to college; and of those who do, few take biology – so the work, if it is to be done at all, must be done in high school and before.

So the task is one of bringing some understanding of genetics to health educators and some idea of what genetics has to do with health to biology teachers hoping these teachers would conspire together to a common end. If a student were able to put biology and health education together, he would be able to grasp that health and disease have social and evolutionary dimensions, that our special susceptibilities, whether as a species or as individuals, reside in our genetic make-up, and that disease is the result of the prevalence of conditions which are inappropriate for specific genetic and developmental constitutions. Sometimes this means everyone, sometimes only the possessors of rare mutants, more often something in between.

Such an exposition of the facts of life is one which students might find easier to extrapolate to their own lives and those of their relatives, setting a context in which admonitions in regard to moderation could be taken or rejected as appropriate to one's own genetic and constitutional circumstances, and that is the lesson of preventive medicine with its close relation to genetics.

In carrying out this coordinated effort, the health educators should emphasize the origins of disease in conditions which overwhelm the powers of homeostasis, capabilities which are forged by each individual out of a lifetime of development determined by his genes and special experiences. How to discover genetic susceptibilities and how to design a life that skirts them should be the subject of health education. And a corollary to this study should be the definition of the political and ethical issues raised by a social system that creates and promotes conditions inimical to the well-being of some of its members.

The tasks of the biologists and health educators overlap in part, but repetition, especially in different contexts, is a useful educational device. A start should be made as early as possible, perhaps with such ideas as variability and its ubiquity, classification, and the arrangement of quantitative data in distributions. It should become apparent even to very young children that the extremes of distributions represent individuals who are relatively infrequent and who are sometimes poorly adapted for the context in which the measurement is made. From this it is a short step to disease, and the idea of prevention by means of some change in the conditions which have determined the distribution could be introduced at some appropriate time. As it happens, this introduction to science through measurements, classification, and analysis of distributions is embodied in the Process Approach to Science for elementary school children, a series which has been widely tried out during the past decade. Later, probability and the idea of personal risk should be taken up and, when cognitive development allows, perhaps in high school, the principles of genetics should follow.

In all this there should be emphasis on the continuity between normality and abnormality, so that the latter should be seen as one end, or possibly both, of a continuous distribution and as variation rather than as a typological discontinuity. Such a biological and evolutionary view of disease, and of one's own position in many distributions, ought to help to provide some orderly insight into the origins of disease, and to serve as a stimulus to take personal and rational action to protect one's own health against forces which can be understood. Furthermore, it should engender the idea that since variability, including individual susceptibility to disease, is characteristic of everyone, one aspect of humanity should be tolerance for differences and acceptance of diversity. And that might be the most valuable preventive medicine of all.

These lessons are perhaps most easily taught in the conventional context of school. But Hurd has suggested that as much as a generation might elapse before genetics will have been translated into the everyday experience of all school children, and in the meantime, decisions will be forced on their parents.[5] So genetics will have to find its way into the lives of the general public by all available means: the news; magazines, especially those devoted to health; television and public lectures. Perhaps such public agencies as health departments will aid in this cause; and the disease-related organizations, most of which are devoted to conditions associated with genes, are a source of support. And the American Academy of Pediatrics Committee on Genetics is also dedicated to education, both in school and out. So I think it is fair to say there is some general recognition that something should be done about increasing the awareness of the place of genetics in health education, and that there is some will to do it. It needs only a focus from which information, stimulus, and leadership can emanate.

One aspirant for this role is the Biological Sciences Curriculum Study (BSCS), an organization which is responsible for the most widely used high school textbooks in the United States. They have also written books for elementary schools and college and have recently undertaken the mission of a curriculum for teaching science to mentally retarded students.

With support from the National Foundation, the BSCS has recently made an assessment of the need for education in human genetics in the United States for people of all ages, and has drawn up a list of usggestions for those who wish to participate in improving the position.[8] Much of what I have said here is drawn from the BSCS report to the National Foundation, a report which was based on questionnaire research, surveys, conferences, interviews, and solicitation of the opinions of knowledgeable people.[9] This organization is in a good position to influence the teaching of biology and genetics in school and college. It can also influence the content and method of teaching of health education in primary and secondary school and can provide or give advice on curricular materials for adult education as well as scripts for radio and television programs. It should also be in a good position to help in organizing genetics for students in school of allied health sciences, a group of critical importance for the successful pursuit of the goals of preventive medicine. Although the BSCS is in a less favorable position to exert much direct influence on medical education, there is much opportunity for collaboration to mutual profit between medical educators and those, like the BSCS, who work with the public. Each needs the other; the development of classroom teaching materials will require the help of physicians, not as such, but as graduates of the only schools of human biology; the medical schools. This need was specifically expressed in a paper which reviewed the use in several textbooks of biology of human traits presumed to be determined by genes at a single locus.[10] Of 57 such traits, the mode of inheritance of only 26 was well established, and even some of them are probably not so simple as they seem, or at least are poor choices to illustrate principles. And the medical establishment will need the help of educators who can bring to the public that enlightenment which will make them informed partners in accomplishing the laudable aims we have discussed in this conference.

Medical Education

I alluded earlier to the want of education for the medical profession as well as the public. Dr. Motulsky touched on the requirements for geneticists to study the problems of human variation, including disease, and Dr. Hsia gave us evidence of the semi-adequacy of this preparation among some primary care physicians – doctors who should be among the best prepared in this most highly developed of all nations. But what of others? There is evidence that others are in worse repair; *e.g.*, general practitioners and family physicians – and no one, to my knowledge, has tested the knowledge, or ignorance, of surgeons.[11] But why should any physician be robbed of the aesthetic pleasure of knowing genetics, and why should not their patients be accorded access to information giving insight into their disorders? In fact, *all* physicians should have a more than superficial familiarity with this discipline since the aims of preventive medicine cannot be fulfilled unless it is universally applied.

What is the reason for this curious condition? I do not pretend to know all the reasons, but some among them must lie in the organization of medicine – its over-compartmentalization, which may be forcing genetics into the position of a medical specialty, muting, thereby, its meaning as a scientific discipline of general application, possessed of a power to illuminate the origins of differences between individuals and species, and of giving insight into the components and shapes of distributions. If the medical students and practitioners perceive that the uses of this discipline are reserved only to one group of specialists, they will, indeed they do, make little effort to have it for themselves. By focusing too narrowly on conditions in which mutant genes and abnormal chromosomes are salient, we support a limiting idea of the role of genetic variability in disease. This over rigid view of genes and disease may be one reason why so little progress has been made in the elucidation of the frequent and chronic multifactorial conditions. When we emphasize one gene, we risk neglecting the wide range of its phenotypic possibilities and of the variable relation of its effects to those of others. So as educators of students who are preparing for many roles in medicine, we should emphasize not just the genes, but variability and distributions. Perhaps genetics would assume an appropriate position in medical education if we were to ask a fundamental medical question in a different way. As it now stands, the question is "What is the cause of a disease, and how do we treat it?" Another way, and I suggest a more humane way, of putting the question is "Why does *this* person have *this* disease, and how do we treat *him*?"

Conclusion

In summary, we must try to find ways to translate the abstractions of genetics into ordinary language and experience. To do so would be to go a long way to reduce the demonology of disease to a list of frailties which are a product of the rapid evolution of the conditions in which we live and the slow evolution of our biological heritage. Such an insight should have two important consequences; it should provide some stimulus for each person to act to protect his own health, and it should give informed citizens the wherewithal to take social and political action to protect the collective health.

REFERENCES

1. S. Scribner and M. Cole, *Science 182*, 553, 1973.
2. I.M. Rosenstock, *Health Educ. Monogr. 2*, 4, 1974.
3. B. Childs, L. Gordis, M.M. Kaback and H.H. Kazazian, Jr., *Amer. J. Hum. Genet. 28*, 537, 1976.
4. R.M. Bannerman, D. Gilleck, R. van Coevering, N.L. Knoblock and G.B. Ingall, *N. Engl. J. Med. 297*, 449, 1977.

5. P.D. Hurd, The historical/philosophical background of education in human genetics in the United States. (in ref. 9).
6. F.M. Hickman, M.H. Kennedy and J.D. McInerny, *Am. Biol. Teacher* (in press).
7. C.R. Scriver, D.E. Scriver, C. Clow and M. Schok, *Am. Biol. Teacher* (in press).
8. Biological Sciences Curriculum Study. Guidelines for Educational Priorities and Curricular Innovations in the Areas of Human Genetics, Genetic Diseases and Birth Defects, 1977.
9. Biological Sciences Curriculum Study. Assessment of Educational Needs in Human Genetics and Birth Defects. Report to the National Foundation, 1977.
10. P. Barnes and T.R. Mertens, *J. Hered.* *67*, 347, 1976.
11. I.M. Rosenstock, B. Childs and A.P. Simopoulos. Genetic screening. A study of the knowledge and attitudes of physicians. National Academy of Sciences, 1975.

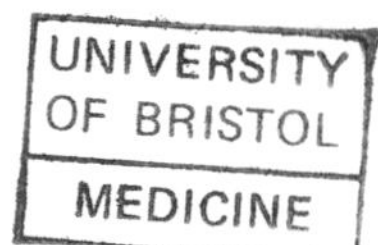